INTERNATIONAL YEARBOOK OF NEPHROLOGY 1992

INTERNATIONAL YEARBOOK OF NEPHROLOGY 1992

Editors

Vittorio E. Andreucci
Department of Nephrology
University of Naples
Naples, Italy

and

Leon G. Fine
University College
Middlesex School of Medicine
The Rayne Institute
London, United Kingdom

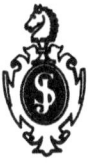

Springer-Verlag
London Berlin Heidelberg New York
Paris Tokyo Hong Kong
Barcelona Budapest

ISBN-13: 978-1-4471-1894-7   e-ISBN-13: 978-1-4471-1892-3

DOI: 10. 978-1-4471-1892-3

British Library Cataloguing-in-Publication Data
A catalogue record for this book is available from the British Library

Library of Congress Data available

Softcover reprint of the hardcover 1st edition 1991

2128/3830-543210 Printed on acid-free paper

PREFACE

The 1992 International Yearbook of Nephrology is the 4th in a successful series of yearly books updating practising nephrologists and nephrologists-in-training on rapidly changing areas of nephrology. We were encouraged to proceed in our editorial venture by reviews of the previous issues which have appeared in various Nephrology Journals. These reviews have pointed to the successful use of the International Editorial Board, the broad range of topics of current interest which have been covered and the comprehensive and practical nature of the reviews.

The principal aim of the Yearbook remains to provide reviews which are more current than those which appear in Nephrology textbooks and which can be in the hands of the readers a few months after the authors have completed the manuscripts. The appointed authors are always experts in the field, who are asked to give an objective review of the topic, up-dating the readers on the world-wide literature and providing them with a complete, accurate and up-to-date list of important recent references.

We have decided to maintain the successful format of the first three issues. Thus, the volume will continue to be divided into sections; each section will continue to have a different primary focus every year, depending upon what is of greatest interest at the time.

The Editorial Board has provided suggestions for topics and authors. We have received more than 150 suggestions and selected from among them the topics and authors for this issue. A number of topics suggested this year will be included in the next issue if they continue to be viewed as current and important.

The Editorial Board of the International Yearbook will be reviewed periodically in order to renew the experts providing the suggestions for relevant topics. However, we continue to invite our readers to suggest topics for upcoming issues of the Yearbook.

We are grateful to the authors for their excellent reviews and for having met the deadline in forwarding their manuscripts. The Yearbook series requires that the entire volume be ready for publication a few weeks after completion of the manuscripts, to avoid the drawback of traditional textbooks whose publication often occurs one to two years after submission of the material.

Vittorio E. Andreucci
Leon G. Fine

CONTENTS

Contributing Authors

Renal Physiology and Pathophysiology

1. Coagulation in renal diseases: the role of the glomerular hemostasis system and implications for therapy.
   Alain Kanfer, Eric Rondeau, Marie-Nöelle Peraldi and Jean-Daniel Sraer   3

2. Central nervous system complications of severe hyponatremia.
   Richard H. Sterns   55

3. The physiologic basis for renal functional reserve testing.
   Francis B. Gabbai, Luca De Nicola and Roland C. Blantz   75

Glomerulonephritis

4. The antiproteinuric effect of angiotensin-converting-enzyme inhibitors in human renal disease.
   Dick de Zeeuw, Jan E. Heeg and Paul E. de Jong   95

Hypertension

5. Insulin resistance in essential hypertension.
   Willa A. Hsueh   117

The Kidney and Diabetes

6. Risk factors and optimal blood pressure level for insulin-dependent diabetic patients.
   Carl Erik Mogensen   141

The Kidney in Pregnancy

7. Treatment of hypertension during pregnancy: drugs to be avoided and drugs to be used.
   Stephen N. Sturgiss, Marshall D. Lindheimer and John M. Davison   163

Hereditary Renal Diseases

8. Prediction of likelihood of polycystic kidney disease in the fetus when a parent has autosomal dominant polycystic kidney disease.
   Patricia A. Gabow and Louise Wilkins-Haug   199

Renal Stone Disease

9. Urinary stones which require adjunctive management for successful extracorporeal shockwave lithotripsy.
   Gerhard J. Fuchs and Anna M. Fuchs   211

Chronic Renal Failure

10. Metabolic and clinical effects of long-term conservative treatment in patients with chronic renal failure.
    Lamberto Oldrizzi, Carlo Rugiu and Giuseppe Maschio   229

Dialysis

11. Treatment of secondary hyperparathyroidism by intravenous calcitriol.
    Francisco Llach   245

12. Non-A, non-B hepatitis in dialysis patients: diagnosis, prevention and treatment.
    Michel Jadoul, Chantal Cornu and Charles van Ypersele de Strihou   253

13. New developments in continuous arteriovenous hemofiltration/dialysis.
    Ravindra L. Mehta   271

Renal Transplantation

14. Ideal immunosuppression after renal transplantation: are steroids needed?
    Timothy H. Mathew   299

Diagnostic Methods in Nephrology

15. Anti-neutrophil cytoplasmic antibodies (ANCA): new tools in the diagnosis and follow-up of necrotizing glomerulonephritis and vasculitis.
    Cees G.M. Kallenberg and Jan W. Cohen Tervaert   313

16. Microscopic examination of the urinary sediment to differentiate high from low renal bleeding.
    G. Berry Schumann and Janet L. Schumann   337

Index   353

CONTRIBUTING AUTHORS

Roland C. Blantz,
Division of Nephrology-Hypertension,
University of California,
San Diego School of Medicine
and Veterans Affairs Medical Center,
3350 La Jolla Village Drive,
La Jolla, CA 92161, USA.

Jan W. Cohen Tervaert,
Department of Clinical Immunology
University Hospital,
Oostersingel 59,
9713 EZ Groningen, The Netherlands.

Chantal Cornu,
Division of Virology,
University of Louvain Medical School,
Cliniques Universitaires St-Luc,
Av. Hippocrate 10,
1200 Bruxelles, Belgium.

John M. Davison,
Department of Obstetrics
and Gynaecology,
University of Newcastle-upon-Tyne,
Princess Mary Maternity Hospital,
Great North Road,
Newcastle-upon-Tyne, UK, NE2 3BD.

Luca De Nicola,
Division of Nephrology-Hypertension,
University of California,
San Diego School of Medicine
and Veterans Affairs Medical Center,
3350 La Jolla Village Drive,
La Jolla, CA 92161, USA.

Paul E. de Jong,
Division of Nephrology,
Department of Medicine,
State University Hospital,
Groningen, The Netherlands.

Dick de Zeeuw,
Division of Nephrology,
Department of Medicine,
State University Hospital,
Groningen, The Netherlands.

Anna M. Fuchs,
UCLA Stone Center,
UCLA School of Medicine,
Division of Urology,
10833 Leconte Ave,
Los Angeles, Ca 90024, USA.

Gerhard J. Fuchs,
UCLA Stone Center,
UCLA School of Medicine,
Division of Urology,
10833 Leconte Ave,
Los Angeles, Ca 90024, USA.

Francis B. Gabbai,
Division of Nephrology-Hypertension,
University of California,
San Diego School of Medicine
and Veterans Affairs Medical Center,
3350 La Jolla Village Drive,
La Jolla, CA 92161, USA.

Patricia A. Gabow,
Denver General Hospital,
University of Colorado
Health Sciences Center,
4200 East Ninth Ave, Box C283,
Denver, CO 80262, USA.

Jan E. Heeg,
Division of Nephrology,
Department of Medicine,
State University Hospital,
Groningen, The Netherlands.

Willa A. Hsueh,
Division of Diabetes,
Hypertension and Nutrition,
Department of Medicine,
University of Southern California
Medical Center,
Los Angeles, CA 90033, USA.

Michel Jadoul,
Division of Nephrology,
University of Louvain Medical School,
Cliniques Universitaires St-Luc,
Av. Hippocrate 10,
1200 Bruxelles, Belgium.

Cees G.M. Kallenberg,
Department of Clinical Immunology,
University Hospital,
Oostersingel 59,
9713 EZ Groningen, The Netherlands.

Alain Kanfer,
Service de Néphrologie A,
Hôpital Tenon,
4 rue de la Chine
75020 Paris, France.

Francisco Llach,
Veterans Affairs Medical Center,
West Los Angeles,
UCLA School of Medicine,
Wilshire & Sawtelle Blvds,
Los Angeles, CA 90073, USA.

Marshall D. Lindheimer,
Departments of Medicine
and Obstetrics and Gynecology,
University of Chicago,
Chicago Lying-in Hospital,
5841 Maryland Avenue,
Chicago, IL 60637, USA.

Giuseppe Maschio,
Division of Nephrology,
University Hospital,
Ospedale Civile Maggiore,
37126 Verona, Italy.

Timothy H. Mathew,
Renal Unit,
The Queen Elizabeth Hospital,
Woodville South
South Australia 5011.

Ravindra L. Mehta,
Division of Nephrology,
Department of Medicine,
University of California,
San Diego UCSD Medical Center H781-D
San Diego, CA 92103, USA.

Carl Erik Mogensen,
Medical Department M
(Diabetes and Endocrinology),
Aarhus Kommunehospital,
DK-8000 Aarhus C, Denmark.

Lamberto Oldrizzi,
Division of Nephrology,
University Hospital,
Ospedale Civile Maggiore,
37126 Verona, Italy.

Marie-Nöelle Peraldi,
Service de Néphrologie A,
Hôpital Tenon,
4 rue de la Chine
75020 Paris, France.

Eric Rondeau,
Service de Néphrologie A,
Hôpital Tenon,
4 rue de la Chine
75020 Paris, France.

Carlo Rugiu,
Division of Nephrology,
University Hospital,
Ospedale Civile Maggiore,
37126 Verona, Italy.

G. Berry Schumann,
Cytopathology and Cytotechnology,
5B2.22 WC Mackenzie
Health Science Centre,
University of Alberta,
Edmonton, Alberta Canada T6G 2RT.

Janet L. Schumann,
Cytopathology and Cytotechnology,
5B2.22 WC Mackenzie
Health Science Centre,
University of Alberta,
Edmonton, Alberta Canada T6G 2RT.

Jean-Daniel Sraer,
Service de Néphrologie A,
Hôpital Tenon,
4 rue de la Chine
75020 Paris, France.

Richard H. Sterns,
Division of Nephrology,
University of Rochester
School of Medicine,
Rochester General Hospital,
1425 Portland Avenue,
Rochester, NY 14621, USA.

Stephen N. Sturgiss,
Department of Obstetrics
and Gynaecology,
University of Newcastle-upon-Tyne,
Princess Mary Maternity Hospital,
Great North Road,
Newcastle-upon-Tyne, UK, NE2 3BD.

Charles van Ypersele de Strihou,
Division of Nephrology,
University of Louvain Medical School,
Cliniques Universitaires St-Luc,
Av. Hippocrate 10,
1200 Bruxelles, Belgium.

Louise Wilkins-Haug,
Maternal-Fetal Medicine,
Harvard Medical School,
Department of OB/GYN,
Brigham and Women's Hospital,
Boston, Massachusetts, USA.

RENAL PHYSIOLOGY AND PATHOPHYSIOLOGY

Chapter 1

COAGULATION IN RENAL DISEASES: THE ROLE OF THE GLOMERULAR HEMOSTASIS SYSTEM AND IMPLICATIONS FOR THERAPY

ALAIN KANFER, ERIC RONDEAU, MARIE-NÖELLE PERALDI AND JEAN-DANIEL SRAER

Service de Néphrologie A, INSERM U 64 and Association Claude Bernard, Hôpital Tenon, Paris, France

INTRODUCTION

A role for the coagulation system in the induction or maintenance of renal diseases, especially glomerulonephritides (GN)[(*)], is at first suggested by the presence of glomerular fibrin deposits and microthromboses in various renal diseases, in humans as well as in laboratory animals (Table 1).

In a majority of patients, deposits of fibrin-related antigen (detected by routine immunofluorescence) were shown to consist at least partly of "true" fibrin, as detected by the use of a monoclonal antibody that discriminates between cross-linked fibrin (resulting from the action of thrombin on fibrinogen), and fibrinogen and other fibrinogen derivatives (1-3).

Fibrin deposits *per se* injure glomeruli in several ways: by occluding glomerular capillaries; by participating in the inflammatory reaction, notably through attraction of monocytes and macrophages (4); and by direct cytotoxicity to glomerular mesangial cells (5). Moreover, thrombin itself can induce proliferative mesangial changes, probably by enhancing synthesis of platelet-derived growth factor (6).

Thus, whatever its pathogenesis, intraglomerular coagulation appears as a nonspecific mechanism of progressive glomerular damage.

Formation of intrarenal fibrin with ensuing extension or dissolution depends upon the respective activities of prothrombotic (procoagulant, antifibrinolytic) and antithrombotic

---

[(*)] For Glossary, see page 54.

3

(anticoagulant, fibrinolytic) activities of the hemostasis system. Studies of systemic blood may disclose activation of the coagulation/fibrinolysis system in nephropathies, for example: consumption coagulopathy in acute renal failure due to acute disseminated intravascular coagulation (7); elevated plasma levels of Factor VIII coagulant activity (8, 9), fibrinopeptide A and high molecular weight fibrinogen complexes in acute or subacute GN and nephrotic syndrome (NS) (10-12). However these data do not yield, by themselves, indications on the local, intrarenal, mechanisms possibly involved in the induction, maintenance or limitation of fibrin deposits.

Table 1. Main experimental and human renal diseases associated with glomerular fibrin deposits.

EXPERIMENTAL DISEASES
       Generalized Shwartzman phenomenon
       Thrombin/thromboplastin-induced acute renal failure
       Glycerol-induced hemoglobinuric acute renal failure
       Aleutian disease
       Nephrotoxic serum nephritis
       Chronic serum sickness
       Murine lupus nephritis
       Mercuric chloride-induced autoimmune glomerulonephritis
       Penicillamine-induced autoimmune glomerulonephritis
       Renal graft rejection
       Toxemia of pregnancy
       Nephropathy following subtotal renal ablation

HUMAN DISEASES
       Disseminated intravascular coagulation-associated acute renal failure
       Bilateral cortical necrosis
       Hemolytic-uremic syndrome
       Extracapillary (crescentic) glomerulonephritis
       Immunoglobulin A nephropathy
       Renal allograft rejection
       Toxemia of pregnancy

An important step forward was taken with the evidence, still in progress, that structural components of the glomerulus pertain to, or are able to interfere with blood hemostasis system (13, 14). This finding was made possible by systematic studies of preparation of isolated glomeruli, and by the application of antibodies specifically directed against platelet antigens or coagulation/fibrinolysis proteins on kidney fragments or extracts. In addition to microscopic renal fibrin deposits, disorders of coagulation in glomerular diseases are characterized, when accompanied by NS, by the onset of deep vein thrombophlebitis, predominantly localized in renal veins; such thromboses increase significantly the morbidity and severity of GN (15, 16).

Accordingly, the present review is intended [1] to provide a comprehensive description of the glomerular hemostasis system; [2] to report its changes, together with those of systemic coagulation/fibrinolysis system, in nephropathies with renal fibrin deposits and/or deep vein thromboses; [3] to emphasize the possible diagnostic and therapeutic importance of these data in human renal diseases.

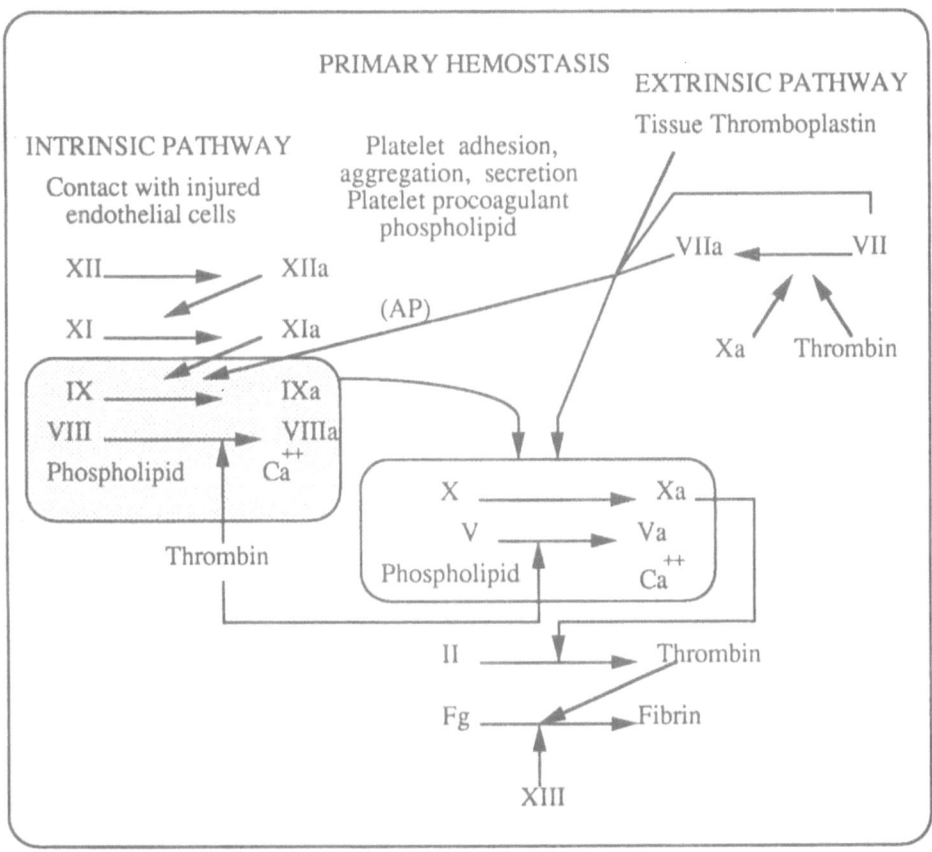

Figure 1. Primary hemostasis, and the intrinsic, extrinsic and alternative (AP) pathways of blood coagulation. The roman numerals denote the plasma coagulation factors with "a" for their activated forms. The activation of endothelium-bound factor XII requires the activation of prokallikrein to kallikrein in presence of high molecular weight kininogen. Collagen-stimulated platelets may also provide a surface for factor XII activation. The prothrombin activation complex (prothrombinase) is constituted by factor Xa (the enzyme) in association with factor Va and calcium, absorbed on phospholipids of either platelet or tissue thromboplastin origin. Thrombin autocatalytically activates factor VIII, factor VII and factor V. Factor XIII stabilizes fibrin which becomes cross-linked. The inhibitors of various steps of the coagulation system are not represented.

PHYSIOLOGY OF GLOMERULAR HEMOSTASIS

Normal blood coagulation and fibrinolysis

PRIMARY HEMOSTASIS AND PLASMA COAGULATION

The main steps of primary hemostasis and blood coagulation are depicted in Figure 1. Some points are worthy of emphasis:

[a] The two pathways of plasma coagulation converge to form prothrombinase, a complex comprising the enzyme factor Xa, associated with factor Va, negatively charged phospholipid (of either tissue thromplastin or platelet origin) and calcium (17, 18). In turn, factor Xa converts prothrombin to thrombin. The latter transforms soluble circulating fibrinogen into an insoluble network of polymeric fibrin, at least cross-linked following the action of circulating factor XIII (19);

[b] Interactions exist between the two classic pathways of plasma coagulation: on the one hand the tissue thromboplastin-factor VII complex is apt to activate not only factor X but also factor IX (20) in the so-called alternative coagulation pathway; on the other hand factors VIII and IX accelerate factor X activation by the thromboplastin-factor VII complex (21);

[c] A hallmark of the successive reactions involved in blood coagulation cascade is their ability to function autocatalytically. Such positive feedback mechanisms are best exemplified by thrombin actions (22): thrombin activates factor V and factor VIII (17), changes platelet membrane conformation making phospholipid available for prothrombinase formation, induces the formation of the proaggregatory platelet thromboxane (Tx) A_2 (23), and may stimulate the synthesis of thromboplastin by endothelial cells (24);

[d] Several natural anticoagulant systems also exist that either limit the formation of thrombin or inhibit its actions. First, by a negative feedback mechanism thrombin, once bound to its cofactor thrombomodulin, a 75 kD glycoprotein of the endothelial cell surface, activates protein C, that in presence of its cofactor protein S, provokes proteolytic degradation and inactivation of non-enzymatic factors V and VIII (25). Second, coagulant action of thrombin can be suppressed: [1] by thrombomodulin itself (25); [2] by its complexing with antithrombin III (AT III) (26); [3] by glomerular basement membrane (GBM) or endothelial cell surface heparan sulfate, which binds the complex AT III-thrombin and accelerates inactivation of the latter (27). Third, an inhibitor that binds to tissue thromboplastin and decreases its activity has recently been evidenced in plasma and called "LACI" (lipoprotein-associated coagulation inhibitor) (28);

6

[e] Current knowledge of blood coagulation derives largely from *in vitro* experiments: accordingly extrapolation to *in vivo* phenomena may be hypothetical.

As far as thrombosis is concerned, we have to assume in the present review that the *in vivo* onset of intravascular thrombosis depends at least in part upon modifications of concentrations and activities of coagulation/fibrinolysis factors, as suggested notably by *in vitro* reproduction of thrombosis in human vessel walls (29, 30), and that experimental data concerning platelets, monocytes, and endothelium functions and interaction are relevant to their behaviour in health and disease.

Table 2. Components of the fibrinolytic system.

MOLECULE	ROLE
Plasminogen	Inactive zymogen of plasmin
Plasmin	Active enzyme with fibrinolytic and proteolytic properties
Tissue-type plasminogen activator (t-PA)	Converts plasminogen into plasmin, fibrin dependency +++, similar to vascular PA
Urokinase-type plasminogen activator (u-PA)	Converts plasminogen into plasmin, fibrin-independency +++
Pro-urokinase, single chain u-PA (SC u-PA)	Inactive proenzyme of u-PA
Streptokinase	Streptococcal protein which converts plasminogen into plasmin
Plasminogen activator inhibitors (PAI)	Endothelial type (PAI-1), placental type (PAI-2), protease nexin
Alpha 2 antiplasmin	rapid, specific inhibitor of plasmin
Urokinase-type plasminogen activator receptor (u-PA-R)	binds u-PA at the cell surface

THE FIBRINOLYTIC SYSTEM. MECHANISMS OF PLASMINOGEN ACTIVATION

The components of the fibrinolytic system have been progressively identified (Table 2). The key enzyme is plasmin, a serine protease derived from the inactive zymogen plasminogen. Plasminogen activation is a highly controlled process which involves specific plasminogen activators and specific inhibitors of these activators (Figure 2).

Plasminogen and plasminogen activators (PA) are serine proteases involved in fibrinolysis and also in extracellular proteolysis for tissue remodeling and cell migration (31, 32). Plasminogen (molecular weight = 90 kD) is a glycoprotein synthesized mainly by hepatocytes. Its gene has been cloned and sequenced, coding for a protein of 791 aminoacids.

Urokinase-type plasminogen activator (u-PA) is a 54 kD serine protease made of 2 polypeptide chains A and B linked by a disulfure bridge. Limited auto-proteolysis of the A chain removes the aminoterminal fragment and results in a 33 kD active form of u-PA. The human gene of u-PA has been cloned and sequenced, encoding for a single-chain inactive form of u-PA (SC u-PA) which is activated by plasmin or kallikrein. Recently a membrane receptor for u-PA (u-PA-R) has been characterized and its gene has been cloned and sequenced (33). It is a highly glycosylated protein anchored to the plasma membrane by a COOH-terminal glycosyl-phosphatidyl-inositol (34) which may give a relative mobility of u-PA bound at the cell surface.

Tissue-type plasminogen activator (t-PA) is also a two chain serine protease synthesized as a single chain of 527 aminoacids. It is biochemically and immunologically different from u-PA. This 70 kD protein is released mainly by endothelial cells. It has 2 kringles domains in its structure which supports its fibrin-binding properties. One of the major difference with u-PA is that the enzymatic activity of t-PA is strikingly increased by fibrin whereas u-PA can convert plasminogen in the absence of fibrin and is not influenced by fibrin. Plasmin, in the vascular bed, is rapidly inhibited by circulating antiplasmin. However, if plasmin is bound at the surface of a fibrin clot, it is protected from inactivation until fibrin is degraded.

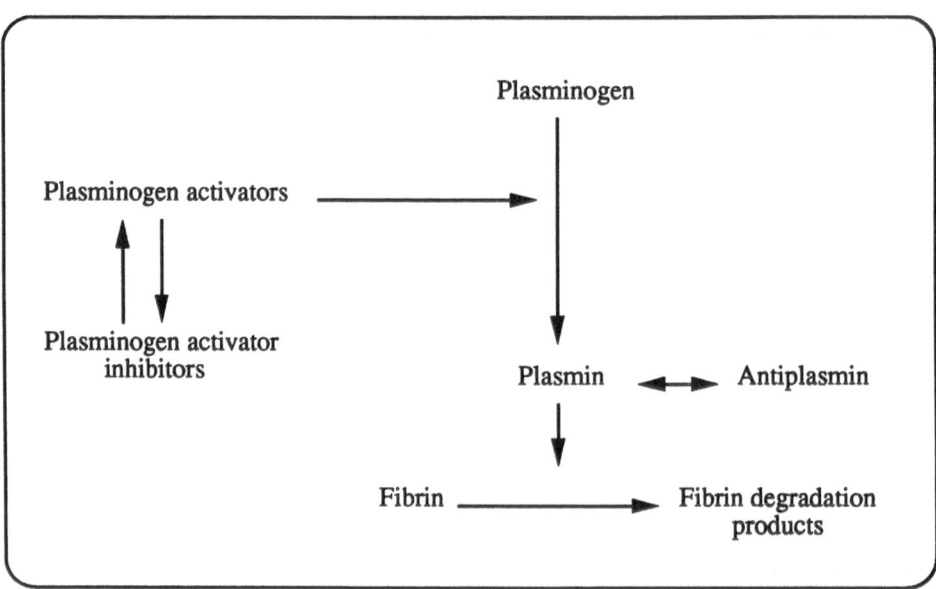

Figure 2. The fibrinolytic system.

The endothelial type plasminogen activator inhibitor (PAI-1) is a rapid and specific inhibitor of both u-PA and t-PA. It is synthesized and released by endothelial cells. Its gene has been cloned and sequenced and encodes for a 50 Kd glycoprotein which has some homology with other protease inhibitors called serine protease inhibitors (SERPIN) (31). PAI-2 is encoded by a different gene, is also a member of the SERPIN family, and was first isolated from placenta. It is also produced by activated monocytes-macrophages (31). PAI-1 can bind u-PA on its cellular receptor and induce endocytosis of the complex PAI-1-u-PA. They do not bind SC u-PA. Protease nexin is a non specific inhibitor of PA, since it inhibits also thrombin, plasmin and other trypsin-like serine proteases (31).

Glomerular hemostasis system

PROCOAGULANTS AND ANTICOAGULANTS

Data concerning procoagulant as well as anticoagulant components are summarized in Table 3. While the presence of all these components in mammalian glomeruli is definitely proved (by immunohistochemical methods or by radioimmunoassay), only for some of them a hemostatic activity has been directly substantiated in glomeruli or glomerular extracts, as detailed below; for other glomerular components such as heparan sulfate and fibronectin (35), von Willebrand factor (36), or thrombospondin (37), hemostatic activity remains putative.

However the activity of prostacyclin and thromboxane A_2, the main glomerular prostanoids in humans, cannot be directly assessed in glomeruli or glomerular cells because of their extremely short life span (less than 4 minutes). Their stable metabolites, 6-keto-PGF$_{1\alpha}$ and thromboxane B_2 respectively, are measured in glomerular supernatants by radioimmunoassay (38-41). Prostacyclin production by cultured human mesangial cells is enhanced by several vasoconstrictive agents: angiotensin II, arginine-vasopressin and platelet activating factor (PAF) (42). *Ex vivo*, thrombin perfusion in the rat increases glomerular thromboxane production (43) while, *in vitro*, thrombin has an opposite effect (44). *In vivo* imbalance of respective productions of prostacyclin and thromboxane in favor of the latter could hypothetically participate in the onset of thrombosis as has been suggested in the hemolytic uremic syndrome (45) and diabetes mellitus (46).

PAF produced by isolated glomeruli and mesangial cells on stimulation by calcium ionophore (47) or endotoxin (48, 49) also provokes irreversible platelet aggregation (47, 48) that occurs even in the absence of thromboxane or adenosine-diphosphate (ADP) (48). Conversely, PAF *per se* is able to increase the production of prostacyclin (and PGE$_2$) by

9

human mesangial cells (42), which may represent an autocrine compensatory feedback mechanism since PAF and prostacyclin have opposite platelet and vascular effects.

Suspension of GBM and type IV collagen (synthesized by epithelial cells) induce irreversible aggregation of platelets mediated by the release of intraplatelet ADP (50, 51); noncollagenous components might also be involved in this phenomenon (51).

Other glomerular lipids including fatty acids are apt to stimulate thromboxane A_2 synthesis by platelets and macrophages (52).

Tissue thromboplastin (tissue factor) is the lipoproteinic cofactor of factor VII that initiates extrinsic coagulation pathway. Significant progresses in the knowledge of structure and action of tissue thromboplastin have been made in the recent years (53). The lipid moiety of thromboplastin is constituted of phospholipids, mainly phosphatidylcholine and phosphatidylethanolamine; phospholipids are necessary to the co-factor function of thromboplastin in the extrinsic coagulation pathway. Human and bovine thromboplastin apoproteins have been purified to homogeneity (53). DNA complementary for thromboplastin apoprotein gene, localized on chromosome 1, has been isolated and cloned (54, 55). The human protein consists of 263 aminoacids (molecular weight: 29.6 kD) with 3 domains: extracellular (219 residues), transmembranar (23 residues), and cytoplasmic (21 residues). Disruption of tissues or cells containing thromboplastin increases procoagulant activity, which appears to be due to a change in membrane conformation depending on cytosolic calcium concentration (56).

The mechanisms of thromboplastin initiated coagulation are currently analyzed as follows, according to Nemerson (53) and Zur and Nemerson (57): [1] thromboplastin *per se* has no enzymatic activity; [2] the presence of thromboplastin is necessary for the enzyme factor VIIa to activate factor X to Xa (and factor IX to IXa): specifically, the substrate, factor X, binds to the complex thromboplastin-factor VIIa, but not to either of these two factors. Most probably thromboplastin, as cofactor, provokes a conformational change in factor VIIa favoring its enzymatic activity; [3] factor VII is a vitamin K-dependent single-chain protein of 406 aminoacids (53 kD) that is converted to a disulfide linked two chain form, factor VIIa, of the same molecular weight. This transformation is achieved by factor Xa and thrombin (another example of positive feedback mechanism) and also by factors XIIa and IXa; [4] factor VII, the zymogen, has an intrinsic enzymatic activity, found to be approximately 1% that of factor VIIa, and competes with factor VIIa for binding to thromboplastin.

Thus the following subtle working of thromboplastin-factor VII interaction is suggested: tissue injury makes thromboplastin available for binding to factor VII, the enzymatic activity of which activates factor X to Xa; in turn factor Xa autocatalytically provokes the transformation of VII to VIIa, which corresponds to a 100-fold enhancement in activity. On the other hand factor VII itself may participate in the regulation of the extrinsic coagulation pathway (in addition to the inhibitor LACI mentioned above). In case of mild tissue injury with relatively low local concentrations of thromboplastin, factor VII competes efficaciously with factor VIIa and, because of its weak enzymatic activity, limits the extension of clotting. On the contrary, in case of extensive tissue injury, large concentrations of thromboplastin allow its binding to both low activity factor VII and high activity factor VIIa, with subsequent dramatic acceleration of the clotting process (58). Finally, the ability of given cells to express procoagulant activity correlates strictly with their number of receptors for factor VII, normally much higher in non vascular than in vascular cells (which certainly participates in the non thrombogenicity of endothelial cells) (59).

The presence of thromboplastin in the mammalian kidney cortex was considered as long as twenty years ago (60). However, only recently the thromboplastinic nature of the cortical procoagulant activity and its glomerular origin have been unequivocally demonstrated. Isolated glomeruli from normal rat (61), rabbit (62-64) or human (52) kidney contain procoagulant activity, evidenced in platelet-poor plasma with the following properties: activity depends on presence of both factors VII and X, but not on that of factor VIII coagulant activity (note that quantitative analysis of receptors for factor VII in glomeruli or glomerular cells has not been reported); activity is suppressed by phospholipase C, an inhibitor of the phospholipid component of tissue thromboplastin; and activity is maximum after mechanical disruption of glomeruli.

Glomerular thromboplastin activity can be quantified, with the expected positive correlation between activity and protein concentration of glomerular suspensions (61). Immunohistochemical methods and activity measurements have shown that thromboplastin is produced by normal epithelial and mesangial cells (65, 66); in the latter cycloheximide blocks the synthesis of thromboplastin activity (66). Moreover mesangial thromboplastin synthesis is stimulated by cell incubation with tumor necrosis factor (TNF) and bacterial lipopolysaccharide (LPS) (66). It is likely that, in some conditions, glomerular endothelial cells also produce thromboplastin as endothelial cells of other origins on stimulation by thrombin (24), interleukin 1 (IL-1) (67), TNF (68), endotoxin (24), antigen antibody complexes (69) and platelets (70); in the absence of stimulation, these cells have no or only quite little coagulant activity. Noteworthily, as IL-1 (71) and TNF (72) are synthesized by mesangial cells as well as by monocytes/macrophages, they might trigger thromboplastin synthesis by adjacent endothelial cells.

In the near future utilization of molecular probes for thromboplastin will be possible in experimental and in human renal diseases. In the latter, studies of thromboplastin mRNA in renal biopsies by *in situ* hybridization should yield important insights into its role in glomerular fibrin deposition, as suggested by results obtained in measuring procoagulant activity of glomeruli isolated in experimental and human nephropathies (73) (see below).

Adenosine-diphosphatase (ADPase), the presence of which was cytochemically proved in rat GBM, appears to contribute to the nonthrombogenic character of normal glomeruli. Indeed Bakker et al (74) observed that perfusion of platelets and ADP (a potent proaggregatory substance) in rat kidney depleted in glomerular ADPase following chemotherapy or irradiation provoked intraglomerular platelet aggregation, whereas this did not occur in normal kidneys. Later, the same authors reported that glomerular ADPase activity was decreased in pregnant rats with endotoxemia (75).

Thrombomodulin was first found by immunofluorescence in rabbit glomerular endothelium (76), which was later confirmed by an immunoperoxydase technique (77). We extended this finding to isolated rat glomeruli, from which we extracted anticoagulantly active thrombomodulin (He and Kanfer, unpublished results). Endotoxin (78), IL-1 (79) and TNF (80, 81) decrease expression of vascular endothelial thrombomodulin, both *in vitro* and *in vivo*.

COMPONENTS OF THE FIBRINOLYTIC SYSTEM

The presence of plasminogen activators in rat (82) and human kidney (83, 84) has been demonstrated by biochemical and histochemical methods many years ago. The first characterization of t-PA and u-PA by immunological methods was made more recently (85) as was reported the intrarenal localization of u-PA in the mouse kidney (86). More recently, by the combined use of zymographies on tissue sections and *in situ* hybridization, u-PA was found to be synthesized by the epithelial cells lining the straight parts of both proximal and distal tubules. In contrast t-PA was found to be produced by glomerular cells and by epithelial cells lining the distal part of collecting ducts (87).

Tissue type plasminogen activator (t-PA)

One group reported specific analysis of glomerular components of the fibrinolytic system. Supernatant and extracts of human glomeruli isolated from normal kidney contain plasminogen activator (PA) activity (88, 89) which is mainly fibrin dependent and inhibited by anti-human t-PA antibody (80% of total activity) whereas a small part is fibrin-independent and blocked by anti-u-PA antibody (10-15% of total activity). Zymographic analysis of these glomerular supernatants showed mainly a 70 kD form of t-PA, small amounts of a 110 kD PAI-1/t-PA complex and traces of 53 kD u-PA. No free PAI-1 was observed by reverse fibrin autography (90). Thus most of the PA activity of the glomerulus is due to t-PA. By immunofluorescence methods using a monoclonal anti-t-PA antibody (EA delta 12 D) (88), we localized t-PA in the glomerular capillary tuft probably in the endothelial and mesangial cells and at the luminal surface of endothelial cells of renal arterioles.

Release of PA from isolated glomeruli is time-dependent and is increased *in vitro* by calcium addition and alcalosis (89). As these regulatory factors could interfere with phospholipase A_2 activity, we tested the effect of arachidonic acid and some of its metabolites.

Polyunsaturated fatty acids were found to increase PA activity of isolated glomeruli *in vitro* and this effect was independent of cyclooxygenase or lipoxygenase pathways, the two major routs of arachidonic acid metabolism.

Urokinase type plasminogen activator (u-PA)

The presence of small amounts of u-PA in human glomeruli has been reported by our group and others (88, 89, 91). In contrast to t-PA, by immunofluorescence on human kidney sections, u-PA was found mainly in the tubular epithelial cells and also in glomerular parietal cells. One group localized u-PA in glomerular endothelial cells by immunofluorescence using a monoclonal anti u-PA antibody (92). By *in situ* hybridization using a specific u-PA cDNA probe, we found that these cells contain u-PA mRNA and thus that u-PA was synthesized at these sites (Figure 3).

Regulation of u-PA synthesis has been studied in LLC-PK1 cells and in human glomerular epithelial cells. In LLC-PK1 cells, a proximal tubule epithelial cell line from a pig kidney, we reported a stimulatory effect of polyunsaturated fatty acids which increase the u-PA gene transcription induced by phorbol myristate acetate (PMA), a protein kinase C activator (93). Conversely, nordihydroguaiaretic acid, an inhibitor of lipoxygenase pathway, inhibited the PMA effect on u-PA gene transcription by blunting protein kinase C activation. Thus, at least in this cell model, regulation of u-PA synthesis is dependent on protein kinase C and fatty acids.

In vivo the release of glomerular PA may thus be controlled by hormones or mediators which activate intracellular protein kinase C and by circulating or intracellular fatty acids (94).

13

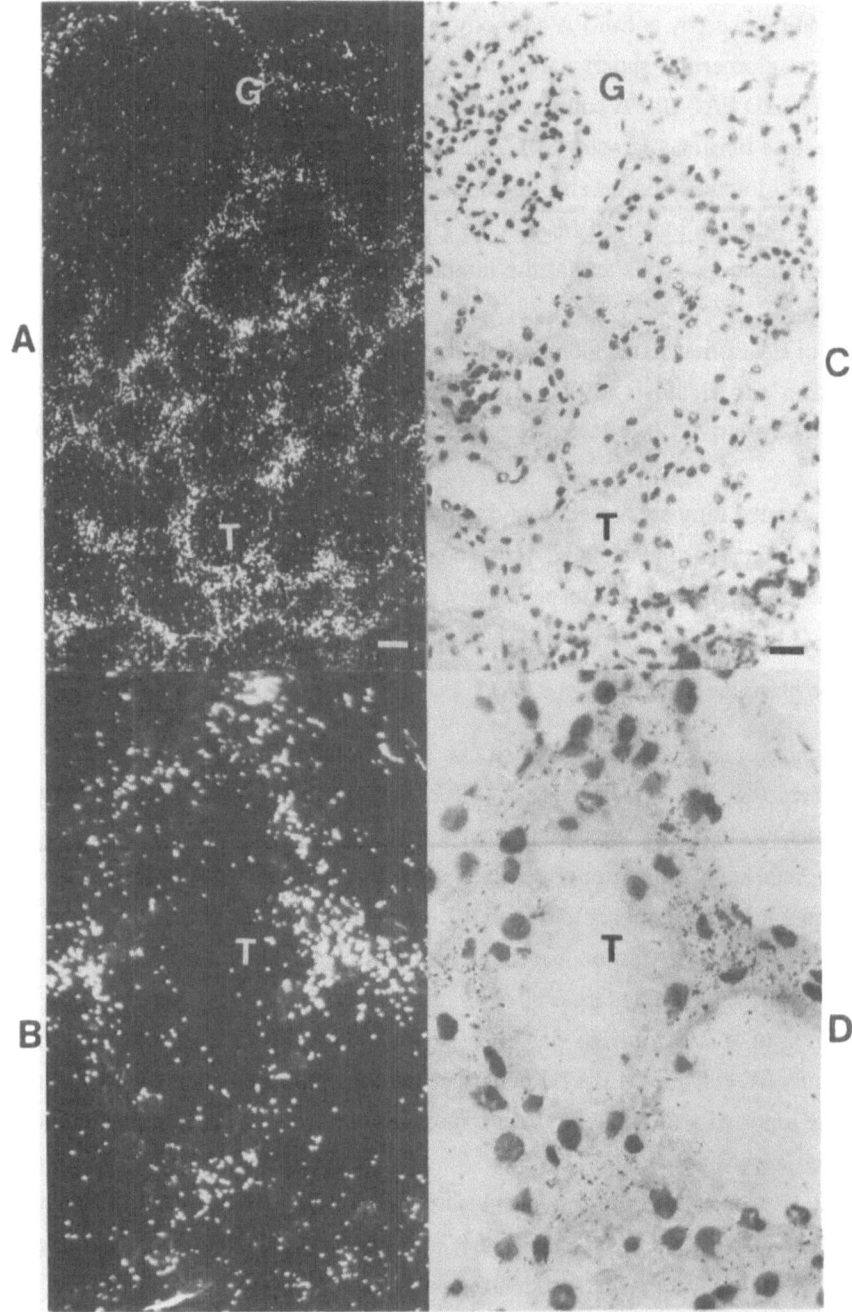

Figure 3.   Localization of urokinase mRNA in normal human kidney by in situ hybridization. A specific urokinase cDNA probe labeled with ^{35}S was used. Histoautoradiographies observed with dark field (A, B) and bright field (C, D) microscopy are shown. Urokinase mRNA is localized in glomerular epithelial cells (G) and in tubular epithelial cells (T). Bar, top 15 μm; bar, bottom 10 μm.

Primary cultures of human glomerular epithelial cells were studied. These cells exhibit some characteristic features of podocytes (CALLA, PHM5), but also contain keratin which is detected *in vivo* in parietal cells and not in podocytes, at least in the adult kidney. They produce SC u-PA, which is released in the extracellular space and which autosaturates u-PA receptors at the cell surface (95). In these cells, activation of protein kinase C by PMA increases u-PA gene transcription whereas activation of protein kinase A by cyclic AMP has an opposite effect. Glomerular epithelial cells also release small amounts of t-PA complexed to PAI-1. PAI-1 is attached to the growth substratum around and under cultured cells. To investigate the pathogenesis of proliferative extracapillary glomerulonephritis, we studied the effects of thrombin on glomerular epithelial cells. We demonstrated a proliferative effect of thrombin, an increased synthesis of u-PA, PAI-1 and t-PA and a decreased u-PA activity related to a direct proteolytic inactivation of SC u-PA by thrombin (96).

Thus thrombin could be responsible for glomerular fibrin deposition, cell proliferation and decreased local fibrinolytic activity. Furthermore thrombin was found to decrease the number of u-PA-R at the cell surface suggesting that the cell surface proteolytic activity is also decreased.

It has been shown that u-PA may play a role in the shape-change produced by agents which elevate intracellular cyclic AMP. Thrombin which inactivates SC u-PA prevents these shape-changes. The role of these u-PA mediated shape-changes *in vivo* remains to be determined (97).

Human glomerular endothelial cells are not currently cultured. However it has been reported that cultured microvascular endothelial cells from human kidney, most of which being of glomerular origin, release large amounts of SC u-PA and that this production is increased by PMA and thrombin (98). It was not modified by dexamethasone and TGF ß (transforming growth factor ß). No PAI-1 was detected. In contrast endothelial cells from umbilical vein produced t-PA and PAI-1 but not u-PA. Thus a heterogeneity of endothelial cells concerning their PA production is observed.

PAI-1 is synthesized by human mesangial cells in culture and is found in the conditioned culture medium as a 110 Kd t-PA/PAI-1 complex and as a 50 kD free form. A large excess of PAI-1 is released compared to t-PA which is never found in a free form (99). PAI-1 and t-PA synthesis are stimulated by activators of protein kinase C, such as PMA or thrombin (100). An increased gene transcription is required for this effect to appear. Protein kinase A activation potentiates the increase of t-PA mRNA induced by PMA but prevents that of PAI-1 mRNA. A post transcriptional effect of protein kinase A is also likely since 8 bromocyclic AMP inhibits both PMA-stimulated t-PA and PAI-1 releases. Interestingly this is a specific way of regulation not found in endothelial cells which also release PAI-1 and t-PA. It may correspond to a tissue-specific control and indicates that specific studies of glomerular cells are needed. PAI-1 is also found attached to the growth substratum of mesangial cells where it can be removed by exogenously added free t-PA (Peraldi et al, unpublished results). It could play a role in the control of cell migration or expansion in the extracellular matrix and in the regulation of glomerular extracellular matrix turn over. Species specificity is likely since rat mesangial cells in culture, although studied after many passages, synthesize mainly u-PA and not t-PA (97).

In conclusion, taken together these data indicate that plasminogen activators, t-PA and u-PA, and PAI-1 but not PAI-2 are produced by renal cells (Table 3). They may play a role in physiological conditions of intravascular fibrinolysis, t-PA being the main PA involved at the endothelial cell surface. The physiopathological role of u-PA in the kidney is still unknown. One can speculate that it is required to induce a proteolytic activity in the lumen of proximal and distal tubules for peptides clivage before reabsorption or for digestion of tubular casts. PA seems to be involved also in the turnover of extracellular matrix and could play a role in embryogenesis, compensatory hypertrophy and/or glomerulosclerosis.

Interaction of glomerular hemostasis components with blood borne leukocytes

The infiltration of glomeruli by blood borne cells in numerous human or experimental GN with fibrin deposits suggests that interaction of these cells and glomerular structural (resident) cells or components operate in the genesis of lesions. The multiple *in vitro* interactions of glomerular constituents on platelet have already been mentioned (Table 3). Hereafter we describe the established *in vitro* interactions of glomerular components with monocytes/macrophages and polymorphonuclear leukocytes.

Incubation with isolated normal glomeruli induces rat peritoneal macrophages to enhance their production of both prostacyclin and thromboxane (101). Moreover this effect is abolished and ever reversed by incubation of the combined preparations with thrombin, which provokes a marked decrease in the macrophage synthesis of both prostanoids (43). Incubation with human GBM-antiGBM complexes (obtained *in vitro*) stimulate human monocyte synthesis of TNF and IL-1 (102). Reciprocally, IL-1 generated *ex vivo* by macrophages extracted from nephritic rat glomeruli are apt to augment *in vitro* endothelial cell thromboplastin activity (103). Thus resident glomerular cells and monocytes/macrophages are mutually capable to enhance their respective procoagulant activity.

16

Table 3. Glomerular hemostasis system.

	GLOMERULAR LOCALIZATION	FUNCTIONS
PROCOAGULANTS		
Collagen	Glomerular basement membrane	Platelet aggregation; contact activation
Platelet activating factor (PAF)	Glomeruli; cultured mesangial cells	Platelet aggregation
Lipid extract (fatty acids)	Glomeruli	Platelet thromboxane synthesis
von Willebrand factor	Cultured endothelial cells	Platelet adhesion to vessel wall
Fibronectin	Extracellular matrix	Platelet adhesion
Thromboxane A$_2$	Glomeruli ; cultured epithelial cells	Platelet aggregation
Thrombospondin	Cultured mesangial cells	Platelet aggregation
Tissue thromboplastin	Glomeruli ; cultured mesangial and epithelial cells	Activation of the extrinsic coagulation pathway
ANTICOAGULANTS		
Heparan sulfate	Glomerular basement membrane; extracellular matrix	Thrombin inactivation
Adenosine diphosphatase	Glomerular basement membrane; endothelial and epithelial cells	Inhibition of platelet aggregation
Prostacyclin (PGI$_2$)	Glomeruli; cultured mesangial cells	Inhibition of platelet aggregation
Thrombomodulin	Endothelial cells	Thrombin inhibition; cofactor of protein C activation
PROFIBRINOLYTIC FACTORS		
t-PA	Endothelial cells	Fibrinolysis
	Mesangial cells	matrix remodeling
u-PA	Epithelial cells	Fibrinolysis
	Endothelial cells in culture	Matrix remodeling
ANTIFIBRINOLYTIC FACTOR		
PAI-1	Mesangial cells in culture	Inhibition of plasmin generation and matrix degradation
	Epithelial cells	

Polymorphonuclear leukocytes, when induced to generate reactive oxygen metabolites, double mesangial cell prostanoid production, notably that of thromboxane and prostacyclin (104). Such metabolites can also directly injure endothelial cells and provoke the exposure of collagen to intracapillary circulating blood, rendering it available for platelet aggregation and/or contact activation in the plasma coagulation intrinsic pathway (105).

Few data are available concerning the effects of blood-borne cells on the fibrinolytic activity of renal cells. Platelets, which may accumulate in the kidney during intravascular coagulation, vasculitis or crescentic glomerulonephritis, are known to release PAI-1 upon activation and aggregation. Activated monocytes or macrophages are known to synthesize u-PA (106, 107) and one inhibitor, PAI-2 (108, 109). LPS stimulation increases u-PA secreted into the medium, bound of human monocytes *in vitro* to the cell surface and found intracellularly (110). The surface bound u-PA is not inhibited by PAI-1 or PAI-2 and may thus influence the ability of monocytes to migrate in and interact with an inflammatory microenvironment. Cytokines, produced by infiltrating inflammatory cells, are also known to modulate the synthesis of fibrinolytic components. Recently we demonstrated that TNFα increases the synthesis of PAI-1 by human mesangial cells in culture (Meulders et al, unpublished results) as previously reported in HT 1080 cells (111). In human umbilical vein endothelial cells, TNFα and IL-1 were shown to decrease t-PA and to increase PAI-1 release in a dose-dependent manner and this effect was associated with an increase in the steady-state level of PAI-1 mRNA (112).

Renal diseases

Glomerular fibrin deposits are found mainly in four circumstances (Table 1): [1] acute renal failure (ARF) due to bilateral cortical necrosis (BCN) or acute tubular necrosis (ATN); [2] the hemolytic uremic syndrome; [3] several types of GN of immunologic origin, and [4] renal allograft rejection. The mechanisms of fibrin deposit and/or formation, on the one hand, and the pathophysiologic role of intraglomerular coagulation, on the other hand, will be considered in each of these circumstances. They have been more extensively studied in animal than in human subjects, due for instance to the obvious difficulties of studying glomerular procoagulant or fibrinolytic activity in human renal diseases, which have been performed in only a very small number of patients.

Intravascular coagulation and acute renal failure

EXPERIMENTAL ACUTE RENAL FAILURE

Glomerular and/or arteriolar acute thromboses occur during disseminated intravascular coagulation (DIC), defined as thrombin formation in systemic circulation. DIC can be induced directly by infusion of procoagulant agents such as thrombin, thromboplastin, or liquoid, or indirectly by the injection of two doses of bacterial endotoxin in the generalized Shwartzman phenomenon (GSP) in rabbits or rats. Injection of immune complexes can also induce DIC. Glycerol administration induces DIC in rats or rabbits through intravascular hemolysis with release of an erythrocytic procoagulant phospholipid (for review see Ref. 7). Pretreatment of the animals by heparin prevents renal damage of the GSP, supporting a pathogenic role of intrarenal coagulation in this model (113). Experimentally renal thromboses following pure thrombin-induced DIC are rapidly cleared. The persistence of glomerular thromboses, leading to severe renal lesions, which may range from moderate tubular necrosis to complete cortical necrosis, results from factors, other than DIC *per se*, that are apt to maintain local coagulation activation or to inhibit fibrinolytic system (114). For example, we have demonstrated that glomerular fibrinolytic activity increases after thrombin infusion in rats and therefore may account for the transient character of glomerular capillary thrombi; on the contrary, inhibition of fibrinolytic activity by epsilon-aminocaproic acid (EACA) allows their maintenance (115).

During GSP the first injection of endotoxin decreases the cortical fibrinolytic activity (116); drugs induced reduction of this activity before endotoxin injection enhances the severity of renal thrombotic lesions (114). Furthermore a single endotoxin injection is effective in EACA-pretreated males and in gravid females in which systemic fibrinolytic activity is physiologically reduced (114). Similarly, the injection of EACA in glycerol-treated animals enhances the severity of renal lesions, essentially because of the presence of extensive glomerular thromboses (117). In addition to fibrinolysis inhibition, involvement of vasoconstrictor factors in the development of renal thrombotic lesions after DIC is suggested by the following features: [1] inhibition of the renin-angiotensin system by sodium overload or saralasin prevents renal failure and lesions during DIC induced by thrombin (118) while this remains uncertain for glycerol ATN (119, 120); [2] chemical blockade of alpha-adrenergic response produces the same preventive effect as renin-angiotensin inhibition during GSP (121), and [3] glomerular production of TxA_2 is increased in DIC induced by glycerol (122) or thrombin (44). In our laboratory, we have shown that in glycerol model, procoagulant activity was decreased and fibrinolytic activity was increased in glomeruli isolated from rats killed one to four hours after glycerol injection (Delarue et al, unpublished data). Such changes point to an adaptation of glomerular hemostasis components to systemic activation of coagulation in this model. On the contrary, in rabbit GSP endotoxin injection induces an enhancement of glomerular procoagulant activity likely to participate in the onset of glomerular thromboses (123).

HUMAN ACUTE RENAL FAILURE: ACUTE TUBULAR NECROSIS (ATN),
BILATERAL CORTICAL NECROSIS (BCN)

In human BCN, a rare situation, glomerular and intra-arteriolar microthrombosis are found in the majority of the patients. It is likely that this thrombosis is of pathophysiologic importance since microthromboses are constant and extensive in total BCN with irreversible anuria, whereas they are mild or even sometimes absent in patchy cortical necrosis with partial recovery of renal function. Arteriolar and extrarenal thromboses are associated with glomerular thrombi, strongly suggesting that glomerular fibrin deposits originate from systemic activation of the coagulation system; such a mechanism is obvious when DIC, accompanied by overt consumption coagulopathy, is associated with acute renal failure, a situation observed in anuric patients with postpartum BCN (124). In contrast, glomerular fibrin is seldom found in ATN, as exemplified by our own findings (5% of our cases) (125) and those of others (126, 127), although Clarkson et al (127) reported a much higher prevalence of glomerular intracapillary thrombosis (about 50% of the cases) in this setting. However fibrin deposits are relatively frequent and abundant in some particular etiologic circumstances associated with ATN such as acute pancreatitis (128), snake bite and obstetric complications (7).

Table 4.   Main causes of association between disseminated intravascular coagulation and acute tubular necrosis (ATN) in humans.

Obstetric conditions
        Abruptio placentae
        Amniotic embolism
        Intrauterine fetal death
        Pre-eclamptic toxemia, Eclampsia
        Puerperal sepsis
        Septic abortion
Septicemias
Intravascular hemolytic anemias
Acute leukemias
Disseminated cancers
Acute pancreatitis

In spite of the usual absence of histologic markers of intraglomerular coagulation in ATN, a pathogenetic role for intrarenal coagulation in this condition is suggested by its frequent association with DIC and/or with an increase in serum and urine fibrin degradation products (7). First, overt DIC occurs in about 5% to 30% of patients with presumed or histologically confirmed ATN. Table 4 indicates the main etiologic circumstances of such an association. Interestingly, in some conditions during which the onset of acute tubular necrosis is not preceded by shock, infection, or administration of nephrotoxins, DIC appears as the main or even sole triggering factor of ATN, for example: pregnancy or the postpartum period, acute leukemias, and acute pancreatitis. Second, increase in urine concentration of fibrin degradation products is found in the majority of patients with acute tubular necrosis, even in the absence of DIC. Since urine fibrin degradation products are of high molecular weight with very low renal clearance, they are likely to correspond to the intrarenal lysis of fibrin deposits, presumably following the action of renal t-PA, inasmuch as urine-urokinase activity is strikingly diminished in renal failure (129).

Similar etiologic circumstances may lead either to bilateral cortical necrosis or to acute tubular necrosis. In the former, glomerular thrombi are generally extensive, while they are rare and mild in the latter. Conceivably, the persistence of microthrombi with renal cortical irreversible ischemia could be due to an insufficient glomerular fibrinolytic activity. Although such an abnormality has not been evidenced in humans, it is however strongly suggested by: [1] the relative frequency of bilateral cortical necrosis during pregnancy, a condition physiologically characterized by diminished fibrinolysis, and [2] the onset of cases of cortical necrosis following the administration of antifibrinolytic drugs (126).

In ATN, the increase in urine fibrin degradation products at the recovery phase, concomitantly with the onset of diuresis, suggests that persistent intrarenal fibrinolytic activity induces ongoing lysis of microthrombi, with accordingly only a minor role for them in ischemia of the renal cortex that must be due mostly to vasoactive phenomena. However we have shown that plasma antiplasmin activity was increased in acute renal failure due to ATN, which could diminish the efficiency of renal fibrinolytic activity in some patients (130). Taken together, these findings lead to the following treatments: in ATN with DIC, in our opinion, heparin may be given in cases of protracted consumption coagulopathy, when no etiologic treatment of underlying disease is attainable, as in some protracted intravascular hemolytic anemias, and in the absence of (risk of) bleeding; also in cases of ATN with reduced systemic fibrinolytic activity, perfusion of plasminogen has been used with rapid improvement of renal function (131). These treatments, although logical, remain empirical because to our knowledge no control studies of their efficiency are available. In any case, antifibrinolytic drugs are absolutely contraindicated.

Role of coagulation and fibrinolysis in glomerulonephritides

EXPERIMENTAL GLOMERULONEPHRITIDES

Anti-GBM glomerulonephritis

Intraglomerular fibrin deposits are almost constant in Masugi's nephritis. More than twenty years ago, Vassalli and Mac Cluskey noted that such deposits are located in the capillary tufts, in the heterologous phase of the disease, and then in Bowman's space during the autologous phase, when crescents are forming (132). Fibrin deposits have been reported in all species: rabbit (132), rat (133, 134), and mouse (135). The mechanisms of intraglomerular fibrin deposition are still unclear. While platelet depletion with antiserum does not alter fibrin deposition (136, 137), a role for platelet aggregation in glomerular coagulation is suggested in some studies by the protective effect of thromboxane inhibition. However the effects of inhibition of thromboxane synthesis in anti-GBM GN remain controversial: it was found to be beneficial in a short term study in rat disease (138) but contradictory results with either beneficial (139) or deleterious effects were reported in rabbit disease (140). On the other hand, fibrin deposition could involve activation of intrinsic or extrinsic coagulation pathway. In favor of a role of the intrinsic pathway is the evidence, provided by immunofluorescence studies, of factor VIII (141) and factor XII deposits (142). In rabbit anti-GBM GN, factor XII (a 80 kD protein) was not detected in glomerular capillaries but early in the disease in Bowman's space, where it appears to be activated, presumably by collagen and fragments of the altered glomerular basement membrane (142). Thus a role for factor XII in ongoing formation of extracapillary fibrin cannot be ruled out. Concerning factor VIII discrepant results have been obtained in rats and rabbits. Factor VIII antigen deposits are detected early in the disease in the glomerular capillary and in crescents in rat anti-GBM GN (141) and therefore may have a pathogenic role in fibrin formation. In contrast, deposits of factor VIII are observed only lately and in marginal amounts in rabbit disease (143).

A role for local activation of extrinsic coagulation pathway in fibrin deposition in capillaries and Bowman's space is strongly suggested in rabbit anti-GBM GN by: [a] the increase in glomerular thromboplastin activity that has been directly evidenced in glomeruli isolated from diseased kidneys (62, 144); [b] the chronologic relationship observed between increased glomerular procoagulant activity and the onset of fibrin deposits in sequential studies (143).

The origin of enhanced procoagulant activity in this disease has been ascribed to the thromboplastin content of invading macrophages, because macrophage depletion returns glomerular procoagulant activity to its control values and prevents fibrin deposits (62). It was also shown that macrophages expressed markedly augmented procoagulant activity compared with blood and alveolar monocytes of the same animals (145).

Macrophages may participate in fibrin deposition not only through their own procoagulant activity but also through their production of IL-1 that can trigger thromboplastin synthesis by adjacent glomerular mesangial or endothelial cells (145). On the other hand, monocytes may reduce crescent formation by phagocytosis and degradation of fibrin (146): therefore, one can hypothesize a dual role of glomerular macrophages which are potentially apt either to induce or to scavenge fibrin deposits.

22

Whatever the mechanism of the fibrin formation, its pathophysiologic importance is certain. Thus, during accelerated models of anti-GBM GN, the thrombotic lesions are extreme, possibly leading to cortical necrosis (134, 147). Both in rats and rabbits, the intensity of glomerular fibrin deposits is clearly correlated, on the one hand, to the intensity of proliferative lesions, and, on the other hand, to the degree of renal failure (132, 133). Some authors have shown that the severity of the proliferative lesions is reduced by pretreatment of the animals by heparin or warfarin which lowers the intensity of fibrin deposits (132, 148-150), but this benefit of heparin is controversial since other studies reported that heparin was ineffective in preventing crescent formation (135, 151). Additional evidence for the importance of coagulation was obtained by Naish et al (152, 153) who showed that treatment with ancrod, a defibrinating agent, markedly reduced glomerular fibrin deposition and inhibited the development of crescents and renal function impairment in rabbits.

The role of the systemic and local fibrinolytic system in the persistence or mitigation of fibrin deposits in anti-GBM GN is still unclear. We have reported increased *ex vivo* glomerular fibrinolytic activity during rat disease (134): this activity was correlated both with the intensity of fibrin deposits and with the number of crescents, which suggests an adaptive, although insufficient, reaction of the endogenous local fibrinolytic system to *in situ* coagulation. On the other hand, in mice (135) and in rabbits (147), early administration of streptokinase decreases the intensity of fibrin deposits, glomerular lesions, and renal failure. Fibrinolysis with streptokinase and defibrination with ancrod, in rabbits with anti-GBM GN, reduced markedly glomerular fibrin deposits and crescent formation and prevented deterioration of renal function in rabbits with anti-GBM GN (154). Recently, a similar beneficial effect was shown with t-PA (155). Although the rabbits had prolonged bleeding time, the authors did not observe signs of systemic fibrinolysis and there were no hemorragic complications. This suggests a major role for fibrinolysis in crescent formation and provides a solid rationale for future studies on the possible role of recombinant t-PA to attenuate crescents and fibrin deposits in human crescentic glomerulonephritis.

Immune complex GN: chronic serum sickness, lupus-like nephritis

Glomerular fibrin deposits associated with extracapillary proliferation have been reported in half of animals in rabbit chronic serum sickness nephritis (151, 156). The mechanism of activation of intraglomerular coagulation is unclear. While again platelet depletion does not prevent fibrin deposits (157), drug-induced inhibition of thromboxane synthetase may have a beneficial effect (158). Wardle (159) has shown an increased renal content of radio-labeled fibrinogen and a decrease of its plasmatic half-life correlated to enhanced circulating fibrin degradation products in rabbits receiving repeated injections of bovine serum albumin. Simultaneously he noted an activation of blood coagulation and a shortened half-life of the labeled antigen (159). Here again, ancrod-induced defibrination prevents fibrin deposits, extracapillary proliferation and impairment of renal function, although the initial immunologically induced events, i.e. IgG, C3 and serum albumin deposits, as well as endocapillary proliferation and leukocyte infiltrates remains unchanged (160).

During acute serum sickness nephritis and Heymann's nephritis, neither fibrin deposits nor extracapillary proliferation is generally reported (151, 153, 161), except when a hypertensive vascular factor is added (162-164). Moreover, during acute serum sickness nephritis, EACA-pretreated animals exhibit important glomerular fibrin deposits (159).

In both autoimmune models of GN in NZB mice (165, 166) and Aleutian disease of minks (167, 168), extracapillary proliferation is present, with numerous crescents and large fibrin deposits. In the lupus-like nephritis of NZB mice, the development of fibrin deposits is strongly linked to the occurrence of DNA-anti-DNA antibody immune complexes (166). The glomerular production of thromboxane is increased in NZB-NZW and MRL mice with lupus-like GN and is correlated with both the degree of renal failure and the intensity of glomerular damage (169). It was also found that splenic macrophage procoagulant activity rose with age and correlated with the development of GN in BxSB lupus mice (170). Another interesting model of immune complex GN was described by Sawtell et al (171) in Balb/c mice, using cationized bovine gammaglobulin as antigen. GN was non proliferative and characterized by conspicuous glomerular capillary thromboses. The factors underlying the development of thrombosis in this model are still unknown.

Rat toxic autoimmune nephritides: Mercuric chloride (HgCl$_2$)-induced GN and
D-Penicillamine-induced GN in Brown Norway rats

Both GN are characterized initially by the appearance of glomerular anti-GBM antibodies, followed by immune complexes; no or only a few blood borne cells, notably macrophages, infiltrate glomeruli. Fibrin deposits are present in glomerular capillaries. It is widely admitted that both chemicals induce a state of polyclonal activation (172). We choose to investigate glomerular procoagulant (thromboplastinic) activity in HgCl$_2$ GN, a self limited disease with an acme marked by heavy proteinuria 20-25 days after the first mercury injection (173). At this phase, some animals exhibit a definite state of DIC and eventually die while less severely ill rats progressively recover (174). Glomeruli were isolated from rats killed at day 12 (latent phase), 20 (acme), 32 and 42 (recovery phase): glomerular procoagulant activity was three fold that of control rats at day 20 whereas at initial or at recovery phases, activity was not different from control values. Conspicuous glomerular fibrin deposits were present in all rats killed at acme of GN, while only some of them have such deposits at the other phases of the disease. Finally we found no correlation between glomerular procoagulant activity and the number of macrophages present in diseased glomeruli (173). These results suggest that [a] immunologically-induced enhancement of glomerular procoagulant activity favor or even trigger local fibrin deposition through activation of extrinsic coagulation pathway; [b] structural glomerular cells themselves, and not only invading macrophages, may participate in the induction of glomerular coagulation.

The mechanisms of fibrin deposition in D-penicillamine-induced autoimmune GN remain to be determined (175).

HUMAN GLOMERULONEPHRITIDES

As compared to animal studies, only a few data on the mechanisms of intrarenal microthromboses in human GN are available. Fibrin deposits were not found to be associated with the presence of platelet aggregates (176), platelet antigens (177) or platelet factor 4 (177) in various GN. Furthermore, in a small group of patients with crescentic GN who had renal venous catheterization, there was no difference between the number of platelets in renal veins and in peripheral blood, indicating no or only little platelet consumption in the kidneys (178). Factor VIII was not immunohistochemically detected in human crescentic GN (179). In contrast, in glomeruli of IgA nephropathy (Berger's disease), which is often accompanied by glomerular fibrin deposits, factor XII (180) and factor VII (181) have been detected, which is not the case in normal glomeruli. Thromboplastinic activity of glomeruli isolated from kidneys of patients who died during the course of crescentic GN was markedly augmented as compared to value obtained in control normal glomeruli (182). Recently, glomerular procoagulant activity was microassayed on kidney fragments obtained by renal biopsies and also found enhanced in necrotic GN, in proliferative lupus GN and in membranous GN: the relevant of this method has to be established (183).

We have recently shown that extracapillary fibrin deposits in human GN contain significant amounts of the PAI-1, not normally detected in glomeruli (184). In agreement with these findings, other authors have observed increased plasma levels of PAI-1 in this setting. Enhanced local or systemic antifibrinolytic activity is probably a factor contributing to the persistence of fibrin deposits (185, 186).

Treatments of GN with fibrin deposits by antiplatelet or anticoagulant agents have given overall rather disappointing results. In extracapillary GN with fibrin deposits (whatever the underlying disease) heparin appears, at best, as an adjuvant to immunosuppressive drugs and/or plasma exchanges, or to treatment of underlying disease (for instance visceral abscesses) (187). However, some data obtained in humans as well as in laboratory animals have lead to therapeutic attempts, undertaken in limited numbers of patients. For instance, non controlled therapeutic assays with the defibrinating agent ancrod have given encouraging results in severe lupus nephritis (185) and in other types of GN (186), which have to be confirmed. Another drug, Defibrotide, with profibrinolytic and prostacyclin-stimulating activity, was recently shown to ameliorate the course of glomerulonephritic patients (188). The importance of such treatments is underlined by the fact that in lupus and other GN, glomerular sclerosis, and ultimately renal failure may be related to glomerular thrombosis, at least partly (185, 186, 189, 190).

Hemolytic uremic syndrome (HUS)

The term hemolytic uremic syndrome (HUS) refers to a clinical disorder characterized by the association of a Coombs negative microangiopathic hemolytic anemia, thrombocytopenia and acute renal failure. The typical histopathologic lesion is a thrombotic microangiopathy with swollen endothelial cells and a widened subendothelial space which produce a thickened capillary wall and a reduced capillary lumen. Fibrin-like material and lipids can be demonstrated in the subendothelial space. Thrombi may occlude the capillary lumen. The mesangium is expanded and there may be mesangiolysis. The medium-size blood vessels present also intimal cell proliferation, thickening of the wall and narrowing of the lumen. Immunofluorescence studies reveal extensive fibrin deposits in the walls of blood vessels and in glomeruli. Some deposits of IgM and C3 may be positive. It is possible to observe a predominance of glomerular injury or a predominance of arteriolar injury, but association between the two is often seen. Intrarenal clotting may be so severe as to lead to cortical necrosis.

EXPERIMENTAL MODELS OF HEMOLYTIC UREMIC SYNDROME (HUS)

Very few experimental models of HUS exist. The first one has been obtained by infusing Mitomycin directly in the renal artery of Lewis rats (191). Renal tissue, examined from one hour up to one month later, showed various degrees of lesions, from early endothelial damage to cortical necrosis, according to the dose injected. However, other studies using systemic administration of Mitomycin in rats and in rabbits did not succeed to induce HUS.

A rabbit model of HUS with renal cortical necrosis can be obtained by injection of LPS from Shigella species (192). However, rabbits made leukopenic with busulfan were protected from the development of cortical necrosis. Rabbits with modified generalized Shwartzman phenomenon exhibit leukopenia after LPS infusion. Additional mechanisms might include release of neutrophil enzymes, impairment of chemotaxis, and evidence of lipid peroxydation in renal cortical tissue (192). One polymorphonuclear leukocyte per endothelial cell supplies enough elastase to inhibit thrombin-induced prostacyclin production, and leukocyte elastase may be a mediator of endothelial cell detachment possibly by degradation of fibronectin (193). Therefore, increasing evidence suggests that neutrophils can contribute to endothelial injury. In that model, other factors can play a role: for example, LPS stimulates IL-1 and TNF production by monocytes, which in turn may imbalance the function of endothelial cells (194), towards coagulation, as discussed elsewhere.

HEMOLYTIC UREMIC SYNDROME (HUS) IN HUMANS

Clinical features

HUS is more frequently encountered in children (195) but is not rare in adults (196). The main clinical signs include acute renal failure, microangiopathic anemia with schizocytes and thrombocytopenia which is peripheral, related to shortened platelet life. Serum levels of fibrin degradation products are increased and there is a consumption coagulopathy with hypofibrinogenemia, prolongation of the prothrombin time and decrease in the level of antithrombin III at the very initial phase of the disease or during relapses.

According to most authors now, HUS and thrombotic thrombocytopenic purpura (TTP) describe different clinical expressions of the same disease (45).

Thrombotic microangiopathy is identical in hemolytic uremic syndrome and thrombotic thrombocytopenic purpura, but mainly involves the kidney in disorders previously called HUS and the brain in disorders called TTP.

The main clinical situations in which hemolytic uremic syndrome occurs are resumed in Table 5.

Pathogenesis of microthrombosis in HUS: evidence for a primary role
of endothelial cell injury

The mechanisms involved in the intrarenal coagulation of HUS are various according
to the various etiologic circumstances. The pathophysiology of the disease remains still
unknown but most available morphologic evidence indicate that endothelial cell damage
constitutes the key lesion in TTP-HUS. Several factors can be involved in the injury of
endothelial cells such as hemodynamic modifications, bacterial toxins or immunologically-
mediated lesions.

Recent studies provide evidence that endotoxins may be one of the major factors
triggering vascular endothelial damage in HUS: it has been proven that these toxins induce
the generation of procoagulant activity (197), and, recently, verotoxin has been shown to
be directly cytotoxic for renal endothelial cells (198).

Table 5.   Classification of hemolytic uremic syndrome (HUS).

---

(1) EPIDEMIC POST INFECTIOUS HUS (TYPICAL CHILDHOOD FORM)
      may follow infection due to:
                Shigella
                Salmonella
                Escherichia coli
                Streptococcus Pneumoniae
                Campylobacter jejuni
                Yersinia pseudotuberculosis
                Coxsackie virus echovirus
                Epstein Barr virus
                Human immunodeficiency virus
(2) HEREDITARY HUS (relapsing form in children and young adults)
(3) SECONDARY HUS
            Systemic lupus erythematosus
            Scleroderma
            Malignant hypertension
            Malignancies
            Preexisting glomerular disease
(4) PREGNANCY-ASSOCIATED HUS
(5) HUS ASSOCIATED WITH HYPERACUTE RENAL ALLOGRAFT REJECTION
(6) HUS RELATED TO A TOXIC CAUSE:
            Oral contraceptives
            Cyclosporin A
            Antineoplastic drugs (mainly Mitomycin C)
            Radiation of the kidney
            Cocaine "crack" inhalation

Detailed mechanisms of action of these toxins can be resumed as follows.
Escherichia coli, Shigella Dysenterial serotype I and Streptococcus Pneumoniae all produce
Shiga-like toxins (SLT) (199). The most commonly HUS-associated pathogen is E. coli.

Some E. coli secrete verotoxins (VT),which are cytotoxins that kill verocells *in vitro* (200). VT1 (SLT1) and VT2 (SLT2) are structurally, functionally and immunologically similar to Shiga toxin. Some HUS-associated strains of E. coli produce only STL1, some other only STL2 and many produce both toxins.

Karmali et al (201) demonstrated that some serotypes of E. coli (e.g. 0157, 026, 0111, 0113) are associated with HUS. In 75% of their patients, they could prove infection with a VT-producing organism (202). Other studies gave similar results (203). Outbreaks of E. coli 0157:H7 infection in HUS are frequent and have been reported in many countries. Infection can occur by person to person spread in families, day care centers and nursing homes (204, 205). Low inocula are sufficient in susceptible person. The diagnosis of SLT-associated HUS is often difficult because SLT producing-E. coli may constitute only 0.3% of the enteric flora (206). SLT have not been detected in sera. Shiga toxin is a 71 kD multisubunit complex made of a single 32 kD A-subunit and five 7.7 kDa B-subunits (207). The glycolipid galactose alpha 1,4–galactose ß 1,4–glucose-ceramide (Gb3) is the cell surface receptor for Shiga toxins, SLT1 and SLT2 (208). These cell receptors have a high affinity (Kd 10^{-10} M) for the toxin. Entry of the toxin is facilitated by cell-mediated endocytosis (209). Shiga toxins enter cells within one hour and the "A-subunit" inhibits protein synthesis within 30 minutes. The toxin selectively inactivates 60 S ribosomal subunits by its N-glycosidase activity (210, 211).

Human kidney, mainly the cortex, contains the Gb3 specific receptor for Shiga toxins, which is also present in endothelial and intestinal cells (212). Actively dividing endothelial cells are more sensitive to purified Shiga toxins that are non dividing cells. All members of the Shiga toxin group are cytotoxic to human umbilical vein endothelial cells in a dose- and time-dependent manner (213).

Besides endotoxins, endothelial damage in HUS-TTP may also be immunologically mediated, as in experimental hyperacute allograft rejection. Some studies demonstrated occasional antibodies directed against endothelial cells in sera from TTP patients. A recent study (214) showed that over 90% of patients, essentially children, with HUS have a cytotoxic antibody that reacts with cultured human umbilical vein endothelium. Frequency of these autoantibodies in adults is about half that in children.

Consequences of the endothelial cell injury

Whatever the precise initial mechanism is, four major consequences of endothelial cell damage have been substantiated: [1] inadequate endothelial-cell production of prostanoids PGI_2 and TxA_2; [2] the presence in the circulation of substances capable of inducing intravascular platelet clumping; [3] the role of unusually large vWF multimeric forms found in patients with the chronic relapsing form of HUS-TTP; [4] defective fibrinolysis may be due to defective production of plasminogen activators in endothelial cells.

Several authors have demonstrated a deficit in PGI_2 in patients with HUS: Remuzzi et al (215) reported in 1978 that vascular specimens from patients with HUS-TTP had reduced ability to form PGI_2. This observation was supported by other studies (216, 217). The 6 keto $PGF_{1\alpha}$ level was low or undetectable in patients with HUS-TTP (218). In one study, plasma 6 keto $PGF_{1\alpha}$ was undetectable during the acute phase of the disease but returned to normal levels when clinical remission was achieved (219). A family with recurrent HUS episodes was affected by a genetic deficiency in prostacyclin synthesis stimulating factor (220). Chen et al (221) reported accelerated serum PGI_2 degradation in a patient with chronic TTP. The capacity of serum to bind PGI_2 was also diminished in several chronic TTP patients compared to normal persons (222). This decreased serum binding of PGI_2 may reduce the availability of PGI_2 at damaged vascular sites.

On the other hand, vascular damage is expected to stimulate rather than to inhibit PGI_2 synthesis, and the reason why patients with HUS should have depressed vascular PGI_2 is not yet clarified. Two hypotheses can be proposed according to Remuzzi: first, repeated stimulation of endothelial cells by toxin, for example, can "exhaust" the vessel wall capacity to produce PGI_2 as suggested by a recent study (223). Second, experimental evidence indicates that PGI_2 synthetase is inhibited by the lipid peroxydes formed during the activation of the arachidonic acid cascade following endothelial cell injury (224).

In this context, some authors have noted that HUS patients lack a plasma factor that regulates endothelial PGI_2 production (225, 226). This factor has been partially characterized: it is a stable substance with a molecular weight of 300 to 400 daltons, that protects the vascular PGI_2 forming system from exhaustion during persistent endothelial injury (227). This PGI_2-regulating plasma factor behaves as a reducing cofactor for cyclooxygenase, maybe by delaying its inactivation in chronically damaged blood vessels. In HUS, remission can follow infusions of fresh frozen plasma. This suggests that normal plasma provides the missing PGI_2 stimulating factor (228).

This theory about a deficiency in PGI_2 synthesis has been recently refuted: Stuart et al (229) did not find any PGI_2 deficiency in children with HUS. Furthermore, in a recent study, different mechanisms of platelet activation were found in the two main subgroups of HUS, i.e. typical (in children) and atypical HUS (230). Platelet activation was a common feature of both forms. However, there was a defect in PGI_2 production only in atypical HUS while this was not found in typical HUS. Furthermore, platelet activation may be due to an insensitivity to PGI_2, rather than to a deficient production of PGI_2 (231). More recently, it was found that TxA_2 biosynthesis was markedly elevated in the acute phases of HUS (232), while concomitantly renal PGI_2 and systemic PGI_2 formation were elevated in 50% of the patients. The authors conclude that the enhanced synthesis of TxA_2 is consistent with increased platelet activation whereas the increased PGI_2 biosynthesis reflects predominantly renal endothelial cell damage. Finally, another argument against PGI_2 deficiency is the failure of infusion of a PGI_2 analog to improve the course of the disease.

A platelet agglutinating factor is detected in the plasma of some patients during episodes of TTP (233): plasma samples from patients with acute TTP induces *in vitro* clumping of washed platelets from both normal donors and patients during remission. Platelet clumping is inhibited by the addition of normal plasma, and does not require platelet release of TxA_2 or active platelet metabolism (it is not dependent on neither calcium nor magnesium). The platelet agglutinating factor (234) is a protein of 37 kD. Its function is inhibited by human IgG but not inhibited by hirudin, the heparin-antithrombin III complex, or aspirin. The 37 kD protein is not present in controls or in patients with autoimmune thrombocytopenia or DIC. Binding of this protein to platelets is not influenced by the coincident presence of monoclonal antibodies to the glycoproteins GPI and GPIIb/IIIa (234).

von Willebrand Factor (vWF) is a multimeric glycoprotein found in platelets, endothelial cells and plasma. Circulating multimers, formed by disulfide linkage, range in molecular weight from 1 to 2.10^6 daltons. Only higher molecular weight polymers support platelet adhesion to subendothelium and promote formation of platelet thrombi. Two receptors on platelets bind vWF: glycoprotein Ib and glycoprotein IIb/IIIa (235). Contradictory results concern the role of vWF in HUS. In one study, ultralarge vWF multimers were present during remissions, whereas they were not detected during relapses of HUS (236). However, in another study, an increased concentration of ultralarge multimers was found in some patients with recurrent episodes of HUS (237); these multimers disappeared with clinical remission. Patients with abnormal multimers have required more blood transfusions (238). Moreover, it was suggested that the presence of ultralarge multimers may predict thrombotic episodes (239). The presence of unusually large vWF multimers in the plasma of relapsing TTP-HUS patients during remission might indicate that endothelial cells of these patients were unable to process the very large multimers. The presence of ultralarge multimers preceded an acute exacerbation of the disease, which was followed by an increase in light multimers and fragments (240). Some of the ultra-large multimers may bind to platelets and may be processed by plasmin, calpaïn or neutrophil proteases. Serum elastase and its inhibitor α-1-antitrypsin are markedly elevated in typical HUS. Elastase cleaves vWF *in vitro*, and there may be a correlation between high serum elastase and high levels of low-molecular-weight vWF (241).

Thrombosed skin vessels from 3 patients with TTP had greatly impaired fibrinolytic activity. In contrast, plasminogen activity was normal in uninvolved vessels. Systemic plasma fibrinolytic activity was found to be normal, suggesting that the loss of fibrinolytic activity was due to a local vascular defect. No such effect was seen in intravascular thrombosis of other types, notably DIC (242). This local loss of t-PA may play an important role in the formation of microthrombi. Kwaan (243) extended this study to 12 patients with TTP and suggested that the absence of local fibrinolytic activity may be the result of either primary endothelial damage or of secretion by platelets of fibrinolysis inhibitors. The latter explanation may also account for the presence of an activity capable of inhibiting fibrinolysis in the plasma of children with HUS (244). However, by the fibrin plate method using human kidney biopsies, fibrinolytic activity of renal cortex was found normal in patients with HUS (84).

In the plasma, decreased levels of circulating t-PA and increased levels of PAI-1 were reported in patients with TTP-HUS (245). The increased level of PAI-1 may play an important role in the pathogenesis and in the persistence of glomerular fibrin deposits. We found that the positive fluorescence obtained with antifibrin antibodies at the site of thrombosis was associated with a positive fluorescence with anti PAI-1 antibodies in kidney biopsies obtained from patients with vascular nephropathies (among them, 5 patients had thrombotic microangiopathy)(184).

Treatment

The clinical course of HUS has been significantly improved in recent years because of more efficient management at the acute phase of the disease, mainly with dialysis and antihypertensive drugs.

Today, the most widely accepted etiopathogenic treatment is repeated fresh plasma infusion, with the probably justified objective of restoring normal plasma antiaggregant properties. There are numerous reports of remission following plasma infusion (228, 246, 247). The most favorable results in treating HUS/TTP have been obtained using combined aspirin and dipyridamole with infusion of fresh plasma or plasma exchanges (248). The latter have been used successfully (249), but it remains unclear whether beneficial effects reflect removal of the insulting agent or replacement of an essential depleted activity. So far, there is no decisive arguments showing that plasma exchange is superior to fresh plasma infusion in HUS treatment. Evaluation of efficacy has been difficult, owing to sample sizes and non randomized therapy administration. Furthermore, it has to be kept in mind that about 75 percent of children with typical cases of HUS recover with supportive care only (250).

The other treatments appear today less important. Heparin (251), dipyridamole and aspirin (252, 253) have been extensively used. The overall results are difficult to interpret because almost all studies involved only small number of patients. However, the prospective study of Vitacco et al (251) did not confirm any useful effect of heparin alone or associated with antiplatelet agents. Thrombolytic therapy with streptokinase or urokinase have been used with conflicting results (254, 255), the main problem being the risk of serious bleeding complications in hypertensive patients. Now that human t-PA obtained by recombinant technology is more and more used in clinical practice, it could be a very effective treatment as in experimental animals. Clinical studies in humans are now required.

Other treatments have been tried in HUS. The results of PGI_2 infusion are so far difficult to evaluate (256, 257). Vitamin E has been used on the basis of low plasma levels (258) and because it could enhance the spontaneously low plasma antioxidant activity detected in HUS patients. The most recent therapeutic agent is infusion of high dose intravenous immunoglobulins, the efficiency of which suggests that the "missing" plasma factor in HUS/TTP is in the immunoglobulin fraction (259). Finally, in spite of these recent advances in therapies intended to reverse microthromboses, the keystone of the treatment of HUS remains symptomatic management of renal failure and of hypertension.

RENAL TRANSPLANTATION

Renal transplant rejection

Vascular thrombosis, interstitial fibrin deposits and sometimes evidence for systemic intravascular coagulation are associated with severe renal allograft rejection. By histochemical method on fibrin slide, it has been shown that the cortical fibrinolytic activity was decreased during renal allograft rejection (84). In 17 human irreversibly rejected renal allografts, which contained interstitial or vascular fibrin deposits, we demonstrated that the glomerular fibrinolytic activity was not decreased compared to control glomeruli from normal kidneys, except in 5 severe cases of rejection where tissue damage was maximal (90). Similar results were obtained by Giroux et al (260) using fibrin slides. Conversely glomerular procoagulant activity (PCA) was always dramatically decreased, which may play an important role in the absence of fibrin within the glomeruli of rejected kidneys.

33

Isolated glomeruli from chronically rejected kidneys synthesized larger amounts of TxB_2 than glomeruli from normal kidneys (261). This disequilibrium between thromboxane and prostacyclin productions could explain the occurrence of hypertension and progressive impairment of renal function. Specific therapeutic approaches such as TxA_2 synthesis inhibitors or receptor antagonists are currently studied in this clinical setting. Platelet activation that can be detected during renal allograft rejection leads to increased generation of platelet factor 3 (262, 263), an increased platelet aggregability (264) and an intrarenal platelet sequestration (265). Increased urine TxB_2 excretion is also compatible with such phenomenon (265b).

Endothelium of renal vasculature seems to be the first target of anti-HLA antibodies or of alloactivated cells during renal allograft rejection associated with subsequent release of thromboplastin, platelet adhesion and activation. Host's monocytes have also a high level of PCA during renal allograft rejection (266) and may participate in the generation of intrarenal thrombosis. As previously discussed, T cell activation during allograft rejection may lead to the release of cytokines which in turn activates procoagulant activity of endothelial cells and monocytes. Interferon gamma, generated by activated lymphocytes, has been shown to enhance macrophage transcription of TNFα, IL-1 and u-PA genes and may thus modulate local fibrinolytic activity. It has been shown that TNFα is generated at the early phase of rejection by infiltrating (267) or by circulating host mononuclear cells (268). Serum TNFα level increases during renal allograft rejection (269). Due to its potent procoagulant (68) and antifibrinolytic (111) stimulating activities, it could play a key role in the hemostatic disorders observed during rejection. Some circulating hemostatic components are also increased during rejection such as inhibitors of kallikrein or of factor XII, plasminogen AT III, and have been proposed as early indicators of kidney transplant rejection (270).

Effects of immunosuppressive therapy

CYCLOSPORIN A

Since the early eighties, organ transplantations, including renal transplantation, have been facilitated by the new immunosuppressive drug, cyclosporin A. However some adverse effects of cyclosporin A were rapidly identified. Renal complications of cyclosporin A range from asymptomatic tubular lesions to severe renal failure (271). Interestingly hemostatic disorders promoted by cyclosporin A may lead in some cases to HUS, occurring *de novo* on the renal graft (272) or as a recurrence of the initial disease

(273). Glomerular and/or arteriolar thrombosis were also reported after bone marrow transplantation (274-276). Elevated plasma vWF (277) and thrombomodulin (278) have been reported in patients treated with cyclosporin A.

Cyclosporin A increases the number and severity of glomerular thrombosis in the rabbit serum sickness (279) and decreases the synthesis of the prostacyclin stimulating factor (279). Prostanoids synthesis is modified in patients treated by cyclosporin A and an increased urinary excretion of TxB_2 has been reported whereas that of PGE_2 and 6-keto-$PGF_{1\alpha}$ were variably altered (280). *In vitro* experiments showed that cyclosporin A has a direct cytotoxic effect on cultured endothelial cells (281) and inhibits PGI_2 synthesis by cultured endothelial cells or smooth muscle cells (282, 283) whereas PGI_2 synthesis by monocytes is increased in the presence of cyclosporin A (284, 284b).

No direct effect of cyclosporin A could be demonstrated on isolated glomeruli or on cortical renal slices (285, 285b). PAF synthesis by mesangial cells was reported after cyclosporin A addition (286). Cyclosporin A also modifies the procoagulant e.g. tissue factor expression, in monocytes/macrophages. However its effect varies according to the experimental protocol. When PCA is induced in macrophages by allostimulated lymphocytes, cyclosporin A inhibits this induction, probably through a decreased release of cytokines by allostimulated lymphocytes (287). Conversely, cyclosporin A increases the PCA of peripheral mononuclear blood cells (288, 289) and endothelial cells (290) stimulated by phorbol myristate acetate, phytohemagglutinin, or lymphokines (290).

Thus cyclosporin A may promote in some patients renal glomerular or vascular thrombosis through different mechanisms including local generation of TxA_2 and PAF, and increased procoagulant activities of circulating renal cells. Deep vein thrombosis and pulmonary embolism are more frequent in patients receiving cyclosporin A than in those receiving other immunosuppressive drugs (291).

ANTI-CD3 MONOCLONAL ANTIBODY (OKT3)

OKT3 is a very potent immunosuppressive antibody binding the CD3 molecule, which is closely linked to the T-cell receptor (292). When this mAb is injected *in vivo*, it induces a severe clinical syndrome related to the release of several cytokines, mainly TNFα (293, 294). Although TNFα and IL-1 induce PCA in endothelial cells (67, 68), as well as "lymphokines" in macrophages (295), and increase the synthesis of PAI-1 in fibroblasts (111) and in human mesangial cells (Rondeau et al, unpublished observations), no consistent clinical data indicate a potential thrombotic effect of this mAb.

35

In vitro studies have shown that antibodies to CD3 can activate T cells in the presence of monocytes (296, 297) and that OKT3 mAb has a potent PCA-inducing effect on peripheral monocytes through its action on T cells (298, 299).

In conclusion, hemostatic disorders and renal vascular thrombosis in renal allograft recipients have been reported. Some of these complications are related to cyclosporin A therapy and should thus be monitored since withdrawal of the drug or lowering the daily dose could prevent further renal damage. On the other hand, these abnormalities may be due to an acute rejection, whether or not circulating preformed anti-HLA antibodies have been detected. In this context, a poor graft survival is expected unless a good response is obtained with intensive immunosuppression. New antithrombotic and/or profibrinolytic drugs would be useful to prevent the severe renal vascular damage which is usually observed in these cases.

CHRONIC RENAL FAILURE AND INTRAGLOMERULAR FIBRIN DEPOSITS: THE ROLE OF GLOMERULAR HEMOSTASIS IN THE NON SPECIFIC PROGRESSION OF RENAL DISEASES

The non specific factors of ineluctable progression of many renal diseases towards renal insufficiency are currently being extensively studied. The experimental model most often used is renoprival nephropathy following subtotal renal ablation in the rat. Pathology of the remnant kidney is basically characterized by progressive glomerular sclerosis, associated with arteriolosclerosis and fibrocellular interstitial lesion. Together with systemic hypertension, hemodynamic factors and glomerular hypertrophy itself, intraglomerular fibrin deposition and thrombosis may have an important role in the onset of glomerular sclerosis (300, 301). Indeed, glomerular fibrin deposits have been found in 20 to 40% of remnant glomeruli, with well formed segmental necrosis and thrombosis in some of the glomeruli (302, 303). Longitudinal studies have shown that necrotizing thrombosis lead to glomerular sclerosis (302). Importance of glomerular fibrin formation is again emphasized by the beneficial effects of anticoagulant or antiplatelet drugs, which, in some studies, markedly reduce the severity of lesions and of functional impairment in treated animals (304-309).

The mechanisms of fibrin deposition in rat renoprival nephropathy remain uncompletely understood. Indirect evidences suggest the involvement of intracapillary platelet aggregation due to the enhanced production of TxA_2. Indeed, its stable metabolite TxB_2 is excreted in excess in the urine of subtotally nephrectomized rats (307, 310) and is synthesized in excess by glomeruli isolated from rat remnant kidneys (311). Moreover specific inhibition of renal and platelet thromboxane synthesis by OKY 1581 was shown to suppress intraglomerular clotting and the development of sclerosis and uremia (307); this effect was obtained in spite of drug-induced enhanced single nephron glomerular plasma flow. However, our own study of rat renoprival nephropathy (303) did not confirm these findings since thromboxane inhibition by OKY 046 for one month had no effect on the course of the disease or on fibrin deposition, which affected about 20% of glomeruli; Zoja et al (312, 313) also failed to show any protective effect of drug-induced selective platelet thromboxane inhibition in this model. In our above mentioned study (303), we also measured procoagulant (thromboplastinic) and fibrinolytic activities of isolated remnant glomeruli one month after subtotal renal ablation. Procoagulant activity dropped to 40% of the control level and fibrinolytic activity rose to 120-130% of this level. In an additional group of non-uremic unilaterally nephrectomized rats, glomerular procoagulant activity was also markedly decreased. These results unexpectedly show that reduction of renal mass in the rat induces changes in glomerular hemostatic properties that tend to have antithrombotic effects: this may constitute an adaptive reaction of a local hemostasis system to fibrin deposition. Further studies of other components of the system should provide insights into the mechanisms triggering glomerular fibrin deposition in renoprival nephropathies.

In other renal diseases in which fibrin deposits represent the predominant pathologic feature, transition to sclerosis is likely to bear close relationships to glomerular thromboses. This is observed not only in extracapillary and lupus GN (189, 190), but also in immune complex GN in mice (171, 314) and rats (315). In human lupus GN, the presence of glomerular thromboses on the initial biopsy was highly correlated with that of glomerular sclerosis on subsequent biopsies (189). The pathogenic role of renal microthromboses is supported by the beneficial effect of anticoagulants in hypertensive rats with Heymann nephritis (315). Finally, the relevance of the above mentioned data, obtained in experimental uremia and in some particular human diseases, to the majority of cases of human chronic renal failure is still largely speculative. Indeed there are so far no systematic histopathologic studies of uremic kidneys as regards intrarenal fibrin deposition or studies of local hemostatic activities.

THROMBOSIS, COAGULATION FACTORS AND NEPHROTIC SYNDROME

Thromboses, localized predominantly in deep veins of the extremities and in renal veins, affect 10-30% of nephrotic patients with pulmonary embolism in about one third of these cases. Nephrotic syndrome (NS) is associated with several disorders of hemostasis altogether tending to induce blood hypercoagulability (for review see Ref 316): thrombocytosis and platelet hyperaggregability; increased plasma levels of factor V and VIII, and of fibrinogen with blood hyperviscosity; decreased plasma levels of two natural anticoagulants, free protein S and AT III; lowered fibrinolytic activity. These disorders are related to urinary losses of anticoagulants (e.g. AT III) and increased hepatic synthesis of procoagulants stimulated by hypoalbuminemia (e.g. fibrinogen). Therefore, as could be expected, intensity of hypercoagulability is related to the degree of hypoalbuminemia. Notably it was recently shown that plasma clot lysis was greatly delayed in nephrotic patients and that *in vitro* correction of this abnormality was achieved by supplementing plasma with albumin up to the normal concentration (4.5 g/dl); furthermore plasminogen binding to the fibrin network increased with albumin concentration (317).

The role of hypercoagulability in the increased incidence of thromboembolic events in NS, including renal vein thrombosis, is not proved, although similar clotting disorders, especially hyperfibrinogenemia and lowered fibrinolytic activity, have been found in large group of nonnephrotic subjects at established risks of venous thrombosis (318, 319). Unfortunately there is no current evidence that one or several particular abnormalities are responsible for thrombogenesis or even able to reliably predict the risk of thrombosis in the individual patient. Thrombogenesis in vessels with usually intact wall implies actual activation of coagulation pathway(s) leading to intravascular thrombin formation (30): this actually may be the case in NS. In fact, signs of thrombin formation, such as increased plasma levels of fibrinopeptide A and high-molecular weight fibrinogen complexes (10-12), are present in the active phases of GN. This corresponds to low grade intravascular coagulation which may also in part account for "paradoxical" hyperfibrinogenemia (320). Thrombin formation with systemic blood coagulation disorders may in fact arise in diseased glomeruli during the nephrotic phase of nephropathies, following immunologically-induced activation of the glomerular hemostasis system. Such mechanism was documented in rat mercuric chloride induced autoimmune GN (173, 174)(see above), but it has to be substantiated in humans by further investigations; it would add a logical link between systemic coagulation disorders and the glomerular lesions underlying nephrotic syndromes. Furthermore, this would account for the preferential localization of thrombosis in renal veins in nephrotic patients, since experimental evidences show that high *in situ* (e.g. intrarenal) concentrations of thrombin are a major factor of *in vivo* venous thrombus constitution (30).

The prevention of venous thrombosis in NS is debated, notably because, as stated above, one cannot reliably predict the patients who are at the highest risk of thrombotic events. Several authors recommend to begin anticoagulant therapy when serum albumin concentration becomes and remains lower than 2 or 1.5 g/dl (321). There is no discussion about the necessity of anticoagulant therapy in established thrombosis: however, the choice of the drug may be difficult. In case of very low plasma AT III concentration, and high alpha-2-macroglobulin concentration, heparin may be inefficient and may even diminish the antithrombin activity of the latter (322). On the other hand, the use of warfarin and other antivitamin K drugs may be difficult in case of variations of albumin concentration, to which they are bound (321). Finally, perfusion of albumin may be indicated in cases of thrombosis associated with low systemic fibrinolytic activity.

CONCLUSION: OVERVIEW ON THE DUAL ROLE OF GLOMERULAR HEMOSTASIS SYSTEM IN NEPHROPATHIES AND THERAPEUTIC PROSPECTS

Results of quantitative or semi-quantitative studies of glomerular procoagulant and fibrinolytic activities are shown in Table 6.

Table 6. Glomerular hemostasis in renal diseases with glomerular fibrin deposition.

Disease	Procoagulant activity	Fibrinolytic activity
Rat DIC (*)	ND	↑
Rabbit DIC (°)	↑	↓
Rat glycerol ARF	↓	↑
Rat HgCl$_2$ GN	↑	ND
Rat antiGBM GN	ND	↑
Rabbit antiGBM GN	↑	ND
Rat renal ablation	↓	↑
Human crescentic GN	↑	→
Human graft rejection	↓	↓

ARF = acute renal failure; DIC = disseminated intravascular coagulation; GBM = glomerular basement membrane; GN = glomerulonephritis; ND = not determined; → = similar to control values.
(*) thrombin-induced
(°) generalized Shwartzman phenomenon

Most of these results have been detailed earlier in this review. The observed changes point to a possible dual role of both activities because they can contribute to the onset of glomerular thrombosis as in rabbit GSP or immune GN, or, on the contrary, homeostatically function so as to mitigate it, as in rat glycerol acute renal failure or renoprival nephropathy. Besides, when examining the role of prothrombotic or antithrombotic factors, species differences must be taken into account. Even in a same animal disease, discrepant results are reported, as for example pharmacologically or diet-induced reduction in thromboxane synthesis that leads either to ameliorated (307, 308), unchanged (303, 312) or aggravated (310) course of rat renoprival nephropathy. Therefore one must exercise caution when extrapolating experimental data to human diseases. It should be reminded that investigations of glomerular hemostasis in humans are scarce in comparison with animal studies, notably because measurements of hemostatic activities demand the handling of large fragments of kidneys; thus in human crescentic GN and graft rejection, the results were obtained on pieces of autopsy or nephrectomy (90, 182). Most available data on the mechanisms of fibrin deposition in human diseases are provided by conventional immunofluorescence.

Further knowledge should be supplied by utilization of novel methods applicable to renal biopsies, such as:

[a]   microassays allowing measurements of glomerular procoagulant activity (183);

[b]   appropriate use of monoclonal antibodies directed against molecules of hemostasis system;

[c]   utilization of the methods of molecular biology, notably in situ hybridization.

Such studies should allow recognition and semi-quantitative assessment of pro/anticoagulant or pro/antifibrinolytic glomerular molecules. This will also indicate whether there is an imbalance between local prothrombotic properties and antithrombotic properties in favor of the former, which could mediate glomerular thrombosis. Interestingly, such imbalance between enhanced thromboplastinic activity and decreased fibrinolytic activity was recently reported in bronchoalveolar lavage product of patients with the adult respiratory distress syndrome (characterized by alveolar fibrin deposition) (323).

Progress in therapy should come from the availability of etiopathogenic treatments directly derived from the knowledge of renal microthrombosis mechanisms, therefore allowing individualization of antithrombotic therapies. In the near future, likely candidates for therapy of nephropathies with fibrin deposits could be: thromboxane inhibitors in diseases with platelet hyperaggregability, e.g. allograft rejection (324), cyclosporin nephrotoxicity (325), lupus nephritis (326); pentoxifylline (327) or genetically engineered proteic inhibitor of factor VII-tissue thromboplastin complex (328), in diseases with activation of the extrinsic coagulation pathway such as extracapillary GN; safe fibrin-selective plasminogen activator therapies (329) in diseases with diminished fibrinolytic activity.

ACKNOWLEDGMENTS

Dr Roger Lacave, Dr Ci-Jiang He, Ms Jacqueline Hagège and Ms Françoise Delarue participated in several studies here reported.

The authors wish to thank Ms Mina Mallet for her expert secretarial assistance.

REFERENCES

1   Takemura T, Yoshioka K, Akano N, Miyamoto H, Matsumoto K, Maki S: Glomerular deposition of cross-linked fibrin in human kidney diseases. Kidney Int, 32: 102-111, 1987.
2. Kamitsuji H, Sakamoto S, Matsunaga T, Taira K, Kawahara S, Nakajima M: Intraglomerular deposition of fibrin/fibrinogen-related antigen in children with various renal diseases. Am J Pathol, 133: 61-72, 1988.
3. Deguchi F, Tomura S, Yoshiyama N, Takeuchi J: Intraglomerular deposition of coagulation-fibrinolysis factors and a platelet membrane antigen in various glomerular diseases. Nephron, 51: 377-383, 1989.
4. Holdsworth SR, Thomson NM, Glasgow EF, Atkins RC: The effect of defibrination on macrophage participation in rabbit nephrotoxic nephritis: studies using glomerular culture and electronmicroscopy. Clin Exp Immunol, 37: 38-43, 1979.
5. Tsumagari T, Tanaka K: Effects of fibrinogen degradation products on glomerular mesangial cells in culture. Kidney Int, 26: 712-718, 1984.
6. Shultz PJ, Knauss T, Mene P, Abboud HE: Mitogenic signals for thrombin in mesangial cells: regulation of phospholipase C and PDGF genes. Am J Physiol, 257: F366-F374, 1989.
7. Kanfer A: Coagulation system in acute renal failure. In "Acute Renal Failure" (Ed VE Andreucci), Martinus Nijhoff Publishing, Boston, 1984, pp 177-188.
8. Ekberg M, Nilsson IM: Factor VIII and glomerulonephritis. Lancet, I: 1111-1113, 1975.
9. Salem HH, Whitworth JA, Koutts J, Kincaid-Smith PS, Firkin BG: Hypercoagulation in glomerulonephritis. Brit Med J, 282: 2083-2085, 1981.
10. Tomura S, Oono Y, Kuriyama R, Takeuchi J: Plasma concentrations of fibrinopeptide A and fibrinopeptide Bβ15-42 in glomerulonephritis and the nephrotic syndrome. Arch Intern Med, 145: 1033-1035, 1985.
11. Alkjaersig N, Fletcher AP, Narayanan M, Robson AM: Course and resolution of the coagulopathy in nephrotic children. Clin Invest, 31: 772-780, 1987.
12. Sagripanti A, Cupisti A, Ferdeghini M, Pinori E, Barsotti G: Molecular markers of hemostasis activation in nephrotic syndrome. Nephron, 51: 25-28, 1989.
13. Sraer JD, Kanfer A, Rondeau E, Lacave R: Glomerular hemostasis in normal and pathologic conditions. Adv Nephrol, 17: 27-55, 1988.
14. Sraer JD, Rondeau E, Kanfer A, Lacave R: Procoagulant and fibrinolytic activity of human glomeruli and glomerular cultured cells. J Nephrol, 1: 45-52, 1990.
15. Cameron JS: Coagulation and thromboembolic complications in the nephrotic syndrome. Adv Nephrol, 13: 75-114, 1984.
16. Bernard DB: Extrarenal complications of the nephrotic syndrome. Kidney Int, 33: 1184-1202, 1988.
17. Ogston D, Bennett B: The blood coagulation cascade. In "Recent Advances In Blood Coagulation" (Ed L Poller), Churchill Livingstone, Edinburgh, 1985, pp 1-10.
18. Zur M, Nemerson Y: Tissue factor pathways of blood coagulation. In "Haemostasis and Thrombosis" (Eds AL Bloom, DP Thomas), Churchill Livingstone, Edinburgh, 1987, pp 148-163.
19. Mosesson MW: Fibrin polymerization and its regulatory role in hemostasis. J Lab Clin Med, 116: 8-17, 1990.
20. Østerud B: Activation pathways of the coagulation system in normal haemostasis. Scand J Haematol, 32: 337-345, 1984.

21. Repke D, Gemmell CH, Guha A, Turitto VT, Broze GJ Jr, Nemerson Y: Hemophilia as a defect of the tissue factor pathway of blood coagulation: effect of factors VIII and IX on factor X activation in a continuous-flow reactor. Proc Natl Acad Sci USA, 87: 7623-7627, 1990.

22. Hemker HC, Lindhout Th: A clotting scheme for 1984. Nouv Rev Fr Hematol, 26: 227-231, 1984.

23. Crawford N, Scrutton MC: Biochemistry of blood platelet. In "Haemostasis and Thrombosis" (Eds AL Bloom, DP Thomas), Churchill Livingstone Edinburgh, 1987, pp 47-77.

24. Brox JH, Østerud B, Bjørklid E, Fenton JW: Production and availability of thromboplastin in endothelial cells: the effects of thrombin, endotoxin and platelets. Brit J Haematol, 57: 239-246, 1984.

25. Esmon NL: Thrombomodulin. Prog Hemost Thromb, 9: 29-55, 1988.

26. Rosenberg RD: Actions and interactions of antithrombin and heparin. N Engl J Med, 292: 146-151, 1975.

27. Marcum JA, Atha DH, Fritze LMS, Nawroth P, Stern D, Rosenberg RD: Cloned bovine aortic endothelial cells synthesize anticoagulantly active heparin sulfate proteoglycan. J Biol Chem, 261: 7507-7517, 1986.

28. Broze GJ Jr, Warren LA, Novotny WF, Higuchi DA, Girard JJ, Miletich JP: The lipoprotein-associated coagulation inhibitor that inhibits the factor VII-tissue factor complex also inhibits factor Xa: insight into its possible mechanism of action. Blood, 71: 335-343, 1988.

29. Thomas DP, Merton RE, Hiller KF, Hockley D: Resistance of normal endothelium to damage by thrombin. Brit J Haematol, 51: 25-35, 1982.

30. Thomas DP: Pathogenesis of venous thrombosis. In "Haemostasis and Thrombosis" (Eds AL Bloom, DP Thomas), Churchill Livingstone, Edinburgh, 1987, pp 767-778.

31. Collen D, Lijnen HR: The fibrinolytic system in man. CRC Crit Rev Oncol Haematol, 4: 249-294, 1986.

32. Blasi F, Vassalli JD, Danø K: Urokinase-type plasminogen activator: proenzyme, receptor, and inhibitors. J Cell Biol, 104: 801-804, 1987.

33. Roldan AL, Cubellis MV, Masucci MT, Behrendt N, Lund LR, Danø K, Appella E, Blasi F: Cloning and expression of the receptor for human urokinase plasminogen activator, a central molecule in cell surface, plasmin dependent proteolysis. EMBO J, 9: 467-474, 1990.

34. Ploug M, Rønne E, Behrendt N, Jensen AL, Blasi F, Danø K: Cellular receptor for urokinase plasminogen activator. J Biol Chem, 266: 1926-1933, 1991.

35. Dousa TP: Glomerular metabolism. In "The Kidney. Physiology/Pathophysiology" (Eds DW Seldin, G Giebisch), Raven Press, New-York, 1985, pp 645-667.

36. Striker GE, Soderland C, Bowen-Pope DF, Gown AM, Schmer G, Johnson A, Luchtel D, Ross R, Striker LJ: Isolation, characterization, and propagation in vitro of human glomerular endothelial cells. J Exp Med, 160: 323-328, 1984.

37. Raugi GJ, Lovett DH: Thrombospondin secretion by cultured human glomerular mesangial cells. Am J Pathol, 129: 364-372, 1987.

38. Sraer J, Foidart J, Chansel D, Mahieu P, Ardaillou R: Prostaglandin synthesis by rat isolated glomeruli and glomerular cultured cells. Int J Biochem, 12: 203-207, 1980.

39. Petrulis AS, Aikawa M, Dunn MJ: Prostaglandin and thromboxane synthesis by rat glomerular epithelial cells. Kidney Int, 20: 469-474, 1981.

40. Sraer J, Ardaillou N, Sraer JD, Ardaillou R: In vitro prostaglandin synthesis by human glomeruli and papillae. Prostaglandins, 23: 855-864, 1982.

41. Ardaillou N, Nivez MP, Striker G, Ardaillou R: Prostaglandin synthesis by human glomerular cells in culture. Prostaglandins, 26: 773-784, 1983.

42. Ardaillou N, Hagège J, Nivez MP, Ardaillou R, Schlondorff D: Vasoconstrictor-evoked prostaglandin synthesis in cultured human mesangial cells. Am J Physiol, 248: F240-F246, 1985.

43. Podjarny E, Rathaus M, Pomeranz A, Shapira J, Bernheim J: Thrombin inhibits the synthesis of prostanoids by isolated glomeruli and peritoneal macrophages in rats. Nephron, 53: 50-53, 1989.

44. Mottin D, Rondeau E, Bens M, Moulonguet Doleris L, Sraer JD: Arachidonic acid metabolites of isolated glomeruli after thrombin induced intravascular coagulation; role of cyclooxygenase and lipoxygenase metabolites. Eur J Clin Invest, 14 (n°2, part 2): 60, 1984.

45. Remuzzi G: HUS and TTP: variable expression of a single entity. Kidney Int, 32: 292-302, 1987.

46. Katayama S, Inaba M, Maruno Y, Omoto A, Kawazu S, Ishii J: Increased thromboxane B_2 excretion in diabetes mellitus. J Lab Clin Med, 109: 711-717, 1987.

47. Schlondorff D, Goldwasser P, Neuwirth R, Satriano JA, Clay KL: Production of platelet-activating factor in glomeruli and cultured glomerular mesangial cells. Am J Physiol, 250: F1123-F1127, 1986.

48. Wang J, Kester M, Dunn MJ: The effects of endotoxin on platelet-activating factor synthesis in cultured rat glomerular mesangial cells. Biochim Biophys Acta, 969: 217-224, 1988.
49. Morell GP, Pirotzki E, Erard D, Desmottes RM, Bidault J, Damais C, Benveniste J: Paf-acether (platelet-activating factor) and interleukin-1-like cytokine production by lipopolysaccharide-stimulated glomeruli. Clin Immunol Immunopathol, 46: 396-405, 1988.
50. Hugues J, Mahieu P: Platelet aggregation induced by basement membranes. Thromb Diathes Haemorrh, 24: 395-408, 1970.
51. Freytag JW, Dalrymple PN, Maguire MJ, Strickland DK, Carraway KL, Hudson BG: Glomerular basement membrane. Studies on its structure and interaction with platelets. J Biol Chem, 253: 9069-9074, 1978.
52. Sraer J, Wolf C, Oudinet JP, Bens M, Ardaillou R, Sraer JD: Human glomeruli release fatty acids which stimulate thromboxane synthesis in platelets. Kidney Int, 32: 62-68, 1987.
53. Nemerson Y: Tissue factor and hemostasis. Blood, 71: 1-8, 1988.
54. Morrissey JH, Fakhrai H, Edgington TS: Molecular cloning of the cDNA for tissue factor, the cellular receptor for the initiation of the coagulation protease cascade. Cell, 50: 129-135, 1987.
55. Spicer EK, Horton R, Bloem L, Bach R, Williams KR, Guha A, Lin TC, Nemerson Y, Konigsberg WH: Isolation of cDNA clones coding for human tissue factor: primary structure of the protein and cDNA. Proc Natl Acad Sci USA, 84: 5148-5152, 1987.
56. Bach R, Rifkin DB: Expression of tissue factor procoagulant activity: regulation by cytosolic calcium. Proc Natl Acad Sci USA, 87: 6995-6999, 1990.
57. Zur M, Nemerson Y: Tissue factor pathways of blood coagulation. In "Hemostasis and Thrombosis" (Eds AL Bloom, DP Thomas), Churchill Livingstone Publishing, Edinburgh, 1987, pp. 148-164.
58. Zur M, Radcliffe RD, Oberdick J, Nemerson Y: The dual role of factor VII in blood coagulation. J Biol Chem, 257: 5623-5631, 1982.
59. Rodgers GM, Broze GJ Jr, Shuman MA: The number of receptors for factor VII correlates with the ability of cultured cells to initiate coagulation. Blood, 63: 434-438, 1984.
60. Glas P, Astrup T: Thromboplastin and plasminogen activator in tissues of the rabbit. Am J Physiol, 219: 1140-1146, 1970.
61. De Prost D, Kanfer A: Quantitative assessment of procoagulant activity in isolated rat glomeruli. Kidney Int, 28: 566-568, 1985.
62. Holdsworth SR, Tipping PG: Macrophage-induced glomerular fibrin deposition in experimental glomerulonephritis in the rabbit. J Clin Invest, 76: 1367-1374, 1985.
63. Wiggins RC, Glatfelter A, Brukman J: Procoagulant activity in glomeruli and urine of rabbits with nephrotoxic nephritis. Lab Invest, 53: 156-165, 1985.
64. Tipping PG, Worthington LA, Holdsworth SR: Quantitation and characterization of glomerular procoagulant activity in experimental glomerulonephritis. Lab Invest, 56: 155-159, 1987.
65. Drake TA, Morrissey JH, Edgington TS: Selective cellular expression of tissue factor in human tissues. Implications for disorders of hemostasis and thrombosis. Am J Pathol, 134: 1087-1097, 1989.
66. Wiggins RC, Njoku N, Sedor JR: Tissue factor production by cultured rat mesangial cells. Stimulation by TNF alpha and lipopolysaccharide. Kidney Int, 37: 1281-1285, 1990.
67. Bevilacqua MP, Pober JS, Majeau GR, Cotran RS, Gimbrone MA Jr: Interleukin 1 (IL-1) induces biosynthesis and cell surface expression of procoagulant activity in human vascular endothelial cells. J Exp Med, 160: 618-623, 1984.
68. Nawroth PP, Stern DM: Modulation of endothelial cell hemostatic properties by tumor necrosis factor. J Exp Med, 163: 740-745, 1986.
69. Tannenbaum SH, Finko R, Cines DB: Antibody and immune complexes induce tissue factor production by human endothelial cells. J Immunol, 137: 1532-1537, 1986.
70. Johnsen ULH, Lyberg T, Galdal KS, Prydz H: Platelets stimulate thromboplastin synthesis in human endothelial cells. Thromb Haemost, 49: 69-72, 1983.
71. Lovett DH, Szamel M, Ryan JL, Sterzel RB, Gemsa D, Resch K: Interleukin 1 and the glomerular mesangium. I. Purification and characterization of a mesangial cell-derived autogrowth factor. J Immunol, 136: 3700-3705, 1986.
72. Baud L, Oudinet JP, Bens M, Noe L, Peraldi MN, Rondeau E, Etienne J, Ardaillou R: Production of tumor necrosis factor by rat mesangial cells in response to bacterial lipopolysaccharide. Kidney Int, 35: 1111-1118, 1989.
73. Brentjens JR: Glomerular procoagulant activity and glomerulonephritis. Lab Invest, 57: 107-111, 1987.

74. Bakker WW, Willink EJ, Donga J, Hulstaert CE, Hardonk MJ: Antithrombotic activity of glomerular adenosine diphosphatase in the glomerular basement membrane of the rat kidney. J Lab Clin Med, 109: 171-177, 1987.

75. Bakker WW, Pelstra K, Timmerman W, Hardonk MJ, Koiter TR, Schuiling GA: Experimental endotoxemia in pregnancy: *in situ* glomerular microthrombus formation associated with impaired glomerular adenosine diphosphatase activity. J Lab Clin Med, 114: 531-537, 1989.

76. Debault LE, Esmon NL, Olson JR, Esmon CT: Distribution of the thrombomodulin antigen in the rabbit vasculature. Lab Invest, 54: 172-178, 1986.

77. Hancock WW: IL-1 and TNF depress glomerular endothelial thrombomodulin expression *in vitro* and *in vivo*. Kidney Int, 38: 557, 1990.

78. Moore KL, Andreoli SP, Esmon NL, Esmon CT, Bang NU: Endotoxin enhances tissue factor and suppresses thrombomodulin expression of human vascular endothelium *in vitro*. J Clin Invest, 79: 124-130, 1987.

79. Nawroth PP, Handley DA, Esmon CT, Stern DM: Interleukin 1 induces endothelial cell procoagulant while suppressing cell-surface anticoagulant activity. Proc Natl Acad Sci USA, 83: 3460-3464, 1986.

80. Conway EM, Rosenberg RD: Tumor necrosis factor suppresses transcription of the thrombomodulin gene in endothelial cells. Mol Cell Biol, 8: 5588-5592, 1988.

81. Moore KL, Esmon CT, Esmon NL: Tumor necrosis factor leads to the internalization and degradation of thrombomodulin from the surface of bovine aortic endothelial cells in culture. Blood, 73: 159-165, 1989.

82. Sraer JD, Boelaert J, Mimoune O, Morel-Maroger L, Hornych H: Quantitative assessment of fibrinolysis on isolated glomeruli. Kidney Int, 4: 350-352, 1973.

83. Myrhe-Jensen O: Localization of fibrinolytic activity in the kidney and urinary tract of rats and rabbits. Lab Invest, 25: 403-411, 1971.

84. Bergstein JM, Michael AF: Cortical fibrinolytic activity in normal and diseased human kidneys. J Lab Clin Med, 79: 701-709, 1972.

85. Sueishi K, Nanno S, Okamura T, Ionuc S, Tanaka K: Purification and characterization of human kidney plasminogen activators dissimilar to urokinase. Biochim Biophys Acta, 717: 327-336, 1982.

86. Larsson LI, Skriver L, Nielsen LS, Grøndahl-Hansen J, Kristensen P, Danø K: Distribution of urokinase-type plasminogen activator immunoreactivity in the mouse. J Cell Biol, 98: 894-903, 1984.

87. Sappino AP, Huarte J, Vassalli JD, Belin D: Sites of synthesis of urokinase and tissue-type plasminogen activators in the murine kidney. J Clin Invest (in press).

88. Angles Cano E, Rondeau E, Delarue F, Hagège J, Sultan Y, Sraer JD: Identification and cellular localization of plasminogen activators from human glomeruli. Thromb Haemost, 54: 688-692, 1985.

89. Rondeau E, Angles Cano E, Delarue F, Sultan Y, Sraer JD: Polyunsaturated fatty acids increase fibrinolytic activity of human isolated glomeruli. Kidney Int, 30: 701-705, 1986.

90. Rondeau E, Delarue F, Kanfer A, Nussaume O, Sraer JD: Profibrinolytic and procoagulant activities of human glomeruli from normal kidneys and rejected renal allografts. Fibrinolysis, 2: 251-257, 1988.

91. Bergstein JM, Riley M, Bang NV: Analysis of plasminogen activator activity of the human glomeruli. Kidney Int, 33: 868-874, 1988.

92. Nakamura M, Takahashi K, Naora H, Tokugoro T: A monoclonal antibody against human urokinase: characterization of the epitope and its localization in human kidney. Cell Struct Funct, 9: 167-179, 1984.

93. Rondeau E, Guidet B, Bens M, Sraer J, Peraldi MN, Ardaillou R, Sraer JD: Nordihydroguaiaretic acid inhibits particulate protein kinase C activity and urokinase messenger RNA accumulation in phorbol myristate acetate-stimulated LLC-PK1 cells. Biochim Biophys Acta, 1055: 165-172, 1990.

94. Grant PJ, Medcalf RL: Hormonal regulation of haemostasis and the molecular biology of the fibrinolytic system. Clin Sci, 78: 3-11, 1990.

95. Rondeau E, Ochi S, Lacave R, He CJ, Medcalf RL, Delarue F, Sraer JD: Urokinase synthesis and binding by glomerular epithelial cells in culture. Kidney Int, 36: 593-600, 1989.

96. He CJ, Rondeau E, Medcalf RL, Lacave R, Schleuning WD, Sraer JD: Thrombin stimulates proliferation and decreases fibrinolytic activity of human glomerular epithelial cells. J Cell Physiol, 146: 131-140, 1991.

97. Glass II WF, Radnik RA, Garoni JA, Kreisberg JI: Urokinase-dependent adhesion loss and shape change after cyclic adenosine monophosphate elevation in cultured rat mesangial cells. J Clin Invest, 82: 1992-2000, 1988.
98. Wojta J, Hoover RL, Daniel TO: Vascular origin determines plasminogen activator expression in human endothelial cells. J Biol Chem, 264: 2846-2852, 1989.
99. Lacave R, Rondeau E, Ochi S, Delarue F, Schleuning WD, Sraer JD: Characterization of a plasminogen activator and its inhibitor in human mesangial cells. Kidney Int, 35: 806-811, 1989.
100. Villamediana LM, Rondeau E, He CJ, Medcalf RL, Peraldi MN, Lacave R, Delarue F, Sraer JD: Thrombin regulates components of the fibrinolytic system in human mesangial cells. Kidney Int, 38: 956-961, 1990.
101. Baud L, Sraer J, Delarue F, Bens M, Balavoine F, Schlondorff D, Ardaillou R, Sraer JD: Lipoxygenase products mediate the attachment of rat macrophages to glomeruli *in vitro*. Kidney Int, 27: 855-863, 1985.
102. Vissers MCM, Fantone JC, Wiggins R, Kunkel SL: Glomerular basement membrane-containing immune complexes stimulate tumor necrosis factor and interleukin-1 production by human monocytes. Am J Pathol, 134: 1-6, 1989.
103. Tipping PG, Lowe MG, Holdsworth SR: Glomerular interleukin 1 production is dependent on macrophage infiltration in anti-GBM glomerulonephritis. Kidney Int, 39: 103-110, 1991.
104. Baud L, Nivez MP, Chansel D, Ardaillou R: Stimulation by oxygen radicals of prostaglandin production by rat renal glomeruli. Kidney Int, 20: 332-339, 1981.
105. Harlan JM: Leukocyte-endothelial interactions. Blood, 65: 513-525, 1985.
106. Unkeless JC, Gordon S, Reich E: Secretion of plasminogen activator by stimulated macrophages. J Exp Med, 139: 834-850, 1974.
107. Vassalli JD, Hamilton J, Reich E: Macrophage plasminogen activator: induction by concanavalin A and phorbol myristate acetate. Cell, 11: 695-700, 1977.
108. Chapman HA Jr, Vavrin Z, Hibbs JB Jr: Macrophage fibrinolytic activity: identification of two pathways of plasmin formation by intact cells and of plasminogen activator inhibitor. Cell, 28: 653-662, 1982.
109. Vassalli JD, Dayer JM, Wohlwend A, Belin D: Concomitant secretion of prourokinase and of a plasminogen activator-specific inhibitor by cultured human monocytes-macrophages. J Exp Med, 159: 1653-1668, 1984.
110. Manchanda N, Schwartz BS: Lipopolysaccharide-induced modulation of human monocyte urokinase production and activity. J Immunol, 145: 4174-4180, 1990.
111. Medcalf RL, Kruithof EKO, Schleuning WD: Plasminogen activator inhibitor 1 and 2 are tumor necrosis factor/cachectin responsive genes. J Exp Med, 168: 751-759, 1988.
112. Schleef RR, Bevilacqua MP, Sawdey M, Gimbrone MA, Loskutoff DJ: Cytokine activation of vascular endothelium. J Biol Chem, 263: 5797-5803, 1988.
113. Corrigan JJ Jr: Effect of anticoagulating and non-anticoagulating concentrations of heparin on the generalized Shwartzman reaction. Thrombos Diathes Haemorrh, 24: 136-145, 1970.
114. Whitaker AN: Acute renal failure in disseminated intravascular coagulation. Progr Biochem Pharmacol, 9: 45-64, 1974.
115. Sraer JD, Delarue F, Dard S, De Seigneux R, Morel-Maroger L, Kanfer A: Glomerular fibrinolytic activity after thrombin perfusion in the rat. Lab Invest, 32: 515-517, 1975.
116. Bergstein JM, Michael AF Jr: Renal cortical fibrinolytic activity in the rabbit following one or two doses of endotoxin. Thrombos Diathes Haemorrh, 29: 27-32, 1972.
117. Wardle N, Wright NA: Intravascular coagulation and glycerin hemoglobinuric acute renal failure. Arch Pathol, 95: 271-275, 1973.
118. Stahl E, Gerdin B, Rammer L: Protective effect of angiotensin II inhibition on acute renal failure after intravascular coagulation in the rat. Nephron, 29: 250-257, 1981.
119. Thiel G, McDonald FD, Oken DE: Micropuncture studies of the basis for protection of renin depleted rats from glycerol induced acute renal failure. Nephron, 7: 67-79, 1970.
120. Bidani AK, Fleischmann LE, Churchill P, Becker-McKenna B: Natriuresis-induced protection in acute myohemoglobinuric renal failure without renal cortical renin content depletion in the rat. Nephron, 22: 529-537, 1978.
121. Bolton WK, Atuk NO: Study of chemical sympathectomy in endotoxin-induced lethality and fibrin deposition. Kidney Int, 13: 263-270, 1978.
122. Sraer JD, Moulonguet Doleris L, Delarue F, Sraer J, Ardaillou R: Prostaglandin synthesis by glomeruli isolated from rats with glycerol-induced acute renal failure. Circ Res, 49: 775-783, 1981.

123. Brukman J, Wiggins RC: Procoagulant activity in kidneys of normal and bacterial lipopolysaccharide-treated rabbits. Kidney Int, 32: 31-38, 1987.
124. Kleinknecht D, Grunfeld JP, Gomez PC, Moreau JF, Garcia-Torres R: Diagnostic procedures and long-term prognosis in bilateral renal cortical necrosis. Kidney Int, 4: 390-400, 1973.
125. Solez K, Morel-Maroger L, Sraer JD: The morphology of "acute tubular necrosis" in man: analysis of 57 renal biopsies and a comparison with the glycerol model. Medicine, 58: 362-376, 1979.
126. Conte J, Delsol J, Mignon-Conte M, Ton That H, Suc JM: Insuffisance rénale aigue et coagulation intravasculaire. In: "Actualités Néphrologiques de l'hôpital Necker" (Eds J Hamburger, J Crosnier, JL Funck-Brentano), Flammarion Médecine Sciences, Paris, 1973, pp. 201-256.
127. Clarkson AR, MacDonald MK, Fuster V, Cash JD, Robson JS: Glomerular coagulation in acute ischaemic renal failure. Quart J Med, 39: 585-599, 1970.
128. Kleinknecht D, Verger D, Mignon F, Richet G: Insuffisance rénale et pancréatite aigue. Signification des dépôts fibrinoides intraglomérulaires. Ann Méd Interne, 121: 17-28, 1970.
129. Vreeken J, Boom-Gaard J, Deggeler K: Urokinase excretion in patients with renal disease. Acta Med Scand, 180: 15-157, 1966.
130. Kanfer A, Vandewalle A, Beaufils M, Delarue F, Sraer JD: Enhanced antiplasmin activity in acute renal failure. Brit Med J, 4: 195-197, 1975.
131. Seitz R, Karges HE, Wolf M, Egbring R: Reduced fibrinolytic capacity and its restoration by plasminogen substitution in acute renal failure. Int J Tiss Reac, 11: 39-46, 1989.
132. Vassalli P, Mc Cluskey RT: The pathogenic role of the coagulation process in rabbit Masugi nephritis. Am J Pathol, 45: 653-673, 1964.
133. Bone JM, Valdes AJ, Germuth FG, Lubowitz H: Heparin therapy in antibasement membrane nephritis. Kidney Int, 8: 72-79, 1975.
134. Giroux L, Verroust P, Morel-Maroger L, Delarue F, Delauche M, Sraer JD: Glomerular fibrinolytic activity during nephrotoxic nephritis. Lab Invest, 40: 415-422, 1979.
135. Briggs JD, Kwaan HC, Potter EV: The role of fibrinogen in renal disease: III Fibrinolytic and anticoagulant treatment of nephrotoxic serum nephritis in mice. J Lab Clin Med, 74: 715-720, 1969.
136. Sindrey M, Marshall TI, Naish P: Quantitative assessment of the effects of platelet depletion in the autologous phase of nephrotoxic serum nephritis. Clin Exp Immunol, 36: 90-97, 1979.
137. Ogawa S, Naruse T: Effects of various antiplatelet drugs and a defibrinating agent on experimental glomerulonephritis in rats. J Lab Clin Med, 99: 428-441, 1982.
138. Lianos EA, Andres GA, Dunn MJ: Glomerular prostaglandin and thromboxane synthesis in rat nephrotoxic serum nephritis. J Clin Invest, 72: 1439-1448, 1983.
139. Macconi D, Benigni A, Morigi M, Ubiali A, Orisio S, Livio M, Perico N, Bertani T, Remuzzi G, Patrono C: Enhanced glomerular thromboxane A_2 mediates some pathophysiologic effect of platelet-activating factor in rabbit nephrotoxic nephritis: evidence from biochemical measurements and inhibitor trials. J Lab Clin Med, 113: 549-560, 1989.
140. Shinkai Y, Cameron JS: Rabbit nephrotoxic nephritis: effect of a thromboxane synthetase inhibitor on evolution and prostaglandin excretion. Nephron, 47: 211-219, 1987.
141. Silva FG, Hoyer JR, Pirani CL: Sequential studies of glomerular crescent formation in rats with antiglomerular basement membrane-induced glomerulonephritis and the role of coagulation factors. Lab Invest, 51: 404-415, 1984.
142. Wiggins RC: Hageman factor in experimental nephrotoxic nephritis in the rabbit. Lab Invest, 53: 335-348, 1985.
143. Tipping PG, Holdsworth SR: The participation of macrophages, glomerular procoagulant activity and factor VIII in glomerular fibrin deposition. Studies in anti GBM antibody-induced glomerulonephritis in rabbits. Am J Pathol, 124: 10-17, 1986.
144. Wiggins RC, Glatfelter A, Brukman J: Procoagulant activity in glomeruli and urine of rabbits with nephrotoxic nephritis. Lab Invest, 53: 156-165, 1985.
145. Tipping PG, Lowe MG, Holdsworth SR: Glomerular macrophages express augmented procoagulant activity in experimental fibrin-related glomerulonephritis in rabbits. J Clin Invest, 82: 1253-1259, 1988.
146. Thomson NM, Holdsworth SR, Glasgow EF, Atkins RC: The macrophage in the development of experimental crescentic glomerulonephritis. Am J Pathol, 94: 223-240, 1979.
147. Tipping PG, Holdsworth SR: Fibrinolytic therapy with streptokinase for established experimental glomerulonephritis. Nephron, 43: 258-264, 1986.
148. Borrero J, Todd ME, Becker CG, Becker EL: Masugi nephritis: the renal lesion and the coagulation processes. Clin Nephrol, 1: 86-93, 1973.

149. Halpern B, Milliez P, Lagrue G, Fray A, Morard JC: Protective action of heparin in experimental immune nephritis. Nature, 205: 257-259, 1965.
150. Klinerman J: Effects of heparin in experimental nephritis. Lab Invest, 3: 495-508, 1954.
151. Border WA, Wilson CB, Dixon FJ: Failure of heparin to affect two types of experimental glomerulonephritis in rabbits. Kidney Int, 8: 140-148, 1975.
152. Naish PF, Penn GB, Evans DJ, Peters DK: The effect of defibrination on nephrotoxic serum nephritis in rabbits. Clin Sci, 42: 643-649, 1972.
153. Naish PF, Evans DJ, Peters DK: The effects of defibrination with ancrod in experimental allergic glomerular injuries. Clin Exp Immunol, 20: 303-309, 1975.
154. Tipping PG, Thomson NM, Holdsworth SR: A comparison of fibrinolytic and defibrinating agents in established experimental glomerulonephritis. Br J Exp Path, 67: 481-491, 1986.
155. Zoja C, Corna D, Macconi D, Zilio P, Bertani T, Remuzzi G: Tissue plasminogen activator therapy of rabbit nephrotoxic nephritis. Lab Invest, 62: 34-41, 1990.
156. Becker GJ, Hancock WW, Stow JL, Glasgow EF, Atkins RC, Thompson NM: Involvment of the macrophage in experimental chronic immune complex glomerulonephritis. Nephron, 32: 227-233, 1982.
157. Lavelle KJ, Murer-Moseman A: The influence of thrombocytopenia on immune complex glomerulonephritis. J Lab Clin Med, 92: 737-749, 1978.
158. Saito H, Ideura T, Takeuchi J: Effects of a selective thromboxane A_2 synthetase inhibitor on immune complex glomerulonephritis. Nephron, 36: 38-45, 1984.
159. Wardle EN: A study of intravascular coagulation in immune complex glomerulonephritis by use of ^{131}I-labelled antigen. Clin Sci Mol Med, 45: 35-43, 1973.
160. Thompson NM, Simpson IJ, Evans DJPeters DK: Defibrination with ancrod in experimental chronic immune complex nephritis. Clin Exp Immunol, 20: 527-535, 1975.
161. Baliah T, Drummond KN: The effect of anticoagulation on serum sickness nephritis in rabbits. Proc Soc Exp Biol Med, 40: 329-341, 1972.
162. Wilens SL: Enhancement of serum sickness lesions in rabbits with pressor agents. Arch Pathol, 80: 590-598, 1965.
163. Okuda S, Onoyama K, Fujimi S, Oh Y, Nomoto K, Omae T: Influence of hypertension on the progression of experimental autologous immune complex nephritis. J Lab Clin Med, 101: 461-471, 1983.
164. Okuda S, Onoyama K, Tsuruda H, Oh Y, Omae T.: Necrotizing vascular lesions in spontaneously hypertensive rats with nephrotic syndrome: hypercoagulability as a contributory factor. J Lab Clin Med, 104: 767-677, 1984.
165. Howie JF, Helyer BJ: the immunology and pathology of NZB mice. Adv Immunol, 9: 215-224, 1967.
166. Lambert PH, Dixon FJ: Pathogenesis of the glomerulonephritis of NZB/W mice. J Exp Med, 127: 507-518, 1978.
167. Henson JB, Gorham JR, Tanaka Y: Renal glomerular ultrastructure in mink affected by Aleutian disease. Lab Invest, 17: 123-130, 1967.
168. McKay DG, Philips LL, Kaplan H: Chronic intravascular coagulation in Aleutian disease of mink. Am J Pathol, 50: 899-909, 1967.
169. Kelley VE, Sneve S, Musinski S: Increased renal thromboxane production in murine lupus nephritis. J Clin Invest, 77: 252-259, 1986.
170. Cole EH, Sweet J, Levy GA: Expression of macrophage procoagulant activity in murine systemic lupus erythematosus. J Clin Invest, 78: 887-893, 1986.
171. Sawtell NM, Weiss MA, Pesce AJ, Michael GJ: An immune complex glomerulopathy associated with glomerular capillary thrombosis in the laboratory mouse. Lab Invest, 56: 256-263, 1987.
172. Druet P, Baran D, Pelletier L, Hirsch F, Druet E, Sapin C: Drug-induced experimental autoimmune nephritis. Concepts Immunopathol, 3: 311-330, 1986.
173. Kanfer A, De Prost D, Guettier C, Nochy D, Le Floch V, Hinglais N, Druet P: Enhanced glomerular procoagulant activity and fibrin deposition in rats with mercuric chloride-induced autoimmune nephritis. Lab Invest, 57: 138-143, 1987.
174. Michaud A, Sapin C, Leca G, Aiach M, Druet P: Involvment of hemostasis during an autoimmune glomerulonephritis induced by mercuric chloride in Brown Norway rats. Thromb Res, 33: 77-88, 1983.
175. Donker AJ, Venuto RC, Vladutiu AO, Brentjens JR, Andres GA: Effects of prolonged administration of D-Penicillamine or captopril in various strains of rats. Clin Immunol Immunopathol, 30: 142-155, 1984.

176. Duffy JL, Cinque T, Grishman E, Churg J: Intraglomerular fibrin, platelet aggregation, and subendothelial deposits in lipoid nephrosis. J Clin Invest, 49: 251-258, 1970.

177. Duffus P, Parbtani A, Frampton G, Cameron JS: Intraglomerular localization of platelet related antigens, platelet factor 4 and ß-thromboglobulin in glomerulonephritis. Clin Nephrol, 17: 288-297, 1982.

178. Conte J, Boneu B, Mignon-Conte M, Suc JM: Exploration of intraglomerular phenomena. In: "Glomerulonephritis. Morphology, Natural History and Treatment" (Eds P Kincaid-Smith, TH Mathew, E Lovell Becker), John Wiley & Sons, New York, 1973, pp. 915-926.

179. Hoyer JR Michael AF, Hoyer LW: Immunofluorescent localization of antihemophilic factor antigen and fibrinogen in human renal diseases. J Clin Invest, 53: 1375-1384, 1974.

180. Yamabe H, Sugawara N, Ozawa K, Kubota H, Fukushi K, Kikuchi K, Onodera K: Glomerular deposition of Hageman factor in IgA nephropathy. Nephron, 37: 62-63, 1984.

181. Matsubara M, Akiu N, Ootaka T, Saito T, Yoshinaga K: Glomerular deposition of coagulation factors VII, VIII and IX in IgA nephropathy: possible coagulation system involvement in IgA nephropathy. Nephron, 53: 381-383, 1989.

182. Tipping PG, Dowling JP, Holdsworth SR: Glomerular procoagulant activity in human proliferative glomerulonephritis. J Clin Invest, 81: 119-125, 1988.

183. Van Zyl-Smit R, Marks T: Procoagulant activity of whole human glomeruli in health and disease. Kidney Int, 37: 446, 1990.

184. Rondeau E, Mougenot B, Lacave R, Peraldi MN, Kruithof EKO, Sraer JD: Plasminogen activator inhibitor in renal fibrin deposits of human nephropathies. Clin Nephrol, 33: 55-60, 1990.

185. Kant KS, Pollak VE, Dosekun A, Glas-Greenwalt P, Weiss MA, Glueck HI: Lupus nephritis with thrombosis and abnormal fibrinolysis: effect of ancrod. J Lab Clin Med, 105: 77-88, 1985.

186. Kim S, Wadhwa NK, Kant KS, Pollak VE, Glas-Greenwalt P, Weiss MA, Hong CD: Fibrinolysis in glomerulonephritis treated with ancrod: renal functional, immunologic and histopathologic effects. Quart J Med, 259: 879-895, 1988.

187. Beaufils M, Morel-Maroger L, Sraer JD, Kanfer A, Kourilsky O, Richet G: Acute renal failure of glomerular origin during visceral abscesses. N Engl J Med, 295: 185-189, 1976.

188. Frasca GM, Vangelista A, Martella D, Dondi M, Bonomini V: Prevention of chronic glomerular uremia in steroid resistant glomerulonephritis. A clinical trial with a new antithrombotic agent. Clin Nephrol, 13: 421-429, 1990.

189. Kant KS, Pollak VE, Weiss MA, Glueck HI, Miller MA, Hess EV: Glomerular thrombosis in systemic lupus erythematosus: prevalence and significance. Medicine, 60: 71-86, 1981.

190. Pollak VE, Glueck HI, Weiss MA, Lebron-Berges A, Miller MA: Defibrination with ancrod in glomerulonephritis: effects on clinical and histologic findings and on blood coagulation. Am J Nephrol, 2: 195-207, 1982.

191. Catell V: Mitomycin-induced Hemolytic Uremic Syndrome. Am J Pathol, 121: 88-95, 1985.

192. Butler T, Rahaman H, Al-Mahmud KA, Islam M, Bardhan P, Kabir I, Rahman MM: An animal model of haemolytic-uremic syndrome in shigellosis: lipopolysaccharides of Shigella Dysenteriae I and S. flexneri produce leukocyte-mediated renal cortical necrosis in rabbits. Br J Exp Pathol, 66: 7-15, 1985.

193. Weksler BB, Jaffe EA, Brower MS, Cole O: Human leucocyte cathepsin G and elastase specifically suppress thrombin-induced prostacyclin production in human endothelial cells. Blood, 74: 1627-1634, 1989.

194. Harlan MD, Harker LA, Reidy MA, Gajdusek CM, Schwartz SM, Striker GE: Lipopolysaccharide-mediated bovine endothelial injury in vitro. Lab Invest, 48: 269-274, 1983.

195. De Chadaverian JP, Kaplan BS: The hemolytic uremic syndrome of childhood. Perspect Pediatr Pathol, 4: 465-473, 1978.

196. Clarkson AR, Lawrence JR, Meadows R: The hemolytic uremic syndrome in adults. Quart J Med, 39: 227-240, 1970.

197. Colucci M, Balconi G, Lorenzet R, Pietra A, Locati D, Donati MB, Semeraro N: Cultured human endothelial cells generate tissue factor in response to endotoxin. J Clin Invest, 71: 1893-1896, 1983.

198. Barley-Maloney L, Obrig T, Daniel T: Human renal microvascular endothelial cells are targets for HUS-associated verotoxin. J Am Soc Neph, 1: 515, 1990.

199. O'Brien A, Holmes RK: Shiga and Shiga-like toxins. Microbiol Rev, 51: 206-220, 1987.

200. Konowalchuk J, Speirs JL, Stavric S: Vero response to a cytotoxin of E. coli. Infect Immunol, 18: 775-777, 1977.

201. Karmali MA, Steele BT, Petric M, Lim C: Sporadic cases of hemolytic-uremic syndrome associated with faecal cytotoxin and cytotoxin-producing E. coli in stools. Lancet, I: 619-620, 1983.

202. Karmali MA, Petric M, Lim C, Fleming PC, Arbus GS, Lior H: The association between idiopathic hemolytic-uremic syndrome and infection by verotoxin-producing E. coli. J Infect Dis, 151: 775-782, 1985.

203. Lopez EL, Diaz M, Grinstein S, Devoto S, Mendilaharzu F, Murray BE, Ashkenazi S, Rubeglio E, Woloj M, Vasquez M, Turco M, Pickering LK, Cleary TG: Hemolytic uremic syndrome and diarrhea: the role of Shiga-like toxins. J Infect Dis, 160: 469-475, 1989.

204. Carter AO, Borczyk AA, Carlson JAK, Harvey B, Hockin JC, Karmali MA, Krishnan C, Korn D, Lior H: A severe outbreak of E. coli 0157:H7-associated hemorrhagic colitis in a nursing home. N Engl J Med, 317: 1496-1500, 1987.

205. Remis RS, MacDonald KL, Riley LW, Phur ND, Wells JG, Davis BR, Blake PA, Cohen ML: Sporadic cases of hemorrhagic colitis associated with E. coli 0157:H7. Ann Intern Med, 101: 624-626, 1984.

206. Brown JE, Echeverria P, Taylor DN, Seriwatana J, Vanapraks V, Lexomboon U, Neill RN, Newland JW: Determination by DNA hybridization of Shiga-like toxins producing E. coli in children with diarrhea in Thailand. J Clin Microbiol, 27: 291-294, 1989.

207. Brown JE, Griffin DE, Rothman SW, Doctor BP: Purification and biological characterization of Shiga toxin from S. Dysenteriae I. Infect Immunol, 36: 996-1005, 1982.

208. Waddell T, Head S, Petric M, Cohen A, Lingwood C: Globotriosyl ceramide is recognized by the E. coli verotoxin. Biochem Biophys Res Commun, 152: 674-679, 1988.

209. Eiklid K, Olsnes S: Entry of Shigella dysenteriae toxin into HeLa cells. Infect Immunol, 42: 771-777, 1983.

210. Saxena SK, O'Brien AD, Ackerman EJ: Shiga toxin, Shiga like toxin II and ricin are all single site RNA N-glycosidases of 28S RNA when microinjected into Xenopus oocytes. J Biol Chem, 264: 596-601, 1989.

211. Obrig TG, Moran TP, Brown JE: The mode of action of Shiga toxin on peptide elongation of eukaryotic protein synthesis. Biochem J, 244: 287-294, 1987.

212. Boyd B, Lingwood C: Verotoxin receptor glycolipid in human renal tissue. Nephron, 51: 207-210, 1989.

213. Obrig TG, Del Vecchio PJ, Karmali MA, Petric M, Moran TP, Judge TK: Pathogenesis of hemolytic-uremic syndrome. Lancet II: 687, 1987.

214. Leung DY, Moake JL, Havens PL, Kim M, Pober JS: Lytic anti-endothelial cell antibodies in hemolytic uremic syndrome. Lancet, II: 183-186, 1988.

215. Remuzzi G, Misiani R, Marchesi D, Livio M, De Gaetano G, Donati MB: Haemolytic uremic syndrome: deficiency of plasma factor(s) regulating prostacyclin activity ? Lancet, II: 871-872, 1978.

216. Levin M, Barratt TM: Haemolytic uremic syndrome. Arch Dis Child, 59: 397-440, 1984.

217. Webster J, Rees AJ, Lewis PJ, Hensby CN: Prostacyclin deficiency in haemolytic uremic syndrome. Br Med J, 281: 271, 1980.

218. Hensby CN, Lewis PJ, Hilgard P, Mufti GJ, Hows J, Webster J: Prostacyclin deficiency in thrombotic thrombocytopenic purpura. Lancet, II: 748-750, 1979.

219. Machin SJ, Defreyn G, Chamone DAF, Vermylen J: Plasma 6-keto $PGF_{1\alpha}$ levels after plasma exchange in thrombotic thrombocytopenic purpura. Lancet, 1: 661, 1980.

220. Jorgensen KA, Pedersen RS: Familial deficiency of prostacyclin production stimulating factor in the hemolytic uremic syndrome of childhood. Thromb Res, 21: 311-315, 1981.

221. Chen YC, McLeod B, Hill ER, Wu KK: Accelerated prostacyclin degradation in thrombotic thrombocytopenic purpura. Lancet, II: 267-269, 1981.

222. Wu KK, Hall ER, Rossi EC, Papp AC: Serum prostacyclin binding defects in thrombotic thrombocytopenic purpura. J Clin Invest, 75: 168-174, 1985.

223. Karch H, Bitzan M, Pietsch R, Stenger KO, Wulffen HV, Heesemann J, Dusing R: Purified verotoxins of E. coli 0157:H7 decrease prostacyclin synthesis by endothelial cells. Microbiol Pathogen, 5: 215-221, 1988.

224. Ham EA, Egan RW, Soderman DD, Gale PH, Kuehl FA Jr: Peroxidase- dependent deactivation of prostacyclin synthetase. J Biol Chem, 254: 2191-2194, 1979.

225. Remuzzi G, Mecca G, Livio M, de Gaetano G, Donati MB, Pearson JD, Gordon JL: Prostacyclin generation by cultured endothelial cells in haemolytic uremic syndrome. Lancet, I: 656-658, 1980.

226. Jorgensen KA, Pedersen RS: Familial deficiency of prostacyclin production stimulating factor in the hemolytic uremic syndrome of childhood. Thromb Res, 21: 311-315, 1981.

227. Deckmyn H, Zoja C, Arnout J, Todislo A, VandenBulcke F, D'Hont L, Hendrikx N, Gresele P, Vermylen J: Partial isolation and function of the prostacyclin regulating plasma factor. Clin Sci, 69: 383-393, 1985.

228. Misiani R, Appiani AC, Edefonti A, Gotti E, Bettinelli A, Giani M, Rossi E, Remuzzi G, Mecca G: Hemolytic uremic syndrome: therapeutic effect of plasma infusion. Br Med J, 285: 1304-1306, 1982.

229. Stuart MJ, Spitzer RE, Walenga RW, Boone S: Prostanoids in the hemolytic uremic syndrome. J Pediatr, 106: 936-939, 1985.

230. Walters MDS, Levin M, Smith C, Nokes TJC, Hardisty RM, Dillon MJ, Barratt TM: Intravascular platelet activation in the hemolytic uremic syndrome. Kidney Int, 33: 107-115, 1988.

231. Bloom A, Hannaford PA, Greaves M, Preston FE, Brown CB: Hemolytic uremic syndrome: demonstration of abnormalities of platelet reactivity and insensitivity to prostaglandin I_2. Clin Nephrol, 23: 85-88, 1985.

232. Tönschoff B, Momper R, Kühl PG, Horst S, Schärer K, Seyberth HW: Increased thromboxane biosynthesis in childhood hemolytic uremic syndrome. Kidney Int, 37: 1134-1141, 1990.

233. Lian ECY, Savaraj N: Effects of platelet inhibitors on the platelet aggregation induced by plasma from patients with thrombotic thrombocytopenic purpura. Blood, 58: 354-359, 1981.

234. Lian ECY: Pathogenesis of thrombotic thrombocytopenic purpura. Semin Haematol, 24: 82-94, 1987.

235. De Gaetano G, Bertele V, Maggi A: The physiology of primary hemostasis. In: "Heamostasis and the Kidney" (Eds G Remuzzi, EC Rossi), Butter Worths, London, 1986, pp 3-18.

236. Moake JL, Rudy CK, Troll LH, Weinstein MJ, Colaninno NM, Azacar J, Seder RH, Hong SL, Deykin D: Unusually large plasma factor VIII: von Willebrand factor multimers in chronic relapsing thrombotic thrombocytopenic purpura. N Engl J Med, 307: 1432-1435, 1982.

237. Rose PE, Enayat SM, Sunderland R, Short PE, Williams CE, Hill FGH: Abnormalities of factor VIII related protein multimers in the hemolytic uremic syndrome. Arch Dis Child, 59: 1135-1140, 1984.

238. Gill JC, Sheth KJ, Endres-Brooks J: Predictive value of von Willebrand factor in hemolytic uremic syndrome. Blood, 72: 1096, 1988.

239. Helmsworth M, Ragin CS, Sherbotie J, Kaplan BS: Abnormal factor VIII von Willebrand multimers in patients with hemolytic uremic syndrome or thrombotic thrombocytopenic purpura may predict thrombotic episodes. Pediatr Nephrol, 3: C182, 1989.

240. Moake JL, Mc Pherson PD: Abnormalities of von Willebrand factor multimers in thrombotic thrombocytopenic purpura and hemolytic uremic syndrome. Am J Med, 87: 3-15, 1989.

241. Kaplan BS, Mills M: Elevated serum elastase and alpha-1-antitrypsine levels in hemolytic uremic syndrome. Clin Nephrol, 30: 193-196, 1988.

242. Kwaan HC, Gallo G, Potter E: The nature of the vascular lesion in thrombotic thrombocytopenic purpura. Ann Intern Med, 68: 1169-1170, 1968.

243. Kwaan HC: The pathogenesis of thrombotic thrombocytopenic purpura. Semin Thromb Haemost, 5: 184-198, 1979.

244. Bergstein JM, Kuederli U, Bang NU: Plasma inhibitor of glomerular fibrinolysis in the hemolytic uremic syndrome. Am J Med, 73: 322-327, 1982.

245. Glas-Greenwalt P, Kont KS, Pollack VE: Severely depressed fibrinolysis in 12 patients with thrombotic thrombocytopenic purpura. Thromb Haemost, 54: 213-214, 1985.

246. Rizzoni G, Claris-Appiani A, Edefonti A, Facchin P, Franchini F, Gusmano R, Pavanello L, Perfumo F, Remuzzi G: Plasma infusion for hemolytic uremic syndrome in children: results of a multicenter controlled trial. J Pediatr, 112: 284-290, 1988.

247. Loirat C, Sonsino E, Hinglais N, Jais JP, Landais P, Fermanian J: Treatment of childhood hemolytic uremic syndrome with plasma. A multicentre randomized controlled trial. Pediatr Nephrol, 2: 279-285, 1988.

248. Bukowski RM: Thrombotic thrombocytopenic purpura: a review. Prog Hemost Thromb, 6: 287-337, 1982.

249. Bukowski RM, King JW, Hewlett JS: Plasmapheresis in the treatment of thrombotic thrombocytopenic purpura. Blood, 50: 413-417, 1977.

250. Levin M, Barratt TM: Hemolytic uremic syndrome. Arch Dis Child, 59: 397-400, 1984.

251. Vitacco N, Avalos JS, Gianantonio CA: Heparin therapy in the hemolytic uremic syndrome. J Pediatr, 83: 271-275, 1973.

252. Arenson GB, August CS: Preliminary report: treatment of the hemolytic uremic syndrome with aspirin and dipyridamole. J Pediatr, 86: 957-961, 1975.

253. Thorsen CA, Rossi EC, Green D, Carone FA: The treatment of hemolytic uremic syndrome with inhibitors of platelet function. Am J Med, 66: 711-716, 1979.

254. Monnens L, Kleynen F, Van Munster P, Schretlen F, Bonnerman A: Coagulation studies and streptokinase therapy in the hemolytic uremic syndrome. Helv Paediatr Acta, 27: 45-54, 1972.
255. Stuart J, Winterborn MH, White RHR: Thrombolytic therapy in hemolytic uremic syndrome. Br Med J, 3: 217-221, 1974.
256. Fitzgerald GA, Maas RL, Stein R, Oster JA, Roberts LJ: Intravenous prostacyclin in thrombotic thrombocytopenic purpura. Ann Intern Med, 95: 319-322, 1981.
257. Johnson JE, Mills GM, Batson AG, Cato AE, Thornsvard CT: Ineffective epoprostenol therapy for thrombotic thrombocytopenic purpura. JAMA, 250: 3089-3091, 1983.
258. Powell HR, McCredie DA, Taylor CM, Burke JR, Walker RG: Vitamin E treatment in haemolytic uraemic syndrome. Arch Dis Child, 59: 401-404, 1984.
259. Lian ECY, Mui PTK, Siddiqui FA, Chiu AYY, Chiu LLS: Inhibition of platelet aggregating activity in thrombotic thrombocytopenic purpura plasma by normal adult Immunoglobulin G. J Clin Invest, 73: 548-555, 1984.
260. Giroux L, Boury F, Smeesters C, Corman J, Daloze PM: Modifications of glomerular fibrinolysis in human renal graft rejection. J Surg Res, 31: 253-258, 1981.
261. Friedlander G, Moulonguet-Doléris L, Kourilsky O, Nussaume O, Ardaillou R, Sraer JD: Prostaglandin synthesis by glomeruli isolated from normal and chronically rejected human kidneys. Contrib Nephrol, 41: 20-22, 1984.
262. Kanfer A, Delarue F, Languille T: Transient platelet factor 3 activation during human renal allograft rejection. Transplantation, 18: 78-81, 1974.
263. Anderson M, Dewar P, Fleming LB, Hacking PM, Morley AR, Murray S, Swinney J, Taylor RMR, Uldall PR, Wardle, EN: A controlled trial of dipyridamole in human renal transplantation and an assessment of platelet function studies in rejection. Clin Nephrol, 2: 93-99, 1974.
264. Frampton G, Parbtani A, Marchesi D, Duffus P, Livio M, Remuzzi G, Cameron JS: *In vivo* platelet activation with *in vitro* hyperaggregability to arachidonic acid in renal allograft recipients. Kidney Int, 23: 506-513, 1983.
265. Grino JM, Torras J, Martin-Comin J, Mora J, Sabate I, Castelao AM, Roca M, Alsina J: [111]indium-oxine labelled platelets in the diagnosis of renal allograft rejection during cyclosporin A therapy. Proc EDTA-ERA, 22: 1183-1186, 1985.
265b Foegh ML, Winchester JF, Zmudka M, Helfrich GB, Cooley C, Ramwell PW, Schreiner GE: Urine i-TXB$_2$ in renal allograft rejection. Lancet, II: 431-434, 1981.
266. Halloran PF, Aprile MA, Haddad GJ, Robinette MA: Procoagulant activity in renal transplant recipients. Transplantation, 39: 374-377, 1985.
267. Lowry RP, Blais D: Tumor necrosis factor-alpha in rejecting rat cardiac allografts. Transplant Proc, 20: 245-247, 1988.
268. Meulders Q, Rondeau E, Delarue F, Lacave R, Sraer JD: Interleukine-2 stimulation of tumor necrosis factor alpha synthesis by peripheral blood mononuclear cells in renal allograft rejection. Transplant Proc, 22: 1987-1988, 1990.
269. Maury CPJ, Teppo AM: Raised serum levels of cachectin/tumor necrosis factor alpha in renal allograft rejection. J Exp Med, 166: 1132-1137, 1987.
270. Schrader J, Gallimore MJ, Eisenhauer T, Isemer FE, Schoel G, Warneke G, Brüggemann M, Scheler F: Parameters of the kallikrein-kinin, coagulation and fibrinolytic systems as early indicators of kidney transplant rejection. Nephron, 48: 183-189, 1988.
271. Neild GH, Reuben R, Hartley RB, Cameron JS: Glomerular thrombi in renal allografts associated with cyclosporin treatment. J Clin Path, 38: 253-258, 1985.
272. Van Buren D, Van Buren CT, Flechner SM, Maddox AM, Verani R, Kahan BD: *De novo* hemolytic uremic syndrome in renal transplant recipients immunosuppressed with cyclosporine. Surgery, 98: 54-62, 1985.
273. Leithner C, Sinzinger H, Pohanka E, Schwarz M, Kretschmer G, Syre G: Recurrence of haemolytic uraemic syndrome triggered by cyclosporin A after renal transplantation. Lancet, I: 1470, 1982.
274. Atkinson K, Biggs JC, Hayes J, Ralston M, Dodds AJ, Concannon AJ, Naidoo D: Cyclosporin A associated nephrotoxicity in the first 100 days after allogenic bone marrow transplantation: three distinct syndromes. Br J Haematol, 54: 59-67, 1983.
275. Powles RL, Kay HEM, Clink HM, Barrett A, Depledge MH, Sloane J, Lumley H, Lawler SD, Morgenstern GR, McElwain TJ, Dady PJ, Jameson B, Watson JG, Leigh M, Hedley D, Filshie J, Robinson B: Mismatched family donors for bone-marrow transplantation as treatment for acute leukaemia. Lancet, I: 612-615, 1983.

276. Shulman H, Striker G, Deeg HJ, Kennedy M, Storb R, Thomas ED: Nephrotoxicity of cyclosporin A after allogeneic marrow transplantation: glomerular thromboses and tubular injury. N Engl J Med, 305: 1392-1395, 1981.

277. Brown Z, Neild GH, Willoughby J, Somia JS, Cameron JS: Factor VIII related antigen (FVIIIRAg) levels in renal allograft recipients taking cyclosporine (CS). Thromb Haemost, 54: 292, 1985.

278. Yoshida M, Kozaki M, Ioya N, Kaji N, Tamaki T, Hiraishi S, Ishii H, Kazama M, Fukutomi K, Nagasawa T: Plasma thrombomodulin levels as an indicator of vascular injury caused by cyclosporine nephrotoxicity. Transplantation, 50: 1066-1069, 1990.

279. Neild GH, Ivory K, Williams DG: Cortical infarction in rabbits with serum sickness following cyclosporin A therapy. Proc EDTA, 20: 662-668, 1983.

280. Perico N, Benigni A, Zoja C, Delaini F, Remuzzi G: Functional significance of exaggerated renal thromboxane A$_2$ synthesis induced by cyclosporin A. Am J Physiol, 251: F581-F587, 1986.

281. Zoja C, Furci L, Ghilardi F, Zilio P, Benigni A, Remuzzi G: Cyclosporin-induced endothelial cell injury. Lab Invest, 55: 455-462, 1986.

282. Brown Z, Neild GH: Cyclosporine inhibits prostacyclin production by cultured human endothelial cells. Transplant Proc, 19: 1178-1180, 1987.

283. Lindsey JA, Morisaki N, Sitts J, Zager RA, Cornwell DG: Fatty acid metabolism and cell proliferation: IV. Effect of prostanoid biosynthesis from endogenous fatty acid release with cyclosporin A. Lipids, 18: 566-569, 1983.

284. Whisler RL, Lindsey JA, Proctor KVW, Morisaki N, Cornwell DG: Characteristics of cyclosporine induction of increased prostaglandin levels from human peripheral blood monocytes. Transplantation, 38: 377-381, 1984.

284b. Sraer J, Bens M, Ardaillou R: Dual effects of cyclosporine A on arachidonate metabolism by peritoneal macrophages. Phospholipase activation and partial thromboxane-synthase blockage. Biochem Pharmacol, 38: 1947-1954, 1989.

285. Duggin GG, Baxter C, Hall BM, Horvath JS, Tiller DJ: Influence of cyclosporine A on intrarenal control of GFR. Clin Nephrol, 25: S43-S45, 1986.

286. Rodriguez-Puyol D, Lamas S, Olivera A, Lopez-Farré A, Ortega G, Hernando L, Lopez-Novoa JM: Actions of cyclosporin A on cultured rat mesangial cells. Kidney Int, 35: 632-637, 1989.

287. Helin HH, Edgington TS: Cyclosporin A regulates monocyte/macrophage effector functions by affecting instructor T cells: inhibition of monocyte procoagulant response to allogenic stimulation. J Immunol, 132: 1074-1076, 1984.

288. Carlsen E, Prydz H: Enhancement of procoagulant activity in stimulated mononuclear blood cells and monocytes by cyclosporine. Transplantation, 43: 543-548, 1987.

289. Carlsen E, Mallet AC, Prydz H: Effect of cyclosporin A on procoagulant activity in mononuclear blood cells and monocytes in vitro. Clin Exp Immunol, 60: 407-416, 1985.

290. Carlsen E, Stinessen MB, Prydz H: Differential effect of alpha-interferon and y-interferon on thromboplastin response in monocytes and endothelial cells. Clin Exp Immunol, 70: 471-478, 1987.

291. Vanrenterghem Y, Lerut T, Roels L, Gruwerz J, Michielsen P, Gresele P, Deckmyn H, Collucci M, Arnout J, Vermylen J: Thromboembolic complications and haemostatic changes in cyclosporin-treated cadaveric kidney allograft recipients. Lancet, I: 999-1002, 1985.

292. Clevers H, Alarcon B, Wileman T, Terhorst C: The T cell receptor/CD3 complex: a dynamic protein ensemble. Annu Rev Immunol, 6: 629-662, 1988.

293. Abramowicz D, Schandene L, Goldman M, Crusiavy A, Vereerstraten P, De Pauw L, Wybran J, Kinnaert P, Dupont E, Toussaint C: Release of tumor necrosis factor, interleukin-2, and gamma-interferon in serum after injection of OKT3 monoclonal antibody in kidney transplant recipients. Transplantation, 47: 606-608, 1989.

294. Chatenoud L, Ferran C, Reuter A, Legendre Ch, Gevaert Y, Kreis H, Franchimont P, Bach JF: Systemic reaction to the anti-T cell monoclonal antibody OKT3 in relation to serum levels of tumor necrosis factor and interferon-alpha. N Engl J Med, 320: 1420-1421, 1989.

295. Geczy CL, Hopper KE: A mechanism of migration inhibition in delayed-type hypersensitivity reactions. II. Lymphokines promote procoagulant activity of macrophages in vitro. J Immunol, 126: 1059-1065, 1981.

296. Van Wauwe JP, De Mey JR, Goossens JG: OKT3: a monoclonal anti-human T lymphocyte antibody with potent mitogenic properties. J Immunol, 124: 2708-2713, 1980.

297. Chang TW, Kung PC, Gingras SP, Goldstein G: Does OKT3 monoclonal antibody react with an antigen-recognition structure on human T cells ? Proc Natl Acad Sci USA, 78: 1805-1808, 1981.

298. Hancock WW, Rickles FR, Ewan VA, Atkins RC: Immunohistological studies with A1-3, a monoclonal antibody to activated human monocytes and macrophages. J Immunol, 136: 2416-2420, 1986.

299. Itaka M, Iwatani Y, Row VV, Volpé R: Induction of monocyte procoagulant activity with OKT3 antibody. J Immunol, 139: 1617-1623, 1987.

300. Brenner BM: Hemodynamically mediated glomerular injury and the progressive nature of kidney disease. Kidney Int, 23: 647-655, 1983.

301. Klahr S, Schreiner G, Ichikawa I: The progression of renal disease. N Engl J Med, 318: 1657-1666, 1988.

302. Schwartz MM, Bidani AK, Lewis EJ: Glomerular epithelial cell function and pathology following extreme ablation of renal mass. Am J Pathol, 126: 315-324, 1987.

303. Ruedin P, Mougenot B, Ruedin D, Rondeau E, Sraer JD, Lacave R, Kanfer A: Fibrin deposition and adaptive changes in glomerular procoagulant and fibrinolytic activities in rat renoprival nephropathy. J Exp Path, 71: 269-278, 1990.

304. Purkerson ML, Hoffsten PE, Klahr S: Pathogenesis of the glomerulopathy associated with renal infarction in rats. Kidney Int, 9: 407-417, 1976.

305. Purkerson ML, Joist JH, Greenberg JM, Kay D, Hoffsten PE, Klahr S: Inhibition by anticoagulant drugs of the progressive hypertension and uremia associated with renal infarction in rats. Thromb Res, 26: 227-240, 1982.

306. Olson JL: Role of heparin as a protective agent following reduction of renal mass. Kidney Int, 25: 376-382, 1984.

307. Purkerson ML, Joist JH, Yates J, Valdes A, Morrison A, Klahr S: Inhibition of thromboxane synthesis ameliorates the progressive kidney disease of rats with subtotal renal ablation. Proc Natl Acad Sci USA, 82: 193-197, 1985.

308. Purkerson ML, Joist JH, Yates J, Klahr S: Role of hypertension and coagulation in the progressive glomerulopathy of rats with subtotal renal ablation. Mineral Electrolyte Metab, 13: 370-376, 1987.

309. Ichikawa I, Yoshida Y, Fogo A, Purkerson ML, Klahr S: Effect of heparin on the glomerular structure and function of remnant nephrons. Kidney Int, 34: 638-644, 1988.

310. Scharschmidt LA, Gibbons NB, McGarry L, Berger P, Axelrod M, Janis R, Ko YH: Effects of dietary fish oil on renal insufficiency in rats with subtotal nephrectomy. Kidney Int, 32: 700-709, 1987.

311. Stahl RAK, Kudelka S, Paravicini M, Schollmeyer P: Prostaglandin and thromboxane formation in glomeruli from rats with reduced renal mass. Nephron, 42: 252-257, 1986.

312. Zoja C, Benigni A, Livio M, Bergamelli A, Orisio S, Abbate M, Bertani T, Remuzzi G: Selective inhibition of platelet thromboxane generation with low-dose aspirin does not protect rats with reduced renal mass from the development of progressive disease. Am J Pathol, 134: 1027-1038, 1989.

313. Zoja C, Perico N, Bergamelli A, Pasini M, Morigi M, Dadan J, Belloni A, Bertani T, Remuzzi G: Ticlopidine prevents renal disease progression in rats with reduced renal mass. Kidney Int, 37: 934-942, 1990.

314. Iskandar SS, Gifford DR, Emancipator SN: Immune complex acute necrotizing glomerulonephritis with progression to diffuse glomerulosclerosis. A murine model. Lab Invest, 59: 772-779, 1988.

315. Okuda S, Onoyama K, Tsuruda H, Oh Y, Omae T: Necrotizing vascular lesions in spontaneously hypertensive rats with nephrotic syndrome: hypercoagulability as a contributory factor. J Lab Clin Med, 104: 767-777, 1984.

316. Kanfer A: Coagulation factors in nephrotic syndrome. Am J Nephrol, 10 (Suppl 1): 63-68, 1990.

317. Gandrille S, Aiach M: Albumin concentration influences fibrinolytic activity in plasma and purified systems. Fibrinolysis, 4: 225-232, 1990.

318. Nilsen DWT, Jeremic M, Weisert OK: An attempt at predicting postoperative deep vein thrombosis by preoperative coagulation studies in patients undergoing total hip replacement. Thromb Haemost, 43: 194-197, 1980.

319. Sue-Ling HM, Johnston D, McMahon MJ, Philips PR, Andrew Davies J: Pre-operative identification of patients at high risk of deep venous thrombosis after elective major abdominal surgery. Lancet, 1: 1173-1176, 1986.

320. Cooper HA, Walter Bowie EJ, Didisheim P, Owen CA: Paradoxic changes in platelets and fibrinogen in chronically induced intravascular coagulation. Mayo Clin Proc, 46: 521-523, 1971.

321. Cameron JS: Coagulation and thromboembolic complications in the nephrotic syndrome. Adv Nephrol, 13: 75-114, 1984.

322. Fischer AM, Tapon-Brétaudière J, Bros A, Josso F: Respective roles of antithrombin III and alpha-2-macroglobulin in thrombin inactivation. Thromb Haemost, 45: 51-54, 1981.

323. Idell SI, James KK, Levin EG, Schwartz BS, Manchanda N, Maunder RJ, Martin TR, McLarty J, Fair DS: Local abnormalities in coagulation and fibrinolytic pathways predispose to alveolar fibrin deposition in the adult respiratory distress syndrome. J Clin Invest, 84: 695-705, 1989.

324. Coffman TM, Ruiz P, Sanfilippo F, Klotman PE: Chronic thromboxane inhibition preserves function of rejecting rat renal allografts. Kidney Int, 35: 24-30, 1989.

325. Coffman TM, Smith SR, Creech EA, Schaffer AV, Martin LL, Rakhit A, Douglas FL, Klotman PE: The thromboxane synthetase inhibitor CGS 13080 improves renal allograft function in patients taking cyclosporine. Kidney Int, 37: 604, 1990.

326. Pierucci A, Simonetti BM, Pecci G, Mavrikakis G, Feriozzi S, Cinotti GA, Patrignani P, Ciabattoni G, Patrono C: Improvement of renal function with selective thromboxane antagonism in lupus nephritis. N Engl J Med, 320: 421-425, 1989.

327. De Prost D, Ollivier V, Hakim J: Pentoxifylline inhibition of procoagulant activity generated by activated mononuclear phagocytes. Mol Pharmacol, 38: 562-566, 1990.

328. Girard TJ, MacPhail LA, Likert KM, Novotny WF, Miletich JP, Broze GJ Jr: Inhibition of factor VIIa-tissue factor coagulation activity by a hybrid protein. Science, 248: 1421-1424, 1990.

329. Haber E, Quertermous T, Matsueda GR, Runge MS: Innovative approaches to plasminogen activator therapy. Science, 243: 51-56, 1989.

GLOSSARY

ADP :	Adenosine diphosphate
ARF :	Acute renal failure
ATN :	Acute tubular necrosis
AT III :	Antithrombin III
BCN :	Bilateral cortical necrosis
DIC :	Disseminated intravascular coagulation
EACA :	Epsilon aminocaproic acid
GBM :	Glomerular basement membrane
GN :	Glomerulonephritis
GSP :	Generalized Shwartzman phenomenon
HUS :	Hemolytic uremic syndrome
IL-1 :	Interleukin 1
LPS :	Lipopolysaccharide
NS :	Nephrotic syndrome
PA :	Plasminogen activity
PAF :	Platelet activating factor
PAI-1 :	Plasminogen activator inhibitor type 1
PGI_2 :	Prostacyclin
PMA :	Phorbol myristate acetate
t-PA :	Tissue plasminogen activator
TNF :	Tumor necrosis factor
TTP :	Thrombotic thrombocytopenic purpura
Tx :	Thromboxane
u-PA :	Urokinase
vWF :	von Willebrand factor

Chapter 2

CENTRAL NERVOUS SYSTEM COMPLICATIONS OF SEVERE HYPONATREMIA

RICHARD H. STERNS

Division of Nephrology, Department of Medicine, University of Rochester School of Medicine, Rochester General Hospital, Rochester, New York 14621, USA

The brain has an astonishing ability to adapt to osmotic disturbances: survival has been recorded at serum sodium concentrations ranging from 85 to 272 mmol/l (1). However, because this adaptation takes time, the brain does not take well to abrupt changes (1-3). A sudden onset of severe hypernatremia dehydrates the brain, shrinking it away from its vascular attachments and causing fatal cerebral hemorrhage (4). An acute onset of severe hyponatremia causes cerebral edema, swelling the brain beyond the capacity of the cranial vault and causing fatal herniation (5). Once the brain has adapted to an abnormal osmotic environment, rapid correction of the disturbance may also be injurious. We have long known that overenthusiastic rehydration of patients with chronic hypernatremia may result in cerebral edema and seizures (4). More recently it has been shown that excessively aggressive correction of chronic hyponatremia may cause delayed neurologic deterioration and brain demyelination - a phenomenon that has been dubbed the "osmotic demyelination syndrome"(1-3, 6-9).

This review will focus on the two causes of brain damage in hyponatremia: injury associated with a rapid onset of the electrolyte disorder and injury associated with its rapid correction.

PHYSIOLOGIC ADAPTATIONS OF THE BRAIN TO HYPONATREMIA

The blood-brain barrier resists the permeation of most osmotically active solutes, but it is highly permeable to water. Thus, when the serum sodium concentration falls, a transient osmotic gradient forms between systemic capillary blood and the brain causing water to flow rapidly across the barrier to restore osmotic equilibrium (1-3).

Because of the confines of the skull, an increase in brain water content of more than about 10% is incompatible with life (1-3, 5). If the brain were to behave as a perfect osmometer, swelling in proportion to the change in sodium concentration, only mild hyponatremia could be tolerated; a reduction from 140 to 127 mmol/l (a 10% change) would result in fatal cerebral edema. The fact that humans may survive unharmed with serum sodium concentrations below 100 mmol/l (low enough to cause a 40% increase in brain volume) is living testimony to the brain's ability to resist osmotic swelling.

Two iines of defense protect against cerebral edema in hyponatremia: [1] sodium-rich interstitial fluid is "squeezed" out of the brain through extracellular channels linking the intersitial space with the cerebrospinal fluid (the excess cerebrospinal fluid then enters the systemic circulation), and [2] brain cells regulate their volume by extruding solute (1-3). The first process, which is nearly instantaneous, limits brain swelling to about half of what would be predicted on the basis of ideal osmotic behavior. The second process takes more time, but it ultimately allows the brain to remain viable and minimally edematous at extraordinarily low serum sodium concentrations (1-3).

Potassium, the most prevalent intracellular solute, begins to be lost from the brain after a few hours of hyponatremia and, within about 24 hours, this adaptation becomes maximal. As there is a limit to the amount of potassium that can be lost, other solutes must also contribute to permit survival at extremely low serum sodium concentrations (1-3).

The brain cell normally contains relatively high concentrations of free amino acids, methylamines, and the polyhydric alcohol, myoinositol. The concentration of these organic osmolytes (once known as "idiogenic osmoles") can vary widely without disrupting cellular functions. Accumulation of extra organic osmolytes when the serum sodium concentration rises and depletion of these compounds when it falls allows the brain cell to adapt to severe hypo- and hypernatremia (10, 11).

The brain's adaptation to hyponatremia is thus a continuous one, beginning with the first minutes of the disturbance. The loss of potassium and organic osmolytes from the brain cell progressively reduces the severity of brain edema at a given serum sodium concentration. The precise amount of time required for complete adaptation is uncertain, but it appears to require at least one to two days (1-3) (Figure 1).

Because adjustments in cell solute take time to fully develop, the brain does not take well to rapid osmotic changes. Thus, acute hyponatremia may be fatal at serum sodium concentrations that are well tolerated chronically (5). Similarly, once an adaptation has taken place, rapid correction of the electrolyte disturbance can cause brain dehydration (and injury) because of slow reaccumulation of lost potassium and organic osmolytes by the brain cell (1-3, 11) (Figure 2).

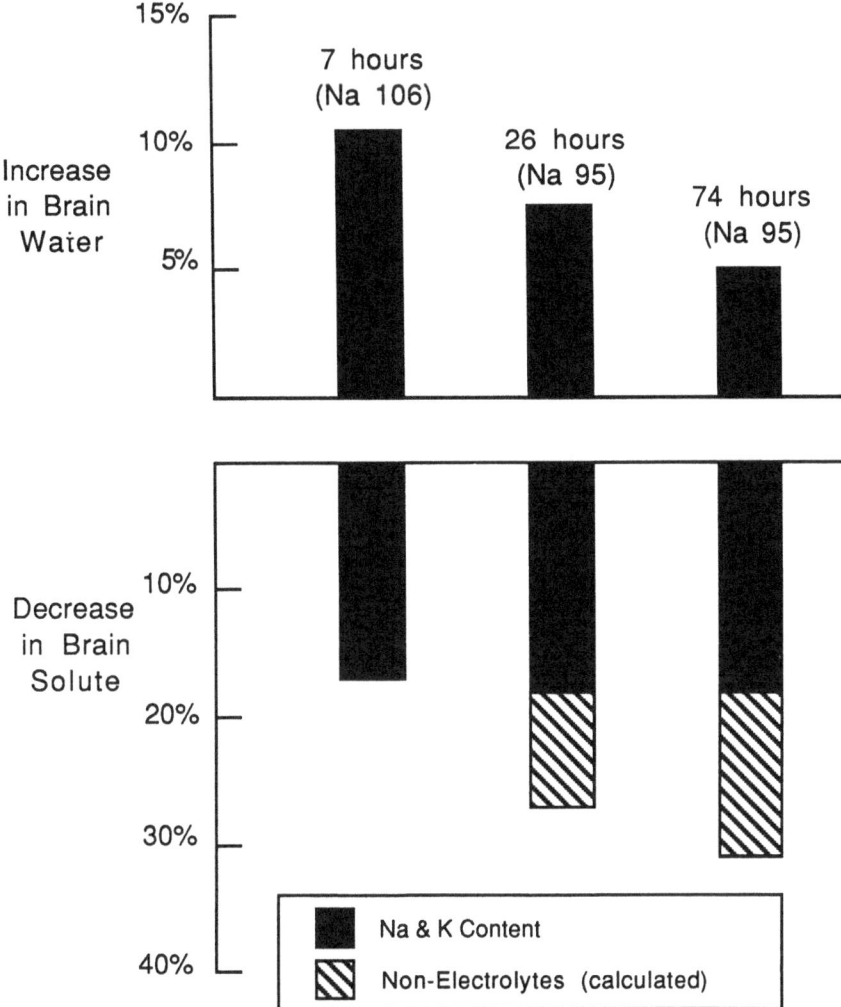

Figure 1. Brain water, sodium, and potassium contents in rats with experimental hyponatremia (2). The calculated losses of non-electrolytes agree well with the losses of organic osmolytes measured by other investigators (11). [Reproduced from Sterns RH, Spital A: Disorders of water balance. In: "Fluids and Electrolytes" (Eds JP Kokko, RL Tannen), Saunders, Philadelphia, 1990, pp 139-194, with permission].

BRAIN INJURY FROM ACUTE HYPONATREMIA

When hyponatremia develops faster than the brain can adapt to the disturbance, cerebral edema accompanied by a syndrome known as "water intoxication" results (5, 12).

The neurologic manifestations of this disorder, which were first recognized in the early 1920's, include headache, nausea, vomitting, weakness, incoordination, tremors, delirium and ultimately seizures. The rapid administration of water was shown to induce some of these symptoms in animals and it was found that the experimental syndrome culminated in convulsions and death associated with cerebral edema (12). Animals could be relieved of their symptoms and in fact saved from death by the administration of concentrated salt solutions.

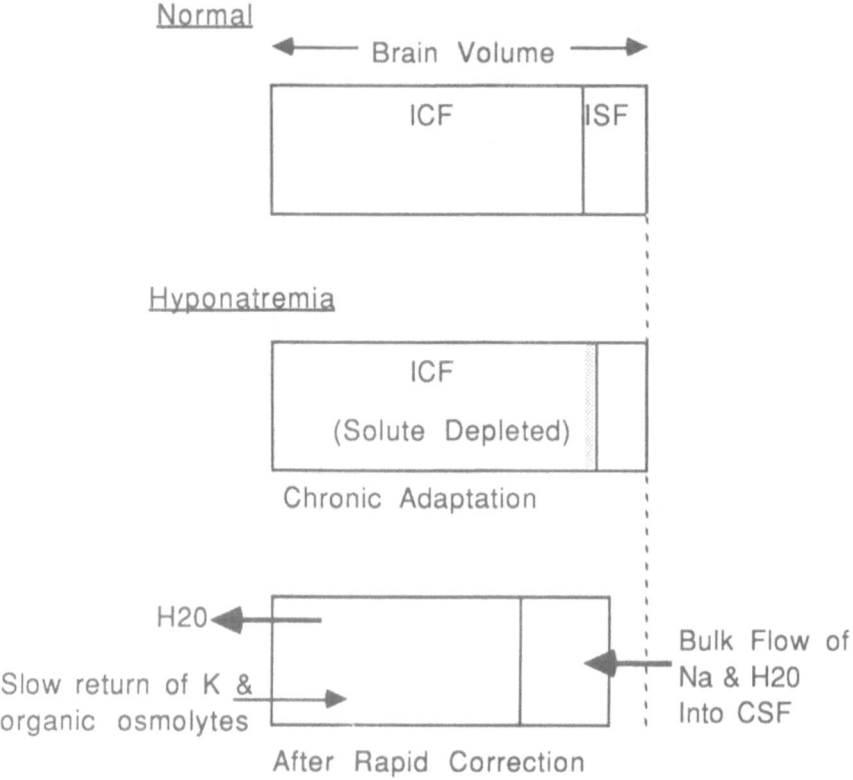

Figure 2. Effect of rapid correction of chronic hyponatremia on brain intracellular (ICF) and interstitial fluid (ISF) volume. The ISF is well defended because of rapid recovery of Na^+-rich fluid via anatomic connections linking the cerebrospinal fluid (CSF) and the brain's interstitial space. However, slow recovery of potassium and organic osmolytes lost in the adaptation to hyponatremia results in cellular dehydration.

Though it is known that an extremely abrupt onset of hyponatremia can be fatal in experimental animals, the precise limits of adaptation have not been conclusively defined. A reduction in sodium concentration to 120 mmol/l over the course of two hours in the rabbit (10 mmol/l/hr) causes seizures, severe cerebral edema and an 80% mortality rate (5). A 5 mmol/l/hr decrease in sodium concentration (to 106 mmol/l in 7 hours) commonly causes seizures in the rat but is not fatal; however, at this rate of onset, brain water content increases by 10%, the approximate limit compatible with survival in this species (2).

HYPONATREMIA AND BRAIN EDEMA IN HUMANS

There are a number of published reports of transtentorial herniation and death caused by acute hyponatremia in humans. The few published cases of fatal cerebral edema have been in patients whose serum sodium concentration was still falling at the time of brain herniation and in whom severe hyponatremia had developed in less than 48 hours (1, 3, 5, 13-21). A recent review of the literature defined the rate of onset of hyponatremia associated with these complications. Deaths and severe sequelae sometimes occur when the serum sodium concentration falls below 120 mmol/l by more than 0.5 mmol/l/hr; these complications become increasingly common when it decreases by more than 1 mmol/l/hr (13) (Figure 3).

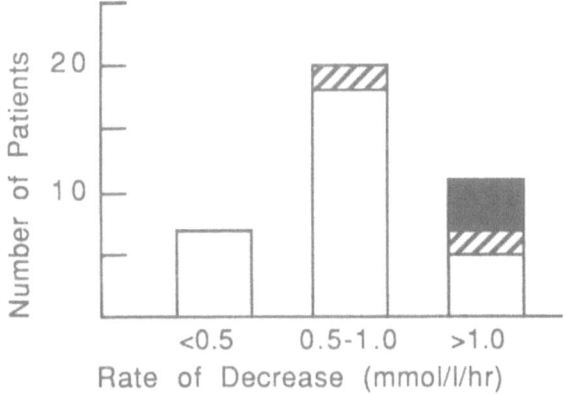

Figure 3. Neurologic sequelae in reported cases with a known rate of onset of acute hyponatremia (13). The speckled bars represent an uncomplicated course; the diagonal stripes represent permanent sequelae; and the solid bars represent deaths from cerebral edema. [Reproduced from Sterns RH, The Management of symptomatic hyponatremia. Seminars in Nephrology, 10 (6): 503-514, 1990 with permission].

Based on this experience and what is known of the rate of adaptation to hyponatremia in animals, we will define hyponatremia as "acute" when the serum sodium has fallen by more than 12 mmol/l/day and has been low for less than 48 hours.

Helwig et al (14) reported the first fatal case of human water intoxication in 1935. A 50 year old woman, who had been given tap water by proctoclysis after a cholecystectomy, developed severe headache, vomiting, and tremor followed within a few hours by convulsions, dilated pupils, and opisthotonos. Despite these symptoms, water continued to be administered and she ultimately died 41 hours after surgery after absorbing a total of 9 liters of water. Post-mortem exam revealed marked cerebral edema. Three years later, the same author reported the first successful treatment of the syndrome in a 64 year old woman who had absorbed 8 liters of water over 39 hours (22). The patient had become totally unconscious, with convulsive movements, cyanosis, Cheyne-Stokes respiration, opisthotonos and bilateral Babinski signs. Cessation of water intake and the prompt administration of 130 ml of 5% saline relieved her acute moribund condition and allowed a complete neurologic recovery.

It is likely that in both of Helwig's patients, severe neurologic symptoms were associated with brain edema. Support for this conclusion is provided by recent reports of computed tomography (CT) of the brain in women presenting with seizures and coma caused by acute hyponatremia. In two patients with reversible symptoms the CT scan showed narrowing of the third ventricle and small lateral ventricles representing diffuse brain edema (23, 24). Compression of the basal cisterns (regarded as an ominous sign) was not present. The scans returned to normal after treatment of hyponatremia and the patients recovered fully. In contrast, in a series of fatal acute hyponatremia CT scans obtained prior to death revealed tentorial herniation, a more severe stage of the same process (15). At autopsy, most patients dying from acute hyponatremia have shown evidence of transtentorial or tonsilar herniation caused by cerebral edema (14, 15-19).

MALE VS FEMALE SUSCEPTIBILITY TO BRAIN INJURY IN ACUTE HYPONATREMIA

Helwig's two female patients are quite representative of subsequent reports of severe acute hyponatremia. Most published cases of iatrogenic water intoxication have been female and young women account for most of the reported fatalities (15, 16, 20, 21). This observation has led some investigators to conclude that women in their reproductive years are less tolerant of hyponatremia than men are (15, 16, 20). The validity of this conclusion is uncertain.

The most striking evidence of a female susceptibility to brain injury is provided by two recent papers which reported 26 previously healthy young women who became severely hyponatremic after routine elective surgery and subsequently suffered permanent neurologic complications (15, 16). Fourteen of the patients undoubtedly died of cerebral edema caused by acute hyponatremia and had documented herniation of the uncus and cerebellum. (As will be discussed later, the cause of brain damage in some of the remaining cases is less certain.) These frightening reports underscore the need for prompt diagnosis and treatment of acute hyponatremia. However, they may not be representative of the usual course of this disorder. Cases were identified over many years from 26 different medical centers. The patients were referred to the authors for review by families, physicians and lawyers and were therefore pre-selected for permanent or fatal brain damage. This experience is considerably different from that found in other reports of acute hyponatremia.

In the 1950's, routine use of hypotonic intravenous fluids after surgery soon led to an understanding of the dangers of this practice. Four series, each collected from individual medical centers provide us with an accurate account of the usual clinical course of acute postoperative water intoxication. Seizures and coma (sometimes with lateralizing neurological signs) developed in 22 patients between 15 and 48 hours after surgery (25-28). Over 75% of these episodes occured in patients over the age of 65 and 82% of the patients were women. The average serum sodium concentration at the onset of seizures was 114 ± 1 mmol/l. Treatment was highly variable, but in the majority of cases improvement was seen after 200 to 300 ml of hypertonic saline. One of the 22 patients (a 68 year old woman) died within 12 hours of her seizure after receiving an additional 3 liters of 5% dextrose in water. The remainder recovered neurologically, but in more severe cases recovery progressed through phases of stupor and confusion, and finally protracted periods in which memory impairment was evident. No permanent neurologic deficits were noted.

There are also several reports of young women who developed severe symptoms of acute water intoxication while receiving oxytocin infusions (1, 3, 29-34). Oxytocin is used in obstetrics to induce labor or abortion and until recently 5% dextrose in water was commonly used as a vehicle. Seizures usually call attention to the hyponatremia and once the oxytocin infusion is stopped, a water diuresis rapidly corrects the disturbance. Like post-operative cases from the 1950's, the vast majority of patients recover uneventfully, despite serum sodium concentrations as low as 100 mmol/l (1, 3, 29, 30). The two reported fatalities experienced a very rapid fall in sodium concentration (to 104 mmol/l within 23 hours and to 116 mmol/l within 26 hours) (33, 34) and had documented cerebral edema at autopsy. Permanent sequelae in surviving patients have only been reported in cases in which hyponatremia was sustained for more than two days before oxytocin was stopped (31, 32). As will be discussed later, these complications may well have been caused by the rapid correction of sustained hyponatremia rather than by the electrolyte disturbance itself.

Pathologic water drinking is fairly common in psychiatric patients and in some cases it can be complicated by severe symptomatic hyponatremia (1, 3, 18, 19, 35-43). In contrast to other causes of acute hyponatremia there is no female predominance. Though the precise onset and duration of hyponatremia is uncertain, a diagnosis of acute hyponatremia can usually be presumed (43). Frantic ingestion of gallons of water can lower the serum sodium concentration rapidly; however, if the urine is dilute (as it usually is), hyponatremia cannot persist for long. Once water intake is interrupted (by sleep or by a convulsion), a spontaneous water diuresis promptly restores a near-normal sodium concentration (1, 3, 36, 38, 40, 43). If patients with seizures and coma are still alive when they reach the hospital, the vast majority recover (1, 3, 35-40, 43). One series of 21 such patients (including seven women aged 31 to 49) all survived without sequelae (40). Fatalities with documented cerebral edema have been reported, however (18, 19, 41), and water intoxication may be responsible for a substantial number of unexplained deaths in psychiatric patients (42); nearly one half of the reported deaths have been men, and about half the women who died were over the age of fifty (35).

A recent report contrasted young female patients dying at serum sodium concentrations of 117 mmol/l with the benign course of male patients whose serum sodium concentrations had fallen to 102 mmol/l within a few hours of prostate surgery (44). This experience is misleading for two reasons. First, the women were selected from many different medical centers because of an adverse outcome (see above) while the males represented the experience of a single medical center. Second, the post-prostatectomy syndrome is not comparable to other causes of post-operative hyponatremia. During prostate surgery isosmolar but electrolyte-free irrigants containing glycine, mannitol or sorbitol may be absorbed systemically. Immediately after surgery, the absorbed solute is confined to the extracellular fluid causing dramatic hyponatremia but a normal plasma osmolality (1, 45).

Animal studies exploring the idea that females are particularly intolerant of hyponatremia have been inconclusive. Female rats have a lower brain content of Na-K ATPase than males (46, 47). However it is unclear how this finding would affect the adaptation to hyponatremia. While one study reported excessive mortality in female rats (without measurements of brain water) (46), two others have shown negligible and identical mortality rates in rats with severe hyponatremia (48, 49). Absolute brain water and solute contents were identical in both sexes with acute (48) or chronic hyponatremia (48, 49), though females did show a slightly greater change in water content and a smaller

62

loss of brain electrolyte relative to their normonatremic controls after three days of the electrolyte disturbance (49).

BRAIN INJURY AFTER RAPID CORRECTION OF CHRONIC HYPONATREMIA

Cerebral edema is mild in experimental animals with severe chronic hyponatremia (2, 11, 50). Likewise, CT scans of patients with profound, sustained hyponatremia show no evidence of brain swelling, including those who present with seizures or other severe neurologic symptoms (51-55). In general, the symptoms of chronic hyponatremia are more subtle, vague, and nonspecific than those of acute water intoxication and they tend to occur at lower serum sodium levels (1-3, 5, 43, 56). Typically, they include anorexia, nausea, emesis, muscular weakness and cramps. The patient may also become irritable and may show striking personality changes, becoming uncooperative, confused or hostile. With extremely low serum sodium concentrations, gait disturbances, stupor, tremulousness and, more rarely, seizures may occur. Chronic hyponatremia has not been known to cause herniation, even when the serum sodium concentration falls below 105 mmol/l (43). However, patients with prolonged hyponatremia are susceptible to iatrogenic complications when their electrolyte disturbance is corrected too rapidly.

RAPID CORRECTION, THE OSMOTIC DEMYELINATION SYNDROME, AND CENTRAL PONTINE MYELINOLYSIS (CPM)

As the serum sodium concentration returns to normal, solutes lost in the adaptation to hyponatremia must be recovered by the brain. Unless this process keeps pace with the rising serum sodium concentration, brain dehydration and injury may result (1-3, 11). For reasons that remain unclear, the clinical manifestations of this injury are delayed, evolving one to several days after treatment in a characteristic fashion that we have called the "osmotic demyelination syndrome" (9). In recent years, over a hundred cases with this clinical syndrome have been reported (1, 3). Most published reports have had pathologic or radiographic evidence of demyelination in the central pons, a finding known as "Central Pontine Myelinolysis" or "CPM" (9, 21, 51-55, 57-62). In the author's experience, confirmed cases of CPM represent a small minority of patients who suffer this injury (9, 43, 63).

In typical cases of the syndrome, hyponatremic symptoms improve during correction of the electrolyte abnormality, but improvement is followed within one to several days by gradual neurologic deterioration (9). A spectrum of neurologic findings distinct from the original hyponatremic symptoms can occur. Mild cases may be manifest by transient behavioral disturbances, seizures, movement disorders or akinetic mutism (1, 3, 43, 63). More severe cases develop clinical features of a pontine disorder (pseudobulbar palsy, quadriparesis and unresponsiveness) (9, 21, 51-55, 57, 59, 60, 62). In its most dramatic form, patients may be awake, but unable to move or communicate and may require ventilator support (9). Marked improvement can occur even after several weeks of severe disability, but some patients are left with significant permanent sequelae (1, 3, 9, 52, 53, 57).

In fatal cases, disruption of myelin with sparing of neurons and axons is usually found in the center of the basal pons - a pathologic finding known as "Central Pontine Myelinolysis" or "CPM"(1, 3, 8, 9, 51, 54, 55, 59-61). Often, histologically similar lesions are found in a symmetrical distribution in extrapontine areas of the brain in which there is a close admixture of grey and white matter (1, 3, 9, 51, 54, 59-61).

Magnetic resonance imaging (MRI) can often demonstrate areas of demyelination in patients who develop this syndrome (21, 53, 57, 58). Lesions appear as areas of hypointensity on T1-weighted images and hyperintensity on T2-weighted images. Pontine myelinolysis appears as an oval shape on saggital images, various shapes on axial images, and a bat-wing configuration on coronal images. Associated lesions are frequently present in the periventricular white matter, basal ganglia, thalamus, and corticomedullary junction bilaterally. Sometimes, the only demonstrable lesions are extrapontine (58). However, a normal MRI scan does not exclude the diagnosis, particularly if it is done too early in the course (57, 58, 61). Typically, no lesions can be documented until three to four weeks after the clinical onset and they may eventually resolve. Milder cases of the syndrome can easily escape detection by MRI.

Patients at greatest risk for the osmotic demyelination syndrome have been hyponatremic for more than two days, usually with very low serum sodium concentrations (105 mmol/l or less) (1, 3, 9, 43, 57). Larger increases in sodium concentration tend to be associated with more severe damage, and most patients with fatal disease have undergone correction by more than 20 mmol/l within one to two days. Almost invariably, correction has exceeded 12 mmol/l during any 24 hour period (1, 3, 9, 13). Alcoholism, severe liver disease and other debilitating illnesses appear to increase the susceptibility to osmotic demyelination, but they are not prerequisites for it (1, 3, 9, 62). Many cases have been reported in patients with no illness other than severe chronic hyponatremia (and its subsequent rapid correction) to explain their neurologic sequelae (1, 3, 9, 13, 51, 53, 57, 59, 61).

EXPERIMENTAL MODELS OF OSMOTIC DEMYELINATION

The osmotic demyelination syndrome has been reproduced in animal models of hyponatremia (2, 6, 7, 64-66). These studies confirm clinical observations suggesting that the syndrome is a complication of the treatment of hyponatremia rather than the electrolyte disturbance itself. The disorder does not develop in animals with uncorrected or slowly corrected hyponatremia. Indeed, rats have been maintained for weeks without morbidity or mortality despite serum sodium concentrations of 110 mmol/l or less (50, 64). However, rapid correction of the electrolyte disturbance in these animals causes seizures, coma, and a high mortality rate (64). As in the human disease, animals initially appear normal after correction of hyponatremia and subsequently deteriorate neurologically a day or two later (2, 6, 7, 64-66). Demyelinating lesions, histologically similar to the human disease are associated with the neurologic abnormalities. In the dog, these lesions have an anatomic distribution that almost exactly mimics CPM in humans (7).

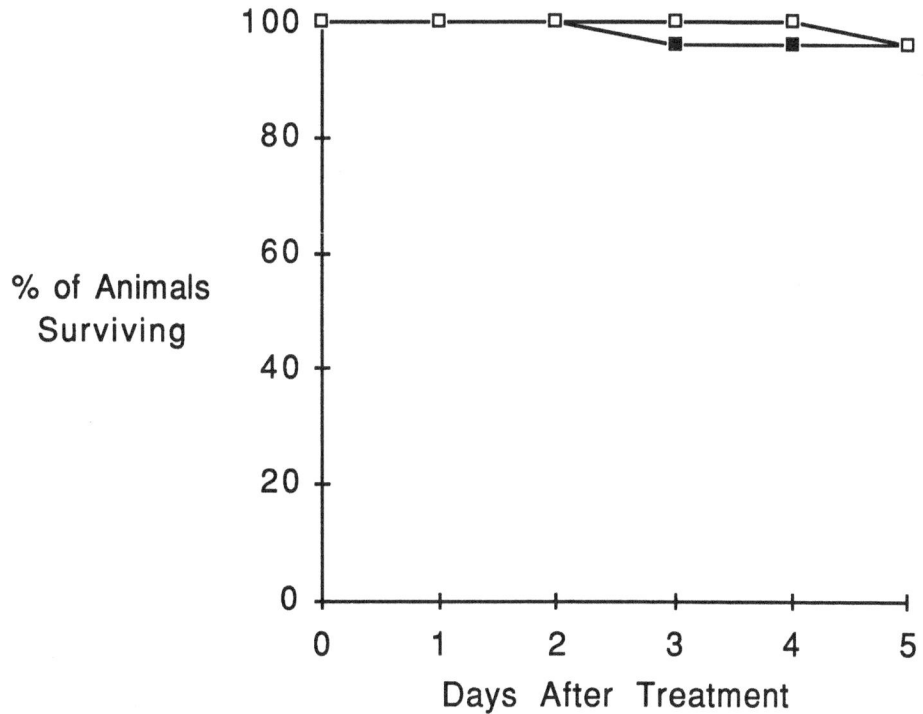

Figure 4. Effect of treatment on survival in rats with acute hyponatremia (serum sodium 95-106 mmol/l for 7-24 hours; n = 24 in both treatment groups). Solid squares represent rapid correction with hypertonic saline; open squares represent slow correction. [Data from Ref. 2. Reproduced from Sterns RH: The treatment of hyponatremia: First, do no harm. Am J Med, 88: 557-560,1990, with permission].

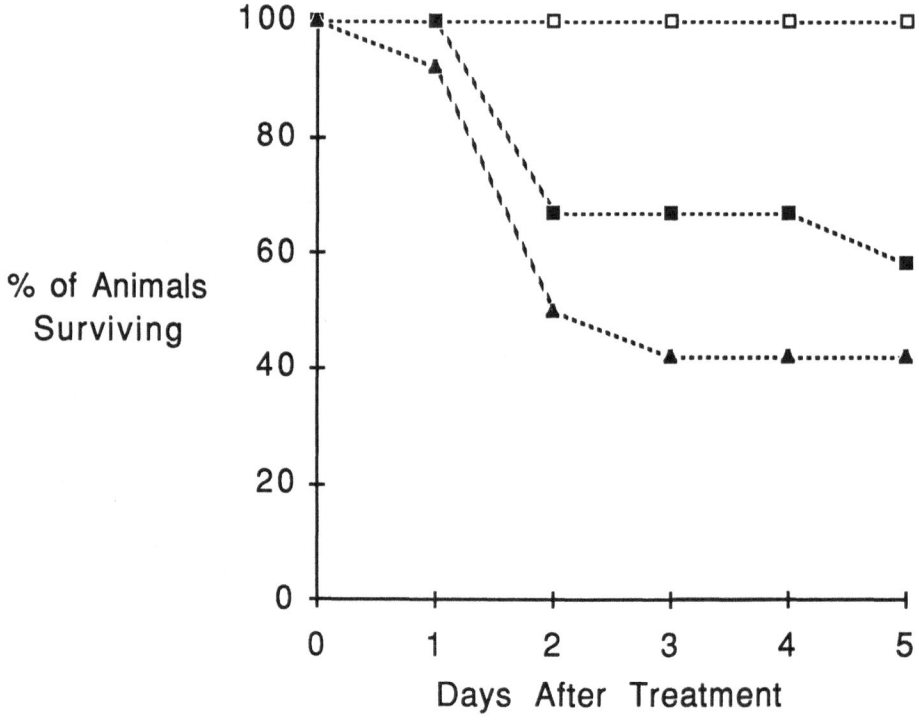

Figure 5. Effect of treatment on survival in rats with chronic hyponatremia (serum sodium 95 mmol/l for three days; n=12 in each treatment group). Solid squares represent rapid correction with hypertonic saline; closed triangles represent rapid correction induced by a water diuresis (withdrawl of DDAVP); open squares represent slow correction. [Data from Ref. 2. Reproduced from Sterns RH: The treatment of hyponatremia: First, do no harm. Am J Med, 88: 557-560,1990, with permission.]

The susceptibility to osmotic demyelination increases with the duration of hyponatremia prior to treatment. Animals that have been hyponatremic for 24 hours or less are relatively resistant to this injury (Figure 4) while lesions are easily produced after three days of hyponatremia (Figure 5) (2, 65, 66); they are most severe in animals undergoing large, rapid increases in sodium concentration. In the rat, the maximal rate of increase over any 4 hour period has been shown to be the most important variable in inducing myelinolysis; lesions begin to be observed when this rate exceeds 1.75 mmol/l/h and become increasingly frequent at higher rates of correction (64). The total increase over a 24 hour period also appears to be important in this species and lesions are most prevalent after correction by 25 mmol/l/day, though smaller increments achieved at a very rapid rate can also produce lesions (64). In the dog the "threshold" for causing the syndrome is approximately 15 mmol/l/day (7). If the initial serum sodium concentration is low enough, correction to the mildly hyponatremic range (120 to 130 mmol/l) can cause the disease in rats, rabbits and dogs (2, 7, 65).

A large, rapid increase in sodium concentration has been shown to cause brain dehydration in animals adapted to hyponatremia for three days (2, 11). The mechanism by which brain dehydration leads to demyelination is not yet understood. Preliminary data in our laboratory suggest that the initial injury may be a mechanical separation of the axon from its surrounding myelin sheath. Ultimately, oligodendrocytes, the cells that provide the sheath, become necrotic. In areas of the brain that are subject to pontine and extrapontine myelinolysis, the vast majority of oligodendrocytes are in close proximity to highly vascular gray matter; in other regions of the brain, these cells are spatially isolated from the circulation, possibly making them less vulnerable to osmotic stress (67).

OSMOTIC DEMYELINATION VS DELAYED POST-ANOXIC ENCEPHALOPATHY

The neurologic manifestations of the osmotic demyelination syndrome bear a superficial resemblance to delayed post-anoxic encephalopathy, a rare disorder which may follow prolonged, ischemic anoxic insults such as carbon monoxide poisoning and cardiopulmonary arrest (68). This has led some investigators to suggest that delayed neurologic deterioration following treatment of hyponatremia results from anoxia caused by cerebral edema and respiratory compromise (16, 20, 69).

The first paper proposing this hypothesis was one of the previously mentioned series of young women with hyponatremic seizures following surgery (16). After treatment with hypertonic saline had raised the serum sodium level above 128 mmol/l, seven of these patients regained consciousness to the point of being able to walk, eat and talk. However, after a mean lucid interval of 58 hours, a progressive clinical course began characterized by decreased alertness, increasing headache, nausea and progressive obtundation. This was followed by recurrence of grand mal seizures and a lapse back into coma. One patient died after two days (and was not autopsied), and the other six remained in a persistent vegetative state. Noting that CT scans failed to disclose evidence of CPM, the author argued that the course of these patients was most consistent with post-anoxic encephalopathy. There was, however, no actual evidence to confirm this suspected diagnosis.

Several features of these cases are consistent with the osmotic demyelination syndrome (61). Seizures first appeared in this group after hyponatremia had been present for two to five days (20), long enough to be classified as "chronic". After the seizures there was a long delay before therapy was initiated (on average 16 hours), allowing further time for adaptation. Hypertonic saline ultimately elevated the serum sodium from 105 ± 2 to 131 ± 1 mmol/l within 41 ± 7 hours after the seizures (16, 20). Because of the delay in therapy, the increase following hypertonic saline may have averaged 26 mmol/l in 25 hours, a rate that is typical for patients with documented severe CPM (69). The biphasic nature of the patients' neurologic symptoms (improvement followed by deterioration two to three days after rapid correction) is the same time course seen in patients with documented CPM, the majority of whom had only mild to moderate symptoms and no seizures before treatment of hyponatremia (9). Delayed post-anoxic encephalopathy typically has a much longer lucid interval (on average 22 days) (61, 62). Normal CT does not exclude a diagnosis of CPM because negative scans are routinely found in patients subsequently proven to have CPM by MRI or autopsy (1, 3, 9, 57, 58, 61).

It remains possible that anoxia may enhance the susceptibility to injury caused by rapid correction of chronic hyponatremia. A recent study found no increase in soluble oxidized proteins after three days of hyponatremia in the rat. However, within 24 hours after rapid correction with 1 M NaCl, there was evidence of protein peroxidation and myelinolysis. This finding suggests that a rapid rise in serum sodium after sustained hyponatremia could potentiate the oxidative stress of reoxygenation after a period of anoxia (70).

MALE VS FEMALE SUSCEPTIBILITY TO BRAIN DAMAGE IN CHRONIC HYPONATREMIA

Series identifying patients with severe chronic hyponatremia (with or without complications) have tended to have a female predominance (43). Diuretic-induced hyponatremia in particular is primarily a disorder of elderly women (43, 71). Chronic hyponatremia caused by diuretics is often corrected rapidly (9, 43); replacement of potassium deficits and recovery of diluting ability after the diuretic is stopped contribute to the increase in serum sodium concentration (1, 3). The lower body water content of elderly females also predisposes to a rapid rise in sodium concentration. Thus, not surprisingly, there have been a large number of cases of documented or probable CPM complicating thiazide-induced hyponatremia; as expected, most of the patients are women (21). However, men with diuretic-induced hyponatremia have developed CPM in rough proportion to the prevalence of the electrolyte disturbance in this sex (1, 3, 9).

Other causes of chronic hyponatremia have been complicated by CPM in approximately equal numbers of men and women (21). A recent survey of patients with serum sodium concentrations of 105 mmol/l or less found a similar incidence of neurologic sequelae in men and women, including women in their child-bearing years (48). No studies have yet explored the possibility that female sex or estrogens alter the susceptibility to experimental myelinolysis.

RAPID VS SLOW CORRECTION OF HYPONATREMIA

Two recent reviews of the literature have shown that when neurologic sequelae complicate chronic hyponatremia the rate of correction has almost invariably exceeded 12 mmol/l/day (9, 13). Therefore, this rate has been defined as the dividing point between rapid and slow correction. Others note that in most cases with severe complications the rate also exceeded 25 mmol/l in the first 48 hours and prefer to call this a "large magnitude" of correction rather than a rapid rate (21, 69).

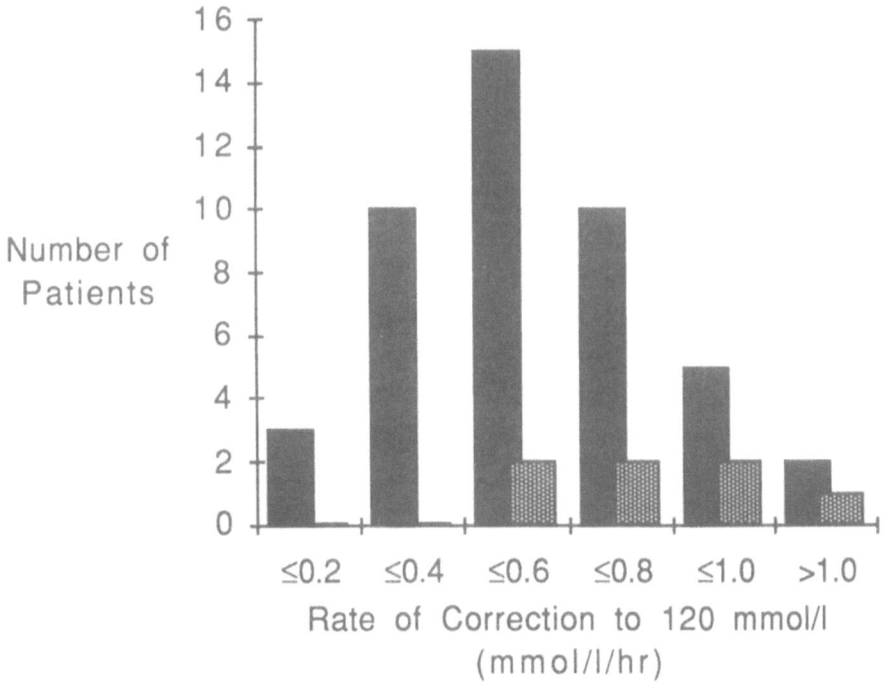

Figure 6. Incidence of delayed neurologic complications after correction of chronic hyponatremia in 54 patients with serum sodium concentrations ≤ 110 mmol/l. Patients corrected to a serum sodium of 120 mmol/l by < 0.55 mmol/l/hr had an uncomplicated recovery. Patients without complications represented by solid bars; patients with post-therapeutic neurologic complications represented by speckled bars. [Reproduced from Sterns RH: Severe symptomatic hyponatremia: treatment and outcome. A study of 64 cases. Ann Intern Med, 107: 656-664, 1987 with permission.]

The benignity of slow correction of severe chronic hyponatremia was demonstrated by a single medical center's experience with serum sodium concentrations of 110 mmol/l or less (43). Among the 64 patients seen with hyponatremia of this severity, the mortality rate was only 8% with all but one of the deaths attributable to severe underlying disease. Most of the patients seen had become hyponatremic at home, drinking conventional volumes of water. Recovery was uneventful in the 54 patients in this group (defined as "chronic") when the serum sodium was elevated to 120 mmol/l by less than 0.55 mmol/l/hr; more rapid rates were associated with an increasing incidence of the osmotic demyelination syndrome, including one fatal case of CPM (Figure 6).

These findings appear to conflict with those of a literature survey which concluded that correction of severe symptomatic hyponatremia by less than 0.7 mmol/l/hr (a rate defined by the authors as "slow") is associated with an extraordinarily high mortality rate (in excess of 60%) (72). The apparent paradox can be explained by the methodology of the review (3, 73). By calculating the correction rate from the time required to reach a sodium concentration of 128 to 130 mmol/l, patients with extremely low serum sodium concentrations who had been corrected by more than 18 mmol/l/day (and sometimes by more than 25 mmol/l in two days) were classified as victims of "slow" correction. None of the fatal cases cited in the review had been corrected by less than 12 mmol/l/day.

Also in support of "rapid" correction of hyponatremia, the same authors reported their personal experience with 33 patients seen in consultation for symptomatic hyponatremia (mean serum sodium was 108 ± 1 mmol/l, including three patients with post-prostatectomy syndrome). All patients were treated with hypertonic saline, increasing the serum sodium concentration by 18 ± 1 mmol/l at an average rate of 1.3 mmol/l/hr. The sodium level was then sustained in the mildly hyponatremic range so that 48 hours after the start of therapy, the absolute change in concentration was 21 ± 1 mmol/l. All of the patients recovered and none developed clinical or radiographic evidence of osmotic demyelination. The authors attributed the favorable outcome in their series to "judiciously rapid correction" in which the serum sodium level was increased to the mildly hyponatremic range while avoiding an increment of more than 25 mmol/l in the first two days of therapy. Ironically, applying these standards to a patient with a serum sodium concentration of less than 105 mmol/l would require "slow" correction using the definitions of their earlier literature review. Moreover as the maximum daily change in sodium concentration was as low as 10 mmol/l, the treatment given to at least some of these patients would be classified as "slow correction" using the 12 mmol/l/day criterion.

It is clear, however, that some patients tolerate extremely rapid correction of hyponatremia by any definition (1, 3, 9, 35, 43, 69). This is especially true of self-induced water intoxication in which correction is often attributable to a spontaneous water diuresis (1, 3, 9, 35, 43). Similarly, patients who have become hyponatremic in the hospital within 48 hours or less seem to tolerate a large, rapid increase in sodium concentration without incident (43). This experience is similar to the findings in experimental models: when hyponatremia is of brief duration, rapid correction is usually well tolerated, but in chronic hyponatremia, the same therapy sometimes leads to osmotic demyelination (2, 66).

THERAPEUTIC APPROACH TO HYPONATREMIA

In practice, the precise duration of hyponatremia is seldom known because most patients develop the electrolyte disturbance outside the hospital. Except for psychotic water drinkers, however, patients who become severely hyponatremic at home can be presumed to have a chronic condition. Even when the patient becomes hyponatremic in the hospital, the duration of the disturbance may be unclear if chemistry determinations have been infrequent. In most cases of uncertainty, it is best to assume that the case is chronic (i.e. of more than two days' duration).

When symptoms demand aggressive action and the duration of the condition is unknown, extreme care must be taken to assure that the amount of correction does not exceed the limits of safety (2, 73, 74). However fear of complications should not inhibit the use of hypertonic saline in the initial phases of therapy. An infusion of 1 to 2 ml/kg/hr of 3% saline will elevate the serum sodium concentration by 1 to 2 mmol/l/hr. This rate of correction appears to be safe, but it need not and should not continue for more than 2 to 4 hours, particularly if neurologic symptoms show some improvement.

A large increase in sodium concentration is not required to reduce cerebral edema in any patient. Because of the confines of the skull, the increase in brain water can never exceed approximately 10% and still be compatible with life. Thus, a 5 to 10% increase in sodium concentration (6 to 12 mmol/l) can be expected to virtually eliminate cerebral edema even in the most extreme case of acute hyponatremia. Clinical experience has shown that increases of this magnitude are effective (1, 3, 22, 25-29, 73, 74). In patients who present with mild to moderate symptoms, the rate of corrections should remain well below 0.5 mmol/l/hr throughout the entire duration of therapy, thereby ensuring that correction cannot exceed 12 mmol/l/day.

The clinician can take comfort from our knowledge of the brain's adaptations to severe hyponatremia. These adaptations are present to some extent in every patient we treat. Thus, it is never necessary to restore a normal serum sodium concentration rapidly.

Nor is it necessary to elevate the serum sodium to a preconceived "safe" level in the mildly hyponatremic range. Our therapeutic efforts should only attempt to supplement - not supplant - what nature has already provided.

REFERENCES

1. Sterns RH, Spital A: Disorders of water balance. In: "Fluids and Electrolytes" (Eds JP Kokko, RL Tannen), Saunders, Philadelphia, 1990, pp 139-194.
2. Sterns RH, Thomas DJ, Herndon RM: Brain dehydration and neurologic deterioration after rapid correction of hyponatremia. Kidney Int, 35: 69-75, 1989.
3. Sterns RH: The Management of symptomatic hyponatremia. Seminars in Nephrology, 10 (6): 503-514, 1990.
4. Ross EJ, Christie SBM: Hypernatremia. Medicine, 48: 441-473, 1969.
5. Arieff AI, Llach F, Massry SG: Neurologic manifestations and morbidity of hyponatremia: Correlation with brain water and electrolytes. Medicine, 55: 121-129, 1976.
6. Kleinschmidt-DeMasters BK, Norenberg MD: Rapid correction of hyponatremia causes demyelination: Relation to central pontine myelinolysis. Science, 211: 1068-1070, 1981.
7. Laureno R: Central pontine myelinolysis following rapid correction of hyponatremia. Ann Neurol, 13: 232-242, 1983.
8. Norenberg MD, Leslie KO, Robertson AS: Association between rise in serum sodium and central pontine myelinolysis. Ann Neurol, 40: 66-69, 1983.
9. Sterns RH, Riggs JE, Schochet SS Jr: Osmotic demyelination syndrome following correction of hyponatremia. N Engl J Med, 314: 1535-1542, 1986.
10. Lien YH, Shapiro JI, Chan L: Effects of hypernatremia on organic brain osmoles. J Clin Invest, 85: 1427, 1990.
11. Thurston JH, Hauhart RE, Nelson JS: Adaptive decreases in amino acids (taurine in particular) creatine, and electrolytes prevent cerebral edema in hyponatremic mice. Rapid correction (experimental model of central pontine myelinolysis) causes dehydration and shrinkage of brain. Metab Brain Dis, 2: 233-241, 1987.
12. Rowntree, LG: The effects on mamals of the administration of excessive quantities of water. J Pharmacol Exp Ther, 29: 135-159, 1926.
13. Cluitsman FHM, Meinders AE: Management of severe hyponatremia: rapid or slow correction? Am J Med, 88: 161-166, 1990.
14. Helwig FC, Schutz CB, Curry DE: Water intoxication. Report of a fatal human case, with pathologic and experimental studies. JAMA, 104: 1569-1575, 1935.
15. Fraser CL, Arieff AI: Fatal central diabetes mellitus and insipidus resulting from untreated hyponatremia: A new syndrome. Ann Intern Med, 112: 113-119, 1990.
16. Arieff AI: Hyponatremia, convulsions, respiratory arrest, and permanent brain damage after elective surgery in healthy women. N Engl J Med, 314: 1529-1535, 1986.
17. Anastassiades E., Wilson R, Stewart JSW, Perkin GD: Fatal brain oedema due to accidental water intoxication. Br Med J, 287: 1181-1182, 1983.
18. Raskind M: Psychosis, polydipsia, and water intoxication. Report of a fatal case. Arch Gen Psych, 30: 112-114, 1974.
19. Peh LH, Devan GS, Low BL: A fatal case of water intoxication in a schizophrenic patient. Br J Psych, 156: 891-894, 1990.
20. Arieff AI: Osmotic failure: Physiology and strategies for treatment. Hosp Pract, 23: 173-194, 1988.
21. Berl T: Treating hyponatremia: damned if we do and damned if we don't. Kidney Int, 37: 1006-1018, 1990.
22. Helwig FC, Schutz CB, Kuhn HP: Water intoxication. Moribund patient cured by administration of hypertonic salt solution. JAMA, 110: 644-645, 1938
23. Berginer VM, Osimani A, BerjinerJ, Barmeir E: CT brain scan in acute water intoxication. J Neurol Neurosurg Psychiatr, 48: 841-842,1985.
24. Kott E, Marcus Y: Acute brain edema due to water loading in a young woman. Eur Neurol, 24: 221-224, 1985.

25. Bartholomew LG, Scholz DA: Reversible post-operative neurological symptoms. Report of five cases secondary to water intoxication and sodium depletion. JAMA, 162: 22-26, 1956.

26. Scott JC Jr, Welch JS, Berman IB: Water intoxication and sodium depletion in surgical patients. Obstet Gynecol, 26: 168-175, 1965.

27. Wynn V, Rob CG: Water intoxication. Differential diagnosis of the hypotonic syndromes. Lancet I: 587-594, 1954.

28. Zimmerman B, Wagensteen OH: Observations on water intoxication in surgical patients. Surgery, 34: 654-669, 1952.

29. Ahmad AJ, Clark EH, Jacobs HS: Water intoxication associated with oxytocin infusion. Postgrad Med J, 51: 249-252, 1975.

30. Feeney JG: Water intoxication and oxytocin. Br Med J, 285: 243, 1982.

31. Lauersen NH, Birnbaum SJ: Water intoxication associated with oxytocin administration during saline-induced abortion. Am J Obstet Gynecol, 121: 2-6, 1975.

32. Morgan DB, Kirwan NA, Hancock KW, Robinson D, Howe JG, Ahmad S: Water intoxication and oxytocin infusion. Br J Obstet, 84: 6-12, 1977.

33. Gupta R, Coen NH: Oxytocin, "salting out", and water intoxication. JAMA, 220: 681-683, 1972.

34. Lillien A: Oxytocin-induced water intoxication. A report of a maternal death. Obstet Gynecol, 32: 171-173, 1968.

35. Cheng JC, Zikos D, Skopicki HA, Peterson DR, Fisher KA: Long-term neurologic outcome in psychogenic water drinkers with severe symptomatic hyponatremia: the effect of rapid correction. Am J Med, 88: 561-566, 1990.

36. Hariprasad MK, Eisinger RP, Nadler IM, Padmanabhan CS, Nidus BD: Arch Intern Med, 140: 1639-1642, 1980.

37. Jose CJ, Perez-Cruet J: Incidence and morbidity of self-induced water intoxication in state mental hospital patients. Am J Psychiatr, 136: 221-222, 1989.

38. Rosenbaum JF, Rothman JS, Murray GB: Psychosis and water intoxication. J Clin Psychiatr, 146: 127-131, 1985.

39. Singh S, Padi MH, Bullard H: Water intoxication in psychiatric patients. Am J Psychiatr, 137: 127-131, 1985.

40. Smith WO, Clark ML: Self-induced water intoxication in schizophrenic patients. Am J Psychiatr, 137: 1055-1060, 1980.

41. Rendell M, McGrane D, Cuesta M: Fatal compulsive water drinking. JAMA 240: 2557-2559, 1978.

42. Vieweg WVR, David JJ, Rowe WT, Wampler GJ, Burns WJ, Spradlin WW: Death from self-induced water intoxication among patients with schizophrenic disorders. J Nerv Mental Dis, 173: 161-165, 1985.

43. Sterns RH: Severe symptomatic hyponatremia: treatment and outcome. A study of 64 cases. Ann Intern Med, 107: 656-664, 1987.

44. Ayus JC, Krothapalli RK, Arieff AI: Sexual difference in survival with severe symptomatic hyponatremia. Kidney Int, 33: 180, 1988 (Abstract).

45. Rothenberg DM, Berns AS, Ivankovich AD: Isotonic hyponatremia following transurethral prostate resection. J Clin Anesth, 2: 48-49, 1990.

46. Fraser CL, Kuchareczyk J, Arieff AI, Rollin C, Sarnacki P, Norman D: Sex differences result in increased morbidity from hyponatremia in female rats. Am J Physiol, 256: R880-R885, 1989.

47. Fraser CL, Sarnacki P: Na$^+$-K$^+$ ATPase pump function in rat brain synaptosomes is different in males and females. Am J Physiol, 157: E284-E289, 1989.

48. Sterns RH, Silver S, Thomas D: Sexual equality in hyponatremia. Kidney Int, 37: 268, 1990 (Abstract).

49. Verbalis JG, Drutarosky MD: Sexual dimorphism of brain adaptation to chronic hyponatremia in rats. Kidney Int, 37: 269, 1990 (Abstract).

50. Verbalis JG, Drutarosky MD: Adaptation to chronic hypoosmolality in rats. Kidney Int, 34: 351-360, 1988.

51. Boon AP, Potter AE: Extensive extrapontine and central pontine myelinolysis associated with correction of profound hyponatremia. Neuropath Appl Neurobiol, 13: 1-9, 1987.

52. DaCunha C, Bertorini TE, Lawrence J, Witherington: Central pontine myelinolysis - a preventable condition. J Tenn Med Assoc, 79: 469-472, 1986.

53. Gerard E, Healy ME, Hesselink JR: MR demonstration of mesencephalic lesions in osmotic demyelination syndrome (central pontine myelinolysis). Neuroradiology, 29: 582-584, 1987.

54. Hazratji SMA, Kim RC, Lee SH, Marasigan AV: Evolution of pontine and extrapontine myelinolysis. J Comput Assist Tomoagr, 7(2): 356-361, 1983.

55. Walker JV, Englander RN: Central pontine myelinolysis following rapid correction of hyponatremia in an alcoholic. Am J Kidney Dis, 12: 531-533,1988.

56. Covey CM, Arieff AI: Disorders of sodium and water metabolism and their effects on the central nervous system. Advances in Nephrology, 13: 1-128, 1978.

57. Brunner JE, Redmond JM, Haggar AM, Kruger MSN, Elias S: Central pontine myelinolysis and pontine lesions after rapid correction of hyponatremia: a prospective magnetic imaging study. Ann Neurol, 27: 61-66, 1990.

58. Miller GM, Baker HL Jr, Okazaki H, Whisnant JP: Central pontine myelinolysis and its imitators: MR findings. Radiology, 168: 795-802, 1988.

59. Tomlinson BE, Pierides AM, Braddley WG: Central pontine myelinolysis. Q J Med, 45: 373-386, 1976.

60. Wright DG, Laureno R, Victor M: Pontine and extrapontine myelinolysis. Brain, 102: 361-385, 1989.

61. Clifford DB, Gado MH, Levy BK: Osmotic demyelination syndrome. Lack of pathologic and radiologic imaging correlation. Arch Neurol, 46: 343-347, 1989.

62. Laureno R, Karp BI: Pontine and extrapontine myelinolysis following rapid correction of hyponatremia. Lancet, I: 1439-1441, 1988.

63. Sterns RH: Neurologic deterioration following treatment for hyponatremia. Am J Kidney Dis, 13: 434-437, 1989.

64. Verbalis JG, Martinez J: Neurological and neuropathological sequelae of controlled correction of hypoosmolality in chronically hyponatremic rats. Kidney Int, 1991 (in press).

65. Illowsky BP, Laureno R: Encephalopathy and myelinolysis after rapid correction of hyponatremia. Brain, 110: 855-867, 1987.

66. Norenberg MD, Papendick RE: Chronicity of hyponatremia as a factor in experimental myelinolysis. Ann Neurol, 15: 544-547, 1984.

67. Riggs JE, Schochet SS: Osmotic stress, osmotic myelinolysis, and oligodendrocyte topography. Arch Pathol Lab Med, 113: 1386-1388, 1989.

68. Plum F, Posner JB, Hain RF: Delayed neurological deterioration after anoxia. Arch Intern Med, 110: 56-63, 1962.

69. Ayus JC, Krothapalli RK, Arieff AI: Treatment of symptomatic hyponatremia and its relation to brain damage. N Engl J Med, 317: 1190-1195, 1987.

70. Mickel HS, Oliver CN, Starke-Reed PE: Protein oxidation and myelinolysis occur in brain following rapid correction of hyponatremia. Biochemical & Biophysical Research Communications, 172 (1): 92-7, 1990.

71. Abramow M, Cogan E: Clinical aspects and pathophysiology of diuretic-induced hyponatremia. Advances in Nephrology, 13: 1-28, 1984.

72. Ayus JC, Krothapalli RK, Arieff: Changing concepts in the treatment of severe symptomatic hyponatremia. Rapid correction and possible relation to central pontine myelinolysis. Am J Med, 78: 897-902, 1985.

73. Sterns RH: The treatment of hyponatremia: First, do no harm. Am J Med, 88: 557-560, 1990.

74. Sterns RH: The management of hyponatremic emergencies. Critical Care Clinics, 7(1): 127-142, 1991.

Chapter 3

THE PHYSIOLOGIC BASIS FOR RENAL FUNCTIONAL RESERVE TESTING

Francis B. Gabbai, Luca De Nicola and Roland C. Blantz

Division of Nephrology-Hypertension, University of California, San Diego School of Medicine and Veterans Affairs Medical Center, La Jolla, California, 92093, USA

Early studies by Pitts demonstrated that protein intake (meat meal) or intravenous administration of amino acid (glycine) to dogs were associated with significant increases in glomerular filtration rate (GFR) and renal plasma flow (RPF) (1, 2). Variations in daily protein intake are also capable of modifying GFR and RPF in both man and experimental animals, with increments in GFR and RPF paralleling the increase in quantity of protein (1-3). Although the acute and chronic effects of protein loading on renal function have been established for nearly 50 years, it is not until recently that major interest has accumulated with respect to the potential role of protein in the progression of renal disease. Pioneer work by Hostetter et al (4) demonstrated in a model of radical subtotal nephrectomy in rats that increased protein intake was associated with hyperfiltration secondary to glomerular hypertension and hyperperfusion. Reducing protein intake in this experimental model decreased hyperfiltration and prevented albuminuria and glomerular sclerosis. Further studies in different experimental models, which include streptozotocin-induced diabetes mellitus, hypertension and partial renal ablation, confirmed previous findings by Hostetter et al and supported the concept that hyperfiltration may play an important role in the progression of kidney disease (5-7). The presence of hyperfiltration in experimental models led many investigators to evaluate the role of hyperfiltration as a mechanism for progression of renal disease in man. Normal pregnancy, early stages of insulin-dependent diabetes mellitus and sickle cell disease are a few clinical conditions associated with absolute increases in GFR (8-10). Since most patients with renal disease have normal or low values of GFR, it is impossible to detect the presence of hyperfiltration by evaluation of absolute GFR values under normal conditions. In order to detect maximum filtration capacity and therefore hyperfiltration in man, Bosch et al proposed in 1983 to measure renal functional reserve (RFR) (11-12). RFR has been defined as the

75

capacity of the kidney to increase RPF and GFR after a protein meal. Lack of an increase in GFR and RPF after protein intake defines maximum filtration capacity and suggests the presence of a hyperfiltering state. Detection of hyperfiltration in man would provide means to evaluate the role of this mechanism in the progression of renal disease as well as the potential beneficial effect of various therapeutic maneuvers. Although the concept that loss of RFR is equivalent to hyperfiltration is quite widely accepted, the significance and specificity of loss of RFR to these events have not been proven. Furthermore, very few experimental data have been obtained to understand the mechanism(s) responsible for the loss of RFR as well as the correlation between loss of RFR and progressive sclerosis.

This paper intends to review the changes in the determinants of the glomerular ultrafiltration process responsible for RFR, the different humoral and intrarenal mechanisms which mediate this response and finally the experience with both human and experimental animal using RFR as a diagnostic tool for determining hyperfiltration.

There remain several important issues that are pertinent and critical to our understanding of mechanisms of RFR and the potential clinical utility of testing RFR. These issues are as follows:

1. What is the normal mechanism which causes increases in GFR after protein or amino acid administration?
2. Does absence of RFR in various pathophysiologic conditions correlate with specific glomerular hemodynamic abnormalities?
3. Are there specific treatments which can restore the normal RFR?
4. Does absence of RFR constitute a valid predictor of risk factors for the progression of renal disease?

RENAL HEMODYNAMICS AND RENAL FUNCTIONAL RESERVE

Several experimental approaches have been utilized to elicit RFR. Oral protein load (OPL), intravenous infusion of mixed or single amino acid solutions and infusion of low dose dopamine have been used in patients and normal volunteers (11-15). Meat meals or milk derived proteins have been used as oral protein load (16-19). Dopamine infusion increases renal plasma flow and GFR; however, since changes in RPF are larger than GFR, filtration fraction (FF) decreases (15, 19, 20). Protein administration elevates both GFR and RPF in parallel with no changes in FF, except under conditions of very high protein intake in which large increases in GFR are associated with an increase in FF (14, 21-30). The absence of changes in FF with protein load compared to the decrease in FF associated with dopamine infusion has been interpreted as an evidence that dopamine and protein elicit RFR through different intrarenal mechanisms. The magnitude of increase in GFR in normal volunteers after i.v. infusion of amino acids or oral protein load (OPL) varies from study to study. A recent review of the literature by Rodríguez-Iturbe (31) demonstrates a range of increases in GFR between 6-40% with a mean increase of 26% after a protein meal and 24% after intravenous amino acid infusion. Differing baseline protein intakes, variable amounts of proteins in the OPL and variations in the salt intake as well as the experimental conditions during the test can certainly account for the big variability in the range of responses to the OPL found from study to study.

The timing of the response has also been variable from study to study. Although the initial observation from Bosch and coworkers noted a maximum increase in GFR 2.5 hrs after the protein intake, most studies using OPL have shown significant increases in GFR and RPF 60 to 180 minutes after protein intake (11, 19, 21, 26, 32, 33). Amino acid infusion elicits a faster GFR response than OPL with significant increases 30-60 minutes after initiation of the infusion although Ruilope and coworkers demonstrated an increase after 2 hours of infusion with a maximal response 6 hrs after initiation (13, 14, 23-25).

Renal plasma flow, transcapillary hydrostatic pressure gradient (ΔP), systemic oncotic pressure and ultrafiltration coefficient (LpA) constitute the four determinants of the glomerular filtration process. Clinical studies have clearly demonstrated that systemic oncotic pressure is not modified during OPL or amino acid infusion, ruling out a role for changes in oncotic pressure as an important determinant of the increase in GFR after protein administration (17, 21). The parallel increase in GFR and RPF certainly suggests an important role for changes in plasma flow. However, it is not possible, by examining changes in RPF alone, to conclude if this is the only determinant responsible for producing an increase in GFR. Under conditions of filtration pressure equilibrium, GFR is plasma flow dependent and increases in RPF could generate a parallel increase in GFR. Under filtration pressure disequilibrium, changes in GFR are not completely plasma flow dependent and increases in ΔP and/or LpA are necessary to increase GFR. Elegant studies by Chan and coworkers (34) using dextran sieving in normal volunteers have proposed that OPL increases GFR through an increase in both ΔP and RPF which overrides a decrease in LpA associated with protein intake.

Intravenous administration of amino acids increases GFR in various animal species. Interestingly, both the dog and the rat show a 25-30% increase in GFR when challenged with i.v. amino acids (35-39). Micropuncture measurements of the determinants of the glomerular ultrafiltration process have demonstrated that i.v. infusion of single (glycine) or mixed amino acids solution in the rat decreases both afferent and efferent resistances and

77

increases single nephron plasma flow (SNPF) and single nephron GFR (SNGFR). Both
ΔP and LpA remain constant (35-37). Similar findings have been demonstrated in the dog,
although the increase in SNGFR is the consequence of increases in both SNPF and ΔP.
The ultrafiltration coefficient was not modified (39).

Table 1.   Mechanisms responsible for increasing GFR with protein administration.

Humoral Mediators
    Growth hormone
    Glucagon
    Insulin-like growth factor 1
    Angiotensin II
    Atrial natriuretic factor
    Prostanoids: PGE_2, PGI_2
    Kinins
    Endothelial-derived relaxing factor (Nitric Oxide)

Tubuloglomerular feedback system

MECHANISMS RESPONSIBLE FOR INCREASING GFR WITH PROTEIN ADMINISTRATION

Table 1 depicts the different mechanisms that have been proposed to explain the
protein-induced kidney vasodilation. Both humoral factors (peptide hormones,
prostanoids, growth factors and more recently endothelial derived relaxing factors) as well
as resetting of the tubuloglomerular feedback system (TGF) have been invoked to explain
the increase in GFR after protein administration.

(1) Humoral factors

(A) GROWTH HORMONE (GH)

There are several clinical observations that constitute evidence that GH plays an
important role in the increase in GFR after protein administration. Protein administration
and more importantly intravenous administration of amino acids (particularly arginine and
glycine) lead to important increases in GH secretion (13). Acromegaly, a disease
characterized by increased GH levels, is associated with elevated GFR and renal
hypertrophy (40). Administration of GH for a period of one week leads to increases in
GFR in normal individuals (41). Patients with panhypopituitarism or GH deficiency do
not increase their GFR after OPL or intravenous amino acid infusion (42, 43).

78

Somatostatin administration which blocks the secretion of several hormones including GH prevents the normal increase in GFR during amino acid infusion in normal individuals (23, 24, 44). Although all of these data would suggest that GH plays a major role in the renal response to proteins, there are important findings which speak against this possibility. There is an important temporal dissociation between the peak increase in GFR and GH after protein or amino acid administration (13, 45, 46). The temporal dissociation as well as the fact that acute GH administration does not increase GFR have suggested that GH does not play an important role in the acute response to protein loading but rather constitutes a more chronic permissive effect (47-49).

(B) GLUCAGON

Protein intake stimulates pancreatic secretion of glucagon (50). Intravenous administration of glucagon produces kidney vasodilation and increases GFR by about 6%. A similar increase in GFR to that observed after a protein meal can be obtained with glucagon administration although the plasma levels of glucagon must be increased several fold higher than the values obtained with a protein meal and i.v. amino acid infusion (51). Interestingly, infusion of glucagon into the portal vein elicits an increase in GFR that cannot be obtained with similar systemic infusion of glucagon (52). These findings have led several investigators to propose the presence of a hepatic factor capable of modifying renal function (53). More recently, Alverstrand and Bergstrom (54) further identified glomerulopressin and demonstrated that glomerulopressin is in fact identical to serotonin. Further studies are necessary to evaluate the potential role of serotonin in the renal response to proteins.

(C) ANGIOTENSIN II (AII)

It is well established that AII plays a very important role in the control of renal circulation. The evidence accumulated suggests that activation of AII (i.e. salt depletion) prevents the increase in GFR after protein administration in normal individuals (14). Measurements of plasma renin activity and AII during protein administration have not demonstrated any specific pattern with increased or normal values associated with protein administration (28, 29). Converting enzyme inhibitors (CEI) restore the response to proteins in some pathophysiologic conditions (14, 55), do not modify or increase the response (28, 55, 56) and sometimes decrease the response in normal individuals (57). Although these findings are difficult to interpret, it seems that AII plays an important role in preventing a normal response rather than directly participating in the normal increase in GFR under normal conditions.

(D) INSULIN-LIKE GROWTH FACTOR 1 (IGF-1)

The correlation between increases in GFR and RPF and IGF-1 level in a patient with GH deficiency raised the possibility that IGF-1 plays an important role in the renal response to proteins (47). Subsequent studies have demonstrated that acute intravenous administration of IGF-1 to starved and to normal rats increases GFR and RPF (58, 59). Recent studies in two healthy human subjects have also demonstrated that intravenous administration of IGF-1 increases RPF and GFR (60). A very provocative explanation for the mechanism by which increases in IGF-1 could lead to renal vasodilation has been proposed by Haylor and coworkers (61). These investigators have demonstrated that blocking nitric oxide synthesis inhibits the vasodilatory response to IGF-1, suggesting that endothelial IGF-1 receptor stimulation produce vasodilation through increases in nitric oxide production.

(E) ATRIAL NATRIURETIC FACTOR (ANF)

Studies in the literature agree that plasma ANF level are not significantly modified by protein administration (28). When increases in plasma ANF have been observed, the plasma level is well below the level required to increase GFR with ANF (62).

(F) PROSTANOIDS

Both prostaglandin E_2 (PGE$_2$) and 6-keto-PGF$_{1\alpha}$ (the active metabolite of PGI$_2$) have been measured in the urine with rather disappointing results since several investigators have not been able to detect any changes during protein administration (17, 21, 27-29, 63, 64). Blocking prostaglandin synthesis with non steroidal anti-inflammatory drugs (NSAID) has also been used to evaluate the role of prostaglandins in the renal response to proteins. The results obtained using NSAID are similar to those obtained with direct measurements of urinary prostaglandins with some authors demonstrating total or partial loss of RFR with NSAID while others demonstrating normal RFR under NSAID treatment (14, 27, 33, 65). Although these findings do not permit specific conclusions regarding the role of PG in the renal response to proteins, they certainly reaffirm the importance of a "standardized protocol" in evaluating RFR as well as the impact of the baseline physiologic conditions (sodium intake, protein intake, etc).

(G) ENDOTHELIAL-DERIVED RELAXING FACTORS (EDRF)

Recent studies have increased our awareness of the role of EDRF in the maintenance of vascular tone. Elegant studies by Moncada's group have demonstrated that the endothelium generates nitric oxide from L-arginine which increases soluble cGMP and produces vasodilation (66). Nitric oxide production has now been recognized in multiple tissues; at the kidney level nitric oxide is produced by the endothelium, mesangial cells and renal epithelial cells (67). The importance of nitric oxide in the renal response to proteins was clearly demonstrated by the studies of King and coworkers (68) in which blocking nitric oxide production with N^G monomethyl-l-arginine (L-NMMA) significantly decreased the renal vasodilation associated with intravenous amino acid infusion. Interestingly, adding amino acids to the perfusate in the isolated perfused kidney produces vasodilation and increases GFR according to Baines et al (69). Adding inhibitors of nitric oxide synthesis to the perfusate significantly decreases GFR and RPF demonstrating that nitric oxide generation is critical to maintain renal vasodilation and perfusion in the isolated perfused kidney preparation (70). These data strongly suggest that increases in nitric oxide production associated with amino acid infusion may be responsible for the renal vasodilatory response after protein administration.

Measuring nitric oxide production is extremely difficult due to its lability. Since nitric oxide stimulates soluble cGMP, various investigators have utilized cGMP production as an index of nitric oxide production. When cGMP is measured as an index of nitric oxide production, several studies in the literature point to nitric oxide as an important mediator of protein induced increases in GFR. Administration of high protein diet to rats for a period of 2 weeks increases GFR and glomerular cGMP production (71). The increase in glomerular cGMP can be suppressed with L-NMMA implying that high protein feeding increases nitric oxide production. A meat meal increases urinary cGMP in humans providing further evidence that nitric oxide constitutes a mediator of the renal vasodilation associated with protein feeding (21).

(H) KININS

Experimental observations suggest that the renal kallikrein-kinin system is also involved in the renal vasodilation induced by protein administration. Bolin and coworkers

(72) demonstrated that in humans acute (oral protein load) or chronic administration of high protein diet increases GFR during a similar time frame that increases in kinin urinary excretion are detected. Administration of a bradykinin antagonist to rats blocks the vasodilatory response to amino acid infusion (73). Since bradykinin induces vasodilation through nitric oxide production, it is intriguing to postulate that the kallikrein-kinin system constitutes another mediator for renal vasodilation after protein administration which acts through the same common pathway of nitric oxide.

(2) Role of the tubuloglomerular feedback (TGF) system

TGF plays a very important role in maintaining the relation of filtration and reabsorption by matching distal tubular NaCl delivery to SNGFR. Increased distal sodium delivery activates TGF which increases afferent resistance thereby decreasing nephron plasma flow, ΔP and SNGFR. In contrast, decreased distal sodium chloride delivery deactivates TGF producing afferent vasodilation and increased plasma flow, ΔP and SNGFR.

The fact that TGF maintains such a tight link between distal tubular delivery and glomerular filtration rate is difficult to accommodate with a 20-30 % increase in GFR after protein administration unless TGF activity is suppressed or reset at a different level after protein administration.

Resetting of the TGF could be achieved through different mechanisms. One such mechanism would be an increase in proximal tubular transport rates leading to a decrease in distal delivery and deactivation of TGF. Deactivation should allow GFR to increase until this increase in GFR compensates for the increase in proximal tubular transport and distal delivery would be restored to values present before the increase in proximal tubular reabsorption. At this time TGF would be operating in a normal manner except that the adjusted SNGFR or GFR would be significantly higher than the baseline GFR. Another explanation for resetting of TGF would be that the increase in GFR and distal delivery do not modify afferent resistance due to a specific effect of the experimental maneuver on either the sensor or the effector limb of the TGF system.

Studies by Woods and coworkers (38) in the dog demonstrated that intravenous infusion of amino acids was associated with a significant increase in the proximal tubular transport as indexed by lithium clearance. This increase in proximal tubular transport mediated by the sodium amino acid co-transport system is responsible for decreasing distal tubular delivery, deactivating TGF and increasing GFR.

Maneuvers capable of suppressing TGF activity were associated with lack of response to amino acids in the studies of Woods et al (38) suggesting a critical role for TGF in the renal response to amino acids. More recently, Brown and Navar (39) have examined the role of TGF during amino acid infusion in the dog with two different experimental maneuvers: blocking distal delivery with a wax block in the late proximal tubule and lowering renal perfusion pressure to minimize TGF activity. None of the two experimental maneuvers prevented the increase in SNGFR during amino acids infusion suggesting to these investigators that TGF is not a major contributor to renal vasodilation during amino acid load.

We have recently evaluated proximal tubular reabsorption during glycine infusion in normal rats, streptozotocin-induced diabetic rats and rats with renovascular hypertension (74, 75). During glycine administration, normal rats showed a significant increase in SNGFR with no changes in fractional reabsorption. In contrast, in both diabetic and hypertensive rats glycine did not modify SNGFR but significantly decreased fractional reabsorption. Administration of converting enzyme inhibitors restored both the glomerular and tubular response to glycine to normal. TGF may not be critical for a normal response to proteins but the presence of abnormal proximal tubular function in pathophysiologic situation may be responsible for activating TGF during glycine and limiting the normal response to proteins.

The role of TGF has also been evaluated in humans during amino acid infusion as well as during oral protein load. As is the case in experimental animals, certain studies support a major role of TGF in the response to protein while others provide contradictory evidence. In support of TGF, several investigators have demonstrated that during amino acid infusion there is no increase in urinary sodium excretion in spite of increased GFR suggesting perfect glomerulotubular balance (14, 64, 65). Using lithium clearance, Claris Appiani and coworkers (76) have demonstrated an increase in proximal tubular reabsorption during amino acid infusion. However, other investigators have not confirmed the increase in proximal tubular reabsorption during protein administration and some have shown significant increases in urinary sodium excretion, although this increase in urinary sodium excretion could be due to decreased tubular transport beyond the distal tubule as suggested by Claris Appiani (13, 24, 26, 28, 29, 63, 76).

In summary it seems that both humoral mediators and resetting of the TGF are necessary requirements for a normal response to proteins. If these two phenomena are directly linked or independent mechanisms await further experimental evidence.

Table 2. Evaluation of renal functional reserve (RFR) under different pathophysiologic conditions

Pathology	CH	Baseline GFR (ml/min)	% Change after CH	Tx	GFR during Tx Pre-Post CH	References
Single Kidney	OPL	80-120	48% (0-150%)			77, 78, 80, 81, 82, 84
	OPL	50-79	46% (18-75%)			12, 77, 82, 85
	DOP	75	2.4% (0-4.8%)			25, 83
	AA	64	11%			25
Chronic Renal Disease	OPL	110-140	6.5% (3-13%)			12, 86
	OPL	70-110	25% (14-45%)			12, 34, 85, 86
	OPL	30-70	23% (0-57%)	CEI	31-37	87, 88
	OPL	<30	21%			88
	AA, D, AA + D	13-115	1-9%			20
Essential Hypertension	OPL	97	0%			90
	OPL	92	0%	M, ßblock, CEI	76-90	32
	OPL	91	18%	CEI	85-112	91
	OPL	74	39%			90
	OPL	60	23%	Nif, Diu	82-80	89
	AA	84	32%	Low salt diet	73-77	55
				Low salt diet + CEI	92-107	55
Tx kidney	AA	79	20%			92
	AA	58-65	0%			24, 92
	OPL	64	0%	CEI	49-58	93
IDDM	OPL	137	0%	Low protein diet	92-129	96
IDDM	OPL	104-125	30% (8-59%)			44, 94, 95
IDDM	AA	165	0%	CEI	148-148	97
IDDM	AA	118	23%	CEI	110-170	56
IDDM	AA	110	17%	CEI	130-130	97
IDDM	AA	102	52%	Insulin	94-141	98
NIDDM	AA	143	43%	Insulin	115-124	99

CH = challenge; Tx = therapy; OPL = oral protein load; AA = amino acid infusion; Dop = dopamine; CEI = converting enzyme inhibitors; % change represents the mean of the values reported in the literature. Shown in parentheses are the range of the responses.
M = minoxidil; ßblock = betablocker; Nif = nifedipine; Diu = diuretics; IDDM = insulin dependent diabetes mellitus; NIDDM = noninsulin dependent diabetes mellitus.

RENAL FUNCTIONAL RESERVE IN PATHOPHYSIOLOGIC CONDITIONS

As depicted in Table 2, RFR has been evaluated in a variety of conditions which include solitary kidney, renal transplant, diabetes mellitus, chronic renal failure, essential hypertension and liver disease. RFR has been examined both in adults as well as children, either normal or with chronic renal failure.

Close analysis of the data in this Table demonstrates that:

- In each of these pathophysiologic conditions, the results generated by individual investigators vary importantly and sometimes are contradictory, with presence or absence of RFR observed in patients with the same type of disease and same baseline GFR.

- There is no consistent pattern of progressive loss of RFR as baseline GFR decreases. Although one would predict that as nephron mass decreases, functioning nephrons should progressively exhibit hyperfiltration and therefore absence of a response to proteins, some authors have demonstrated that patients with GFR of 11-30 ml/min still respond with a 21% increase in GFR after oral protein load (OPL).

- There is no consensus regarding the effect of therapeutic maneuvers, since, for example, under certain circumstances, administration of converting enzyme inhibitors restores RFR, while in others administration of the same agent produces loss of RFR.

Why is there so much discrepancy in the literature with respect to the RFR? As we have previously described, it appears that the lack of a standard protocol constitutes a major reason for many of the discrepancies. Patients are evaluated under different conditions, criteria for interpretation of the results vary from author to author (time after response, maximum response, area under the curve, expression of results as percentage of baseline or absolute values) and types and quantities of protein (OPL vs amino acid infusion, meat meal vs milk products) also vary among investigations.

DOES LOSS OF RENAL FUNCTIONAL RESERVE SIGNIFY THE PRESENCE OF HYPERFILTRATION? EXPERIMENTAL DATA

The concept that loss of RFR is equivalent to the presence of hyperfiltration is widely accepted and has led to numerous clinical studies; but very few experimental studies have analyzed the changes in glomerular hemodynamics associated with loss of RFR.

Since elevated ΔP has been proposed as the major risk factor by which hyperfiltration leads to progression of renal disease, does loss of RFR correlate with glomerular hypertension? Table 3 presents a summary of the data available in the literature. Normal rats (male and female) with normal ΔP increase GFR and SNGFR during intravenous administration of amino acids (35-37). Female rats with normal ΔP but increased GFR and SNGFR due to pregnancy demonstrate further increases in GFR during glycine infusion (36). However, when increased GFR and SNGFR are associated

85

with glomerular hypertension as in the two kidney one clip model or in rats with hypertension and renal ablation, there is a lack of response to glycine infusion, defining loss of RFR (37, 101).

Table 3. Correlation between values of ΔP and presence or absence of renal functional reserve (RFR) (as indexed by % change in SNGFR during amino acid infusion) in different rat experimental models.

Experimental model	ΔP	RFR	Reference
Male Munich-Wistar	N	+ 46%	35
Female Munich-Wistar	N	+ 25%	36
Pregnant Munich-Wistar	N	+ 36%	36
Male Wistar rats	N	+ 75%	37
2K-1C	H	+ 6%	37
SHR (Normotensive)	H?	+ 7%	100
(Hypertensive)	H	0%	
Renal ablation (Normotensive)	N	+ 34%	101
(Hypertensive)	H	0%	
Renal ablation (Normotensive after unclipping)	N	+ 83%	102
2K-1C	H	- 10%	74
2K-1C + CEI	N	+ 15%	74
2K-1C + verapamil	N	- 8%	74
Diabetes Mellitus	N	0%	75
Diabetes Mellitus + CEI	N	+ 43%	75

H = increased ΔP; N = normal ΔP; 2K-1C = Two kidney one clip Goldblatt hypertension model; CEI = converting enzyme inhibitor.

Interestingly, in the model of hypertension and renal ablation the loss of RFR is present prior to the development of important histologic damage which is clearly present 60 days after induction of the experimental model (103). Lowering systemic blood pressure by relieving renal artery stenosis in rats with renal ablation and hypertension normalized ΔP and SNGFR and restored the RFR (102). Spontaneously hypertensive rats also demonstrate loss of RFR; however interpretation of the presence or absence of glomerular hypertension is difficult due to lack of appropriate comparisons to non hypertensive rats in a recent study by Baylis (100). Although the previous data would support the correlation between loss of RFR and glomerular hypertension, we have recently been able to dissociate these two alterations. In two different experimental models (two kidney one clip Goldblatt hypertension treated with verapamil and early stages of poorly controlled experimental diabetes mellitus) we have shown loss of RFR in the presence of normal ΔP (74, 75). These data suggest therefore that although glomerular hypertension is often associated with loss of RFR, one cannot predict the presence of glomerular hypertension by simply examining RFR. There is very little information with respect to the effect of different therapeutic maneuvers on RFR; however, based on our recent studies it would appear that converting enzyme inhibitors can restore the response both in hypertension and experimental diabetes (74, 75).

FUTURE PERSPECTIVES ON THE USE OF RFR

It is very clear that the concept of RFR has stimulated significant interest in the mechanism(s) by which protein administration induces renal vasodilation and significant progress has been made. However the correlation between presence or absence or RFR and its link to progression of renal disease remains unclear.

Based on the findings in both humans and experimental animals it is difficult to demonstrate clearly that loss of RFR is equivalent to hyperfiltration and/or glomerular hypertension. The impact of loss of RFR on kidney function and progression of renal disease has not as yet been addressed. There are no studies on the longterm outcome of renal function in patients or experimental animals exhibiting loss of RFR. The fact that loss of RFR does not always correlate with glomerular hypertension does not invalidate the concept that RFR may represent a marker or a prognostic index of intrarenal conditions favoring progression of renal disease.

ACKNOWLEDGEMENTS

This work was supported by grants from the National Institutes of Health (DK28602), Grant-in-Aid from the American Heart Association, Santa Clara County Chapter and from funds supplied by the Research Service of the Department of Veterans Affairs. We thank Helene Lojwaniuk for secretarial assistance in the preparation of this manuscript.

REFERENCES

1. Pitts RF: The effect of protein and amino acid metabolism on the urea and xylose clearance. J Nutrition, 9: 645-666, 1935.
2. Pitts RF: The effects of infusing glycine and of varying the dietary protein intake on renal hemodynamics in the dog. Am J Physiol, 142: 355-365, 1944.
3. Pullman TN, Alving AS, Dern RJ, Landowne M: The influence of dietary protein on specific renal functions in normal man. J Lab Clin Med, 44: 320-332, 1954.
4. Hostetter TH, Olson JL, Rennke HG, Venkatachalam MA, Brenner BM: Hyperfiltration in remnant nephrons: A potentially adverse reaction to renal ablation. Am J Physiol, 241: F85-F93, 1981.
5. Anderson S, Meyer TW, Rennke HG, Brenner BM: Control of glomerular hypertension limits glomerular injury in rats with reduced renal mass. J Clin Invest, 76: 612-619, 1985.
6. Dworkin LD, Hostetter TH, Rennke HG, Brenner BM: Hemodynamic basis for glomerular injury in rats with desoxycorticosterone-salt hypertension. J Clin Invest, 73: 1448-1461, 1984.

7. Zatz R, Meyer TW, Rennke HG, Brenner BM: Predominance of hemodynamic rather than metabolic factors in the pathogenesis of diabetic glomerulopathy. Proc Natl Acad Sci USA, 82: 5963-5967, 1985.
8. Lindheimer MD, Katz AI: The kidney and hypertension in pregnancy. In: "The kidney" (Ed BM Brenner, FC Rector), WB Saunders, Philadelphia, 1991, pp 1551-1595.
9. Hostetter TH: Diabetic nephropathy. In: "The kidney" (Ed BM Brenner, FC Rector), WB Saunders, Philadelphia, 1991, pp 1695-1727.
10. Diederich D: The kidney and sickle cell disease. In: "The principles and practice of nephrology" (Ed HR Jacobson, GE Striker, S Klahr), BC Decker Inc, Philadelphia, Hamilton, 1991, pp 382-387.
11. Bosch JP, Saccaggi A, Lauer A, Ronco C, Belledonne M, Labman S: Renal functional reserve in humans. Effect of protein intake on glomerular filtration rate. Am J Med, 75: 943-950, 1983.
12. Bosch JP, Lauer A, Glabman S: Short-term protein loading in assessment of patients with renal disease. Am J Med, 77: 873-879, 1984.
13. Hirschberg R, Kopple JD: Role of growth hormone in the amino™acid-induced acute rise in renal function in man. Kidney Int, 32: 382-387, 1987.
14. Ruilope LM, Rodicio J, Garcia Robles R, Sancho J, Miranda B, Granger JP, Romero JC: Influence of a low sodium diet on the renal response to amino acid infusions in humans. Kidney Int, 31: 992-999, 1987.
15. ter Wee PM, Smit AJ, Rosman JB, Sluiter WJ, Donker AJM: Effect of intravenous infusion of low-dose dopamine on renal function in normal individuals and in patients with renal disease. Am J Nephrol, 6: 42-46, 1986.
16. Dhaene M, Sabot JP, Philippart Y, Doutrelepont JM, Vanherweghem JL: Effects of acute protein loads of different sources on glomerular filtration rate. Kidney Int, 32 (suppl 22): S25-S28, 1987.
17. Kontessis P, Jones S, Dodds R, Trevisan R, Nosadini R, Fioretto P, Borsato M, Sacerdoti D, Viberti GC: Renal, metabolic and hormonal responses to ingestion of animal and vegetable proteins. Kidney Int, 38: 136-144, 1990.
18. Jones MG, Lee K, Swaminathan R: The effect of dietary protein on glomerular filtratiom rate in normal subjects. Clin Nephrol, 27: 71-75, 1987.
19. Mansy H, Patel D, Tapson JS, Fernandez J, Tapster S, Torrance AD, Wilkinson R: Four methods to recruit renal functional reserve. Nephrol Dial Transplant, 2: 228-232, 1987.
20. ter Wee PM, Rosman JB, van der Geest S, Sluiter WJ, Donker AJM: Renal haemodynamics during separate and combined infusion of amino acids and dopamine. Kidney Int, 29: 870-874, 1986.
21. Hostetter TH: Human renal response to a meat meal. Am J Physiol, 250: F613-F618, 1986.
22. Castellino P, DeFronzo RA: Effect of plasma amino acid and hormone concentrations on renal plasma flow and glomerular filtration rate. Blood Purification, 6: 240-249, 1988.
23. Castellino P, Giordano C, Perna A, DeFronzo RA: Effects of plasma amino acids and hormone levels on renal hemodynamics in humans. Am J Physiol, 255: F444-F449, 1988.
24. Castellino P, Coda B, DeFronzo RA: Effect of amino acid infusion on renal hemodynamics in humans. Am J Physiol, 251: F132-F140, 1986.
25. ter Wee PM, Geerlings W, Rosman JB, Sluiter WJ, van der Geest S, Donker AbJM: Testing renal reserve filtration capacity with an amino acid solution. Nephron, 41: 193-199, 1985.
26. Viberti G, Bognetti E, Wiseman MJ, Dodds R, Gross JL, Keen H: Effect of protein-restricted diet on renal response to a meat meal in humans. Am J Physiol, 253: F388-F393, 1987.
27. Hirschberg RR, Zipser RD, Slomowitz LA, Kopple JD: Glucagon and prostaglandins are mediators of amino acid-induced rise in renal hemodynamics. Kidney Int, 33: 1147-1155, 1988.
28. Krishna GG, Newell G, Miller E, Heeger P, Smith R, Polansky M, Kapoor S, Hoeldtke R: Protein-induced glomerular hyperfiltration: Role of hormone factors. Kidney Int, 33: 578-583, 1988.
29. Swainson CP, Walker RJ: Renal Haemodynamic and hormonal responses to a mixed high-protein meal in normal men. Nephrol Dial Transplant 4: 683-690, 1989.
30. Rodríguez-Iturbe B, Herrera J, García R: Relationship between glomerular filtration rate and renal blood flow at different levels of protein induced hyperfiltration in man. Clin Sci, 74: 11-15, 1988.
31. Rodríguez-Iturbe B: The renal response to an acute protein load in man: Clinical perspective. Nephrol Dial Transplant, 5: 1-9, 1990.
32. Gabbai F, Herrera-Acosta J: Es la lesion renal por hypertension realmente isquemica? Arch Inst Cardiol Mex, 56: 81-87, 1986.
33. Herrera-Acosta J, Reyes P, Manay GL, Perez-Grovas H: La inhibición de la síntesis de prostaglandinas suprime la reserva functional renal en pacientes con nefropatía lúpica. Rev Invest Clin, 39: 107-114, 1987.

34. Chan AYM, Cheng MLL, Keil LC, Myers BD: Functional response of healthy and diseased glomeruli to a large, protein rich meal. J Clin Invest, 81: 245-254, 1988.

35. Meyer TW, Ichikawa I, Zatz R, Brenner BM: The renal hemodynamic response to amino acid infusion in the rat. Trans Assoc Am Phys, 96: 76-83, 1983.

36. Baylis C: Effect of amino acid infusion as an index of renal vasodilatory capacity in pregnant rats. Am J Physiol, 254: F650-F656, 1988.

37. Gabbai FB, Tapia E, Cermeño JL, Romero L, Bobadilla N, Alvarado JA, Herrera-Acosta J: Evaluation of renal functional reserve of contralateral kidney of two kidney, one clip Goldblatt hypertensive rats. J Hypertension, 4 (suppl 5): S279-S281, 1986.

38. Woods LL, Mizelle HL, Montani J, Hall J: Mechanisms controlling renal hemodynamics and electrolyte excretion during amino acids. Am J Physiol, 252: F303-F312, 1986.

39. Brown SA, Navar LG: Single nephron responses to systemic administration of amino acids in dogs. Am J Physiol, 259: F739-F746, 1990.

40. Ikkos D, Ljunggren R, Luft R: Glomerular filtration and renal plasma flow in acromegaly. Acta Endocrinol, 21: 226-236,1957.

41. Christiansen JS, Gammelgaard J, Orskov H, Andersen AR, Telmer S, Parving HH: Kidney function and size in normal subjects before and during growth hormone administration for one week. Eur J Clin Invest, 11: 487-490, 1962.

42. Kleinman KS, Glassock RJ: Glomerular filtration rate fails to increase following protein ingestion in hypothalamo-hypophyseal-deficient adults. Am J Nephrol, 6: 169-174, 1986.

43. Ruilope L, Rodicio J, Miranda B, Garcia Robles R, Sancho-Rof J, Romero JC: Renal effects of amino acid infusions in patients with panhypopituitarism. Hypertension, 11: 557-559, 1988.

44. Brouhard BH, La Grone LF, Richards GE, Travis LB: Somatostatin limits rise in glomerular filtration rate after a protein meal. J Pediatr, 110: 729-734, 1987.

45. Brouhard BH, Richards GE: Effects of growth hormone on the glomerular filtration response to a protein meal. J Am Coll Nutr, 8: 57-60, 1989.

46. Bergstrom J, Ahlberg M, Alvestrand A: Influence of protein intake on renal hemodynamics and plasma hormone concentrations in normal subjects. Acta Med Scand, 217: 189-196, 1985.

47. Hirschberg R, Kopple JD: Increase in renal plasma flow and glomerular filtration rate during growth hormone treatment may be mediated by insulin-like growth gactor 1. Am J Nephrol, 8: 249-253, 1988.

48. Hirschberg R, Raab H, Bergamo R, Kopple JD: The delayed effect of growth hormone on renal function in man. Kidney Int, 35: 865-870, 1989.

49. Parving HH, Noer J, Mogensen CE, Svendsen PA: Kidney function in normal man during short-term growth hormone infusion. Acta Endocrinol (Copenh), 89: 796-800, 1978.

50. Premen AJ: Protein-mediated elevations in renal hemodynamics: Existence of a hepato-renal axis? Medical Hypotheses, 19: 295-309, 1986.

51. Premen AJ, Hall JE, Smith MJ: Postprandial regulation of renal hemodynamics: role of pancreatic glucagon. Am J Physiol, 248: F656-F662, 1985.

52. Uranga J, Fuenzalida R, Rapoport AL, del Castillo E: Effect of glucagon and glomerulopressin on the renal function of the dog. Horm Metab Res, 11: 275-279, 1979.

53. Alvestrand A, Bergstrom J: Glomerular hyperfiltration after protein ingestion, during glucagon infusion, and in insulin-dependent diabetes is induced by a liver hormone: deficient production of this hormone in hepatic failure causes hepatorenal syndrome. Lancet I: 195-197, 1984.

54. Alverstrand A, Zimmerman L, Bergstrom J: Potential role of a liver-derived factor in mediating renal response to protein. Blood Purification, 6: 276-284, 1988.

55. Juncos LI, Salom MG, Cornejo JC, Romero JC: Renal response to amino acid infusion in essential hypertension. J Am Soc Nephrol, 1: 507, 1990 (Abstract).

56. Slomowitz LA, Hirschberg R, Kopple JD: Captopril augments the renal response to an amino acid infusion in diabetic adults. Am J Physiol 255: F755-F762, 1988.

57. Chagnac A, Gafter U, Zevin D, Hirsch Y, Markovitz I, Levi J: Enalapril attenuates glomerular hyperfiltration following a meat meal. Nephron, 51: 466-469, 1989.

58. Hirschberg R, Kopple JD: Evidence that insulin-like growth factor 1 increases renal plasma flow and glomerular filtration rate in fasted rats. J Clin Invest, 83: 326-330, 1989.

59. Hirschberg R, Kopple JD, Blantz RC, Tucker BJ: Effects of IGF-1 on glomerular hemodynamics in rats. J Am Soc Nephrol, 1: 666, 1990 (Abstract).

60. Guler HP, Eckardt KU, Zapf J, Bauer C, Froesch ER: Insulin-like growth factor 1 increases glomerular filtration rate and renal plasma flow in man. Acta Endocrinol (Copenh), 121: 101-106, 1989.

61. Haylor J, Singh I, El Nahas AM: Nitric oxide synthesis inhibitor prevents vasodilation by insulin-like growth factor 1. Kidney Int, 39: 333-335, 1991.

62. Rodríguez-Iturbe B, Herrera J, Gutkowska J, Parra G, Coello J: Atrial natriuretic factor increases after a protein meal in man. Clin Sci, 75: 495-498, 1988.

63. Vanrenterghem YFCh, Verberckmoes RKA, Roels LM, Michielsen PJ: Role of prostaglandins in protein-induced glomerular hyperfiltration in normal humans. Am J Physiol, 254: F463-F469, 1988.

64. Herrera J, Rodríguez-Iturbe B, Parra G, Coello J, García R, Colina-Chourio J, Sinaiko A: Urinary prostaglandin E and kallikrein activity in glomerular hyperfiltration induced by a meat meal in man. Clin Nephrol, 30: 151-157, 1988.

65. Brouhard BH, La Grone L: Effect of indomethacin on the glomerular filtration rate after a protein meal in humans. Am J Kidney Dis, 13: 232-236, 1989.

66. Moncada S, Palmer RMJ, Higgs EA: Biosynthesis of nitric oxide from L-arginine. A pathway for the regulation of cell function and communication. Biochem Pharmacol, 38: 1709-1715, 1989.

67. Marsden PA, Goligorsky MS, Brenner BM: Endothelial cell biology in relation to current concepts of vessel wall structure and function. J Am Soc Nephrol, 1: 931-948, 1991.

68. King AJ, Troy JL, Downes SJ, Anderson S, Brenner BM: Effects of N-monomethyl-L-arginine (L-NMMA) on the basal renal hemodynamics response and the response to amino acid infusion. Kidney Int, 37: 371A, 1990 (Abstract).

69. Baines AD, Ho P, James H: Metabolic control of renal vascular resistance and glomerulotubular balance. Kidney Int, 27: 848-854, 1985.

70. Ferrario RG, Salvati P: Intrarenal production of endothelium-derived nitric oxide (NO) modulate renal hemodynamics. J Am Soc Nephrol 1: 664, 1990 (Abstract).

71. Don BR, Sechi LA, Schambelan M: Dietary protein modulates glomerular cGMP via endothelium-derived relaxing factor (EDRF): a possible mediator of glomerular hyperfiltration. J AM Soc Nephrol 1: 441, 1990 (Abstract).

72. Bolin P, Jaffa AA, Rust PF, Mayfield RK: Acute and chronic responses of human renal kallikrein and kinins to dietary protein. Am J Physiol, 257: F718-F723, 1989.

73. Jaffa AA, Stewart JM, Vavrek RJ, Rust PF, Mayfield RK: A bradykinin inhibitor prevents the increase in glomerular filtration rate induced by amino acids. Clin Res 37: 492A, 1989.

74. De Nicola L, Blantz RC, Gabbai FB: Renal functional reserve in treated and untreated hypertensive rats. Kidney Int (in press).

75. Gabbai FB, De Nicola L, Blantz RC: Renal functional reserve in rats with recent onset poorly controlled diabetes mellitus. J Am Soc Nephrol 1: 664, 1990 (Abstract).

76. Claris Appiani A, Assael BM, Tirelli AS, Cavanna G, Corbetta C, Marra G: Proximal tubular function and hyperfiltration during amino acid infusion in man. Am J Nephrol, 8: 96-101, 1988.

77. Cassidy MJD, Beck R: Renal functional reserve in live related kidney donors. Am J Kidney Dis, 11: 468-472, 1988.

78. Amore A, Coppo R, Roccatello D, Martina G, Rollino C, Basolo B, Novelli F, Amprimo MC, Cavalli G, Piccoli G: Single kidney function: Effect of acute protein and water loading on microalbuminuria. Am J Med, 84: 711-717, 1988.

79. ter Wee PM, Tegzess AM, Donker AJM: The effect of low dose dopamine on renal function in uninephrectomized patients: special emphasis on kidney donors before and after nephrectomy. Clin Nephrol, 28: 211-216, 1987.

80. Rodríguez-Iturbe B, Herrera J, García R: Response to acute protein load in kidney donors and in apparently normal postacute glomerulonephritis patients: Evidence for glomerular hyperfiltration. Lancet, August 31: 461-464, 1985.

81. Tufro A, Arrizurieta E, Repetto H, Dieguez SM, Picon A: Renal response to a protein meal in children with single kidneys. Clin Nephrol, 34: 17-21, 1990.

82. Rugiu C, Oldrizzi L, Maschio G: Effects of an oral protein load on glomerular filtration rate in patients with solitary kidneys. Kidney Int, 32 (suppl 22): S29-S31, 1987.

83. Wheeler DC, Cosgriff PS, Bennett SE, Walls J: Measurement of renal functional reserve of the single kidney in man. Clin Nephrol, 28: 87-92, 1987.

84. Tapson JS, Mansy H, Marshall SM, Tisdall SR, Wilkinson R: Renal functional reserve in kidney donors. Quart J Med, 60: 725-732, 1986.

85. Zuccala A, Gaggi R, Zucchelli A, Zucchelli P: Renal functional reserve in patients with a reduced number of functioning glomeruli. Clin Nephrol, 32: 229-234, 1989.

86. Molina E, Herrera J, Rodríguez-Iturbe B: The renal functional reserve in health and renal disease in shool age children. Kidney Int, 34: 809-816, 1988.

87. De Santo NG, Capasso G, Anastasio P, Coppola S, Castellino P, Lama G, Bellini L: The renal hemodynamic response following a meat meal in children with chronic renal failure and in healthy controls. Nephron, 56: 136-142, 1990.

88. Krishna GG, Kapoor SC: Preservation of renal reserve in chronic renal disease. Am J Kidney Dis, 17: 18-24, 1991.

89. Notghi A, Anderton JL: Effect of nifedipine and mefruside on renal reserve in hypertensive patients. Postgrad Med J, 64: 856-859, 1988.

90. Losito A, Zampi I, Fortunati I, del Favero A: Glomerular hyperfiltration and albuminuria in essential hypertension. Nephron, 49: 84-85, 1988.

91. Valvo E, Casagrande P, Bedogna V, Dal Santo F, Alberti D, Fontanarosa C, Braggio P, Maschio G: Renal functional reserve in patients with essential hypertension: effect of inhibition of the renin-angiotensin system. Clin Sci, 78: 585-590, 1990.

92. Cairns HS, Raval U, Neild GH: Failure of cyclosporine-treated renal allograft recipients to increase glomerular filtration rate following an amino acid infusion. Transplantation, 46: 79-82, 1988.

93. Bochicchio T, Sandoval G, Ron H, Pérez-Grovas H, Bordes J, Herrera-Acosta J: Fosinopril prevents hyperfiltration and decreases proteinuria in post-transplant hypertensives. Kidney Int, 38: 873-879, 1990.

94. Fioretto P, Trevisan R, Valerio A, Avogaro A, Borsato M, Doria A, Semplicini A, Sacerdoti D, Jones S, Bognetti E, Viberti GC, Nosadini R: Impaired renal response to a meat meal in insulin-dependent diabetes: role of glucagon and prostaglandins. Am J Physiol, 258: F675-F683, 1990.

95. Brouhard BH, La Grone LF, Richards GE, Travis LB: Short term protein loading in diabetics with a ten-year duration of disease. AJCD, 140: 473-476, 1986.

96. Castellino P, De Santo NG, Capasso G, Anastasio P, Coppola S, Capodicasa G, Perna A, Torella R, Salvatore T, Giordano C: Low protein alimentation normalizes renal haemodynamic response to acute protein ingestion in type 1 diabetic children. Eur J Clin Invest, 19, 78-83, 1989.

97. Eisenhauer T, Jungmann E, Warneboldt D, Ansorge G, Scherberich J, Talartschik: Renal functional reserve in type 1 diabetics: Effect of ACE-inhibition. Kin Wochenschr, 68, 750-757, 1990.

98. Tuttle K, Perusek M, DeFronzo R, Kunau R: Increased renal reserve and size regress with strict glycemic control in insulin dependent diabetes mellitus. Kidney Int 37: 261, 1990 (Abstract).

99. Bruton JL, Perusek MC, Lancaster JL, Kopp DT, Tuttle KR: Effects of glycemia on basal and amino acid stimulated renal hemodynamics and kidney size in non-insulin dependent diabetes (NIDD). J Am Soc Nephrol, 1: 623, 1990 (Abstract).

100. Baylis C: Immediate and long term effects of pregnancy on glomerular function in the SHR. Am J Physiol, 257: F1140-F1145, 1989.

101. Herrera-Acosta J, Tapia E, Bobadilla NA, Romero L, Cermeño JL, Alvarado JA, Gabbai FB: Evaluating hyperfiltration with glycine in hypertensive rats with renal ablation. Hypertension, 11 (suppl 1): I33-I37, 1988.

102. Tapia E, Bobadilla N, Romero L, Amato D, Herrera-Acosta: Reduction of arterial pressure after removing the clip restores renal functional reserve in Goldblatt hypertensive rats with renal ablation. Kidney Int, 35: 336A, 1989 (Abstract).

103. Tapia E, Gabbai FB, Calleja C, Franco M, Cermeño JL, Bobadilla NA, Pérez JM, Alvarado JA, Herrera-Acosta J: Determinants of renal damage in rats with systemic hypertension and partial renal ablation. Kidney Int, 38: 642-648, 1990.

GLOMERULONEPHRITIS

Chapter 4

THE ANTIPROTEINURIC EFFECT OF ANGIOTENSIN-CONVERTING-ENZYME INHIBITORS IN HUMAN RENAL DISEASE

DICK DE ZEEUW, JAN E. HEEG AND PAUL E. DE JONG

Division of Nephrology, Department of Medicine, State University Hospital, Groningen, The Netherlands.

Many renal diseases are accompanied by an excess loss of plasma proteins in the urinary space. As such proteinuria has been successfully used as a tool both to detect the presence of renal disease and to evaluate the success of therapeutic interventions on disease activity. The quantity and quality of the urinary protein leakage may in some cases distinguish between the different underlying causes of renal disease. In case of minimal-change disease, protein is usually excreted in considerable quantities, largely confined to albumin, whereas in case of specific renal tubular diseases proteinuria is rather small consisting mainly of low-molecular-weight proteins. However, in general, proteinuria does not differentiate between the multiple causes of renal insults, suggesting a more or less common cause and pathway of urinary protein loss. Indeed, such a common cause may be a loss of the discriminating properties of the glomerular filtration barrier for different macromolecules. In health, this barrier prevents the leakage of plasma proteins to the urinary space by at least two selective mechanisms. Firstly, the filtration pores are of limited size, hindering passage of macromolecules larger than ≈ 55 Angstrom (size selectivity). Secondly, negative charges embedded in the filtration barrier prevent leakage of the main negatively-charged plasma protein, albumin (charge selectivity). Furthermore, proximal tubular protein reabsorption prevents urinary protein leakage of those proteins that escape these restrictive filtration properties.

It is obvious that when any of these protein retaining mechanisms is structurally affected by a renal injury, proteinuria will be the consequence. Toxins or immune reactants have indeed been shown to induce such a mechanical injury to the glomerular capillary barrier, thus altering glomerular permselectivity. However attractive and simple this *mechanical* model may be, alternative pathways for protein leakage have been suggested.

Probably the most important one is the role of altered glomerular hemodynamics in causing a leakage of filtered proteins. This model of *functional* proteinuria is based on the finding that an increase in intraglomerular pressure constitutes a driving force for plasma proteins to pass an anatomically intact filtration barrier. In animal models of renal disease such a rise in intraglomerular pressure has been demonstrated, accompanied by a rise in urinary protein loss. The prevailing hypothesis explaining this rise in glomerular pressure is that a reduction in the number of adequately functioning nephron units (due to any renal insult) prompts the kidneys to increase filtration in the remaining number of (healthy) nephrons, in order to maintain an adequate overall glomerular filtration (1-3). This is achieved through an increase in filtration pressure, either by a decreased preglomerular resistance and/or an increased postglomerular resistance. Although this so-called hyperfiltration prevents excessive loss of glomerular filtration rate, it is at the cost of an increased protein filtration. Experimental evidence for this theory of functional proteinuria comes from elegant micropuncture experiments of Yoshioka et al (4). They demonstrated, in a model of chronic renal disease, that the protein loss found its primary origin not so much in the damaged glomeruli, but in the remaining healthy nephrons. Obviously, direct insults to the pre- or postglomerular adaptation mechanism can also lead to hyperfiltration states, without a concomitant reduction of functioning nephrons. An example of such a functional inadequate adaptation may be found in incipient diabetic disease, which is characterized by supernormal glomerular filtration rates and microalbuminuria (5). Such a functional inadequate adaptation may occur simultaneously with structural abnormalities. Thus, increased protein filtration may be the result of both a mechanically defective glomerular filtration barrier and an altered glomerular hemodynamic profile. Which of these two causes for proteinuria is the most important probably depends on the underlying renal disease.

Since the therapeutic tools to treat or even cure the underlying renal disease are rather limited to date, and since proteinuria often persists even when the renal disease is no longer active, the important clinical question remains whether there is a need to treat proteinuria. Such a symptomatic treatment may be useful in case of massive urinary protein loss (nephrotic syndrome). This condition is usually accompanied by an increased susceptibility to infectious diseases, by hyperlipidemia, and by hypercoagulation. These symptoms are thought to be the result of the loss of specific plasma proteins. The reduction of proteinuria may thus reduce the sometimes life-threatening risks involved with these symptoms. Moreover, both hyperlipidemia and increased coagulation have been associated with an increased glomerular sclerosis and thus loss of nephron units (3). Recently, evidence has accumulated from animal studies to suggest that even the reduction of asymptomatic proteinuria may be of therapeutic relevance. This is based on the theory that an excess amount of filtered proteins may functionally damage several renal cell types, such as glomerular mesangial and epithelial cells, as well as proximal and distal tubular cells, leading to further nephron damage and ultimately to glomerulosclerosis (6). This potentially damaging effect of proteinuria is supported by clinical observations indicating that the degree of proteinuria is positively correlated with the rate of progression of renal function loss over time (7). Thus, although it remains difficult to differentiate between proteinuria originating from mechanically damaged nephrons and proteinuria from intact hyperfiltering nephrons, lowering of urinary protein excretion may well prevent further loss of nephron units.

What are the therapeutic tools available to date to lower urinary protein excretion? Besides the drugs aiming at curing or stabilizing the underlying renal disease process itself, steroid-resistant proteinuria can be reduced by non-steroidal-antiinflammatory drugs (NSAIDs) like indomethacin, as reviewed by Vriesendorp et al (8). The rather high doses needed as well as the many side-effects of NSAIDs have limited their wide-spread use. The discovery of a similar antiproteinuric effect of angiotensin-converting-enzyme (ACE) inhibitors, constitutes a possible better alternative. The aim of this review is to determine the use of ACE-inhibitors in the treatment of human renal disease, with an emphasis on the antiproteinuric effect of these agents.

ANTIPROTEINURIC EFFECT OF ACE-INHIBITORS

As with many newly developed drugs, multiple, frequently unexpected, (side-) effects are discovered in the first clinical studies. ACE-inhibitors are no exception in this respect. This class of drugs was designed as a typical antihypertensive treatment modality with a highly specific mode of action, that is inhibition of the enzyme that converts angiotensin-I to the potent vasoconstrictor angiotensin-II. However, when we started to study the pharmacokinetics of the ACE-inhibitor lisinopril in hypertensive patients with renal insufficiency, in the beginning of 1985, we coincidently discovered that lisinopril reduced urinary protein excretion in the subset of patients that had proteinuria (9). Taguma et al (10) were the first to publish a similar coincidental finding late 1985 in diabetic nephropathy, although in retrospect Herlitz et al (11) had previously found a reduction in proteinuria in some patients with renal failure in lupus erythematosus, without paying specific attention to that finding. Since then, many studies followed (9-27) of which the majority confirmed the antiproteinuric properties of ACE-inhibitors.

Table 1 summarizes the data of these studies. It is intriguing to see that a 50 per cent reduction, on the average, in urinary protein excretion was noted in these studies, irrespective of the type of ACE-inhibitor used, the underlying renal disease, the presence or absence of systemic hypertension, the prevailing degree of renal insufficiency, or the degree of initial proteinuria. Apparently, the treatment is very effective under nearly all different circumstances. However, the degree of the antiproteinuric effect varied considerably, not only within one study, but also between the different studies (Table 1).

Table 1.   Summary of the literature on the effect of ACE-inhibition on proteinuria in patients with different renal diseases.

Ref	# Pat	Renal disease	Pretreatment parameters				Therapy	Dose (mg)	Time	U prot change	Range
			MAP mm Hg	GFR ml/min	Prot g/day	Na-int mmol/d					
11	11	SLE	133	30	4.5	?	captopril +	70	6 mo	-40%	?
10	10	DN	108	25	10.6	70	captopril +	112	8 wk	-48%	+5 to -91%
12	16	DN	112	99	1.5(*)	200	captopril	84	1 wk	-32%	+31 to -81%
9	13	GN	132	26	4.2	50-100	lisinopril	22	3 mo	-61%	+17 to -100%
13	10	GN	116	≈50	4.9	?	captopril +	50	6 mo	-60%	+26 to -100%
14	10	DN	100	130	0.12(*)	ad lib	enalapril	20	6 mo	-44%	?
15	8	GN	98	94	2.8(°)	?	captopril	90	3 mo	-75%	-36 to -97%
16	10	DN	?	≈30	3.7	?	captopril +	37.5	6 mo	+46%	+300 to -45%
17	12	DN	99	101	0.62(*)	?	enalapril	5	6 mo	-55%	?
18	12	GN	101	74	6.0	80	lisinopril	5-10	3 mo	-50%	-17 to -71%
19	20	DN	115	46	2.0	?	enalapril+	5-20	8 wk	-56%	?
20	6	DN	95	84	0.05(*)	150	enalapril	7.9	6 wk	-35%	-8 to -50%
21	9	GN	108	61	3.3	ad lib	captopril	25	4 hr	-20%	+10 to -58%
22	12	DN	79	161	0.11(*)	≈120	captopril	≈60	3 mo	-41%	?
23	20	GN	96	102	3.9	160	benazepril	10	6 mo	-34%	-1 to -84%
24	8	DN	118	83	4.1	90	lisinopril	?	4 mo	-43%	?
25	12	DN	93	125	0.04(*)	ad lib	enalapril	10-20	6 mo	-50%	-20 to -95%
26	10	GN	125	33	5.5	50-100	enalapril +	10-40	1.3 y	-75%	+2 to -97%
27	12	DN	109	95	3.2	?	lisinopril	5-20	3 wk	-41%	?

Ref = reference number; U prot change = the change in urinary protein (albumin) excretion expressed as percentage change compared to pretreatment; MAP = mean arterial pressure; Na-int = estimated dietary sodium intake or, if available, urinary sodium output; SLE = systemic lupus erythematosus; DN =(incipient) diabetic nephropathy; GN = primary glomerular disease.
(*) = albumin (g/day); (°) = protein/creatinine ratio; + = ACE-inhibitor therapy evaluated during use of concomitant antihypertensive or antiproteinuric drugs.

This led us to conclude that it was not possible to predict an effective antiproteinuric response to treatment in an individual patient.

DETERMINANTS OF THE ANTIPROTEINURIC RESPONSE

Several factors may be considered to be responsible for the large inter-individual variation in the antiproteinuric response to ACE-inhibitor therapy. First of all those related to the study protocol, such as: the ACE-inhibitor type, the drug dose, concomitant therapies, and the evaluation time. Secondly, the patient-related pre-treatment variables, such as: the underlying (renal) disease, the blood pressure, glomerular hemodynamic profile, degree of proteinuria, and the hormonal status, in particular the degree of activation of the renin-angiotensin-aldosterone-system (RAAS). Unfortunately, most of the studies carried out to date have either studied small patient numbers and/or have not controlled for the different parameters that might be in play. To identify or refute a role for each of these response-determining factors, one thus has to rely in most cases on comparisons between different studies. The possible bias introduced by these comparisons has to be taken into account in the following paragraphs.

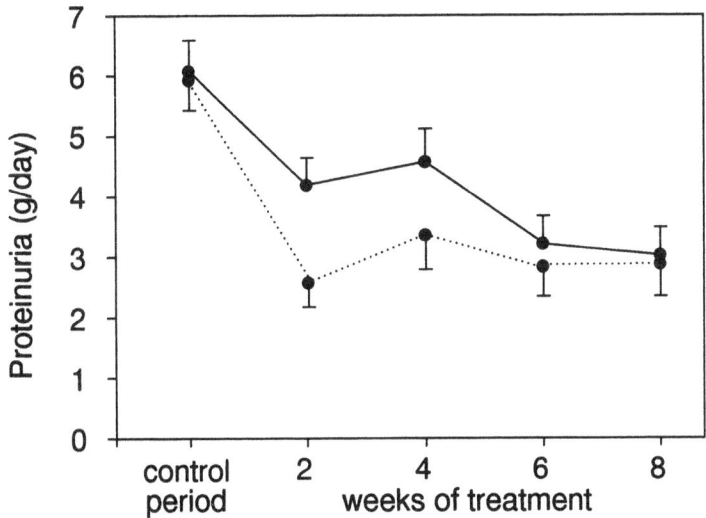

Figure 1. Urinary protein excretion in 12 proteinuric patients during an 8 week follow-up after start of treatment. Patients were evaluated during both lisinopril treatment (solid line) and indomethacin (broken line) therapy. Indomethacin caused a stable antiproteinuric effect within 2 weeks, whereas the antiproteinuric effect of lisinopril reaches maximum after several weeks of treatment [from de Jong PE, Heeg JE, de Zeeuw D: Angiotensin-I converting enzyme inhibition and its antiproteinuric effect in renal disease. In: Proceedings XIth Int Congr Nephrol, Tokyo 1990, Springer Verlag Tokyo, in press, with permission.]

Indeed, no study has made a straight-forward comparison between different ACE-inhibitors. Nevertheless, the several different ACE-inhibitors tested to date do not seem to have marked differences in their antiproteinuric effects (Table 1). In contrast, the dose of the ACE-inhibitor does seem to determine the response. We found that doubling of the lisinopril dose (from 5 to 10 mg), after a stable response plateau had been reached, increased the antiproteinuric response from approx 20 to 50 per cent in the same patients (18). To our knowledge, no data are available on concomitant therapies as response determinants. However, it could certainly be hypothesized that concomitant use of diuretics might increase the response, since these drugs tend to stimulate the RAAS. The latter may lead to an increased antiproteinuric effect (see below). Another possibly important parameter, which might explain discrepancies in response between the different studies, is the time-point at which the antiproteinuric response is evaluated after the start of treatment. We and others (15, 20, 26) found that it takes several weeks before the antiproteinuric effect reaches its maximum and stabilizes (Figure 1) (28). This phenomenon is further illustrated by the fact that although an initial response (within hours) has been clearly documented (21), this response appears to be much lower (around 20% reduction in proteinuria) compared to the more long-term studies. However, a direct comparison in the same study group between the immediate and long-term antiproteinuric response of ACE-inhibiton is lacking.

As far as the patient-related parameters are concerned, the underlying renal disease appears not to play an important role. A spectrum of renal diseases has been studied in both adults and children, with the only exception, to our knowledge, of steroid-sensitive minimal change disease (Table 1). In all different disease states, ACE-inhibitors were able to lower urinary protein excretion. Similarly, the pretreatment blood pressure appears not to play an important role, since hypertensives as well as normotensives show a similar antiproteinuric response profile (Table 1). Pretreatment glomerular filtration rate (GFR), renal blood flow, or filtration fraction also do not appear to play a crucial role in the antiproteinuric response (18, 23). This may be a somewhat surprising finding, since one would expect that, considering the putative mechanism of the antiproteinuric effect of ACE-inhibitors (see below), a hyperfiltering kidney, which is likely to be associated with a high filtration fraction, would be expected to show an increased antiproteinuric response to ACE-inhibition. The absence of a relation between the antiproteinuric response and the pretreatment renal hemodynamic state may be explained by the fact that studies designed to answer this question are lacking. Moreover, the lack of such a relation could be due to the different individual causes for proteinuria, that may be determined by mechanical nephron damage, by renal hemodynamic mechanisms, or by a combination of both. This is illustrated by conflicting data in the literature on the question whether the pretreatment proteinuria determines the antiproteinuric response.

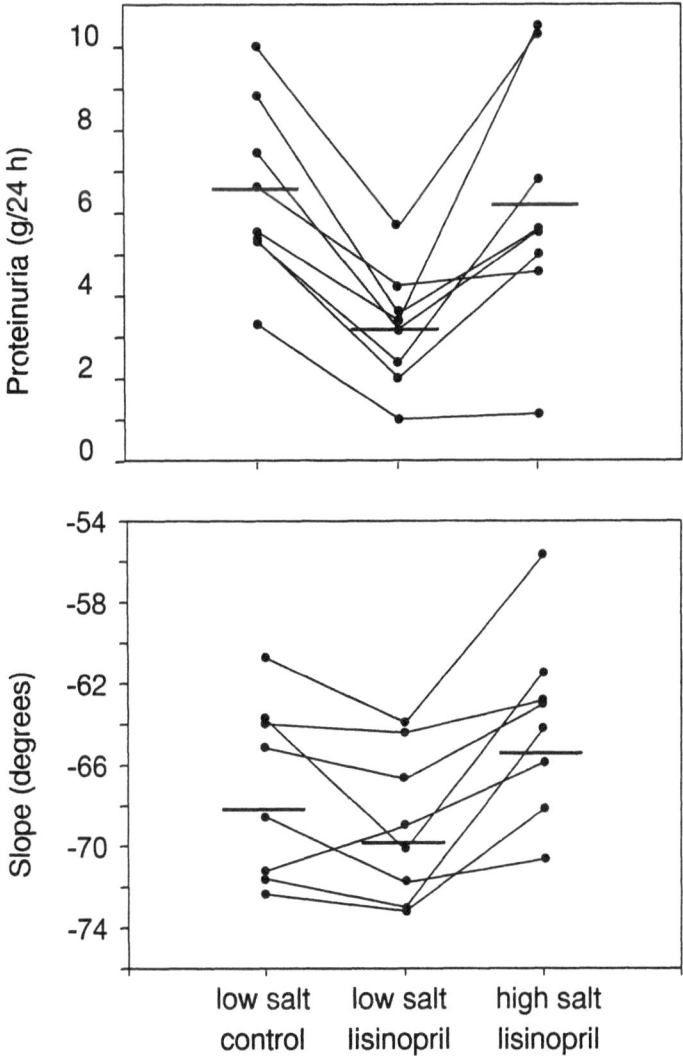

Figure 2.   The effect of dietary sodium intake on urinary protein excretion (top panel) and on protein selectivity (bottom panel) during lisinopril treatment in 8 proteinuric patients. Protein selectivity index is estimated from the changes in slope of the regression line of the fractional renal clearances of albumin, IgG, and α_2-macroglobulin versus molecular weight. High sodium intake during continued treatment with lisinopril offsets both the antiproteinuric effect and the improved protein selectivity [from de Zeeuw D, Heeg JE, Stelwagen T, de Jong R, de Jong PE: The mechanism of the antiproteinuric effect of angiotensin converting enzyme inhibition. Contr Nephrol, vol. 83, S Karger AG, Basel, 1990, pp 160-165, with permission.]

Slomowitz et al (20) found in diabetics that the magnitude of the ACE-inhibition-induced fall in albuminuria correlated with the baseline albumin excretion, whereas many other studies both in diabetic and non-diabetic renal disease failed to detect such relation (9, 13, 18, 23, 25, 27, 29). These findings suggest that the pretreatment level of proteinuria does not determine the antiproteinuric response to an ACE-inhibitor, although exceptions may exist, possibly related to the (hemodynamic) cause of the increased protein excretion.

An important determinant for the antiproteinuric response is the pretreatment activation state of the RAAS.

We demonstrated that the antiproteinuric effect of lisinopril can be completely abolished in a patient when he/she switches from a 50 mmol to a 200 mmol dietary sodium intake, without changing the ACE-inhibitor treatment (Figure 2) (18).

Bedogna et al (23) found that the discriminating factor between good and bad responders was the initial plasma renin activity. These authors moreover found that the good responders showed more marked changes in the fall in systemic blood pressure as well as in the fall in filtration fraction, compared to the non-responders. Since it is known that both systemic as well as renal hemodynamic response to ACE-inhibitor therapy is more exaggerated when given in a RAAS stimulated state (30, 31), the above data suggest that the antiproteinuric response is enhanced by a stimulated RAAS. The latter can be induced either by dietary sodium restriction and/or by diuretic therapy.

In summary, both the dose of the ACE-inhibitor as well as the degree of stimulation of the RAAS appear to be important factors that determine the antiproteinuric response to an ACE-inhibitor. Clearly, more studies controlling for these parameters are needed to exclude a role for any of the other mentioned, and yet unknown, parameters.

MECHANISM OF THE ANTIPROTEINURIC EFFECT

Several mechanisms for the antiproteinuric effect of ACE-inhibitors have been proposed. Some state that the effect may be aspecific and related to the fall in systemic blood pressure, whereas others state that the effect is related to the highly specific effects of ACE-inhibitors on the kidney.

As far as the renal effect is concerned, glomerular hemodynamic changes, in particular a fall in intraglomerular pressure, are suggested to play a key role. However, alternative explanations may also be valid. Besides a potent vasoconstrictor hormone, angiotensin-II is also a potent mitogen. Inhibition of angiotensin-II production might thus result in an antiproliferative effect, which might lead to changes in glomerular permselectivity (3).

Systemic blood pressure

Data for and against a role for a fall in systemic blood pressure to cause the antiproteinuric effect of ACE-inhibitors can be found in the current literature. In diabetic nephropathy it is accepted that lowering of systemic blood pressure with one, or a combination of, antihypertensive agent(s) lowers albuminuria (32, 33). However, Bjorck et al (19) found, when directly compared ACE-inhibitor with β-blocker therapy, that, at any given blood pressure, urinary protein excretion was lower during the ACE-inhibitor treatment compared to the β-blocker therapy (Figure 3).

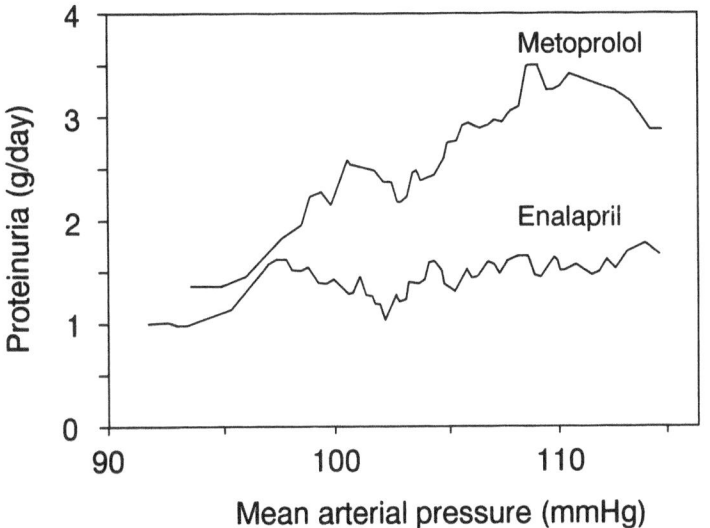

Figure 3.   Relation between mean arterial pressure and proteinuria in 40 diabetic patients randomized to treatment with either enalapril or metoprolol. Lines represent sliding mean values of relation between all simultaneous measurements of mean arterial blood pressures and urinary protein excretion during treatment. At any given blood pressure protein excretion is lower during enalapril treatment compared to metoprolol therapy [from Bjorck S, Mulec H, Johnson SA, Nyberg G, Aurell M: Contrasting effects of enalapril and metoprolol on proteinuria in diabetic nephropathy. Br Med J, 300: 904-907, 1990, with permission.]

Other studies in diabetics reached similar conclusions, based on the fact that albuminuria falls upon ACE-inhibitor treatment without a significant fall in systemic blood pressure occurring (17, 25). We found in non-diabetic renal disease that several conventional treatment modalities such as triple therapy or α-methyldopa had no effect on proteinuria, whereas these patients demonstrated a clear antiproteinuric effect of an ACE-inhibitor (9, 18). Recently, we found in a double-blind study comparing enalapril with atenolol that although the β-blocker did lower proteinuria slightly, enalapril had a far more significant antiproteinuric effect (34). Thus, both in diabetic and non-diabetic patients, a fall in systemic blood pressure can result in a fall in proteinuria. However, the antiproteinuric effect of ACE-inhibitors is considerably greater than that reached with conventional antihypertensive drug regimens, inducing a similar systemic blood pressure fall. This suggests that the antiproteinuric effect of ACE-inhibitors must be found in other factors than the lowering of systemic blood pressure *per se*.

Renal hemodynamics

The most likely explanation for the antiproteinuric effect of ACE-inhibitors to date is a specific effect of these drugs on glomerular hemodynamics. Studies in patients with essential hypertension have clearly demonstrated the specific renal hemodynamic profile of these drugs compared to conventional antihypertensive drugs, consisting of a rise in renal blood flow with a relatively stable glomerular filtration rate, thus inducing a fall in filtration fraction (31, 35, 36). This renal hemodynamic profile is suggested to be the result of a predominantly postglomerular vasodilation (37). Since angiotensin-II is known to predominantly constrict the efferent arteriole, this effect of ACE-inhibitors was no surprise. Moreover, these typical renal hemodynamic effects of ACE-inhibition can be counteracted by systemic infusion of low doses of angiotensin-II (38). An identical renal hemodynamic profile is observed in patients with renal disease and proteinuria: ACE-inhibition induces a rise in renal blood flow, and a fall in filtration fraction. GFR generally remains unaffected (21, 23, 25, 27, 39), although we observed in some studies that GFR may fall slightly but significantly (9, 18, 40). The fact that we found this fall in GFR, whereas others found a relatively stable GFR, might be due to the fact that we studied our patients in a condition of moderate sodium restriction, in contrast to most of the other studies. In case of a stimulated RAAS, maintenance of an already more or less compromised GFR is likely to be more dependent on angiotensin-II induced postglomerular vasoconstriction. Whatever the effect on GFR, a parallel between the antiproteinuric effect of an ACE-inhibitor and the fall in filtration fraction is observed in many studies (9, 18, 21, 23, 25, 27). Moreover, we found that the fall in filtration fraction induced by prolonged ACE-inhibitor treatment, correlated with the degree of the antiproteinuric response (9). The observed parallel changes in both parameters and the correlation between them suggest a causal relationship. Indeed, Yoshioka et al (4) and Pelayo et al (41) showed in animal studies that a reduction in intraglomerular pressure leads to a fall in protein filtration. Although we cannot measure intraglomerular pressure in humans, the fall in filtration fraction at least suggests a postglomerular vasodilation, which would lead to a fall in intraglomerular pressure. The slight fall in GFR may well fit this hypothesis. Moreover, we demonstrated that changes in the antiproteinuric response, induced by either changes in the ACE-inhibitor dose or changes in the dietary sodium intake, are accompanied by parallel changes in renal hemodynamics (18). This again points to the alledged causal relationship between the renal hemodynamic response and the antiproteinuric effect of ACE-inhibition. In addition, a few human studies both in diabetic- and non-diabetic renal disease have demonstrated that the glomerular permselectivity improves during ACE-inhibition, measured with exogenous (dextrans) as well as endogenous (proteins) macromolecules (42-44). We found that permselectivity regained pretreatment levels after switching from a low- to a high sodium intake (Figure 2) (43). These changes in permselectivity may indeed be the effect of changes in intraglomerular pressure.

However, although many, if not all, of the above findings point to a single simple explanation for the antiproteinuric effect of ACE-inhibition, that is a fall in intraglomerular pressure, several confounding findings should be mentioned. First of all, why does the antiproteinuric effect of ACE-inhibitors take a rather long time to reach a maximum (Figure 1), whereas the renal hemodynamic effect occurs within hours and remains relatively stable upon continued treatment? Moreover, if the renal hemodynamic and antiproteinuric effect are causally related, one would expect that angiotensin-II infusion would restore proteinuria to pretreatment levels. However, we recently found that angiotensin-II infusion during several hours did not at all affect proteinuria, which had fallen during 3 months ACE-inhibitor treatment, whereas the hemodynamic effects of ACE-inhibition were completely abolished (45). Combining both these observations, one could argue that the renal hemodynamic effects are either not at all causally related to the antiproteinuric effect of ACE-inhibitors, or in a different way than we are assuming.

Allon et al (21) recently published interesting data on the acute effects of captopril on protein excretion in proteinuric patients. Although they observed a significant reduction in proteinuria by 20 per cent, as well as a fall in filtration fraction by 15 per cent, both parameters were not correlated. Moreover, glomerular permselectivity, estimated by the change in renal clearance of IgG and albumin, did not change at all in this acute study. The authors conclude that the antiproteinuric mechanism of an ACE-inhibitor is unrelated to changes in renal hemodynamics or changes in glomerular permselectivity.

Taken together the currently available data suggest that changes in renal hemodynamics may play a pivotal role in the antiproteinuric effect of ACE-inhibitors. However, within that large body of evidence, cumulative data is building up refuting a direct causal relation. Before dismissing such a causal relation, we have to clarify whether the ACE-inhibition-induced renal hemodynamic changes could in the long-run alter the glomerular structure resulting in a fall in protein excretion. Clearly, more studies are needed to resolve this issue.

Hormonal effects

Because of the rather specific action of ACE-inhibitors inhibiting the formation of angiotensin-II, it logically followed that the mechanism of the antiproteinuric effect of this class of drugs would be associated with these effects on the RAAS. Indeed, high levels of circulating angiotensin-II have been shown to induce proteinuria in different animal studies (46-51). Moreover, specific inhibition of the angiotensin-II receptors by saralasin, offsets this proteinuric action of angiotensin-II (48, 51). In humans, the relation between angiotensin-II and proteinuria is more complex. High renin states, such as in case of renovascular hypertension, have indeed been associated with proteinuria (52-54). Removal of the cause for the high renin state by "removal" of the renal artery stenosis or ACE-inhibition therapy, resulted in a decrease or even disappearance of the proteinuria. These data suggest that angiotensin-II may indeed play a role in the cause of increased protein excretion, and that inhibition of this hormone is the mechanism by which ACE-inhibitors exert their antiproteinuric effect in man.

However, infusion of angiotensin-II in humans did, surprisingly, not lead to increased proteinuria. Loon et al (55) infused pressor doses of angiotensin-II in proteinuric patients without observing any increase (rather a decrease) in urinary protein excretion. We similarly found that subpressor doses of angiotensin II had no effect on protein excretion (45). Moreover, as stated above, angiotensin-II infusion could not offset the antiproteinuric effect of an ACE-inhibitor in this study. Thus, although some of the above data clearly define angiotensin-II as a key hormone explaining the antiproteinuric mechanism of ACE-inhibition, several human studies argue against this hypothesis. However, these latter studies used a protocol in which angiotensin-II was infused for only several hours. It could well be that the proteinuric effect of angiotensin-II, as well as the antiproteinuric effect of angiotensin-II synthesis inhibition, is the result of another important characteristic of this hormone besides its hemodynamic effect, that is its mitogenic effect. It may well be that the reduction in the (tissue) angiotensin-II levels, induced by the ACE-inhibitors, leads to a structural modification in the glomerular filtration barrier, which in turn explains the reduction in protein filtration (56). Certainly, the relatively long time needed for ACE-inhibitors to reach their maximal antiproteinuric effect may well support this hypothesis. Conversely, to demonstrate a proteinuric effect of angiotensin-II, or to offset the ACE-inhibitor-induced antiproteinuric effect with angiotensin II infusion, one would possibly need to infuse the hormone for longer time periods.

Alternatively, the antiproteinuric effect of ACE-inhibitors may not be mediated through angiotensin-II at all. It is known that ACE-inhibition has clear effects on other hormone systems such as the kinin and prostaglandin system.

Firstly, the converting enzyme also facilitates the breakdown of the vasodilator bradykinin. An excess of this latter hormone may explain the antiproteinuric effect. Indeed, Hutchison et al (57) found that inhibition of bradykinin production prevented the antiproteinuric action of the ACE-inhibitor in proteinuric rats. Whether these results can be extrapolated to the human situation remains to be investigated. Studies in patients with proteinuria using the recently developed specific angiotensin-II receptor antagonists may clarify this issue.

Another explanation for the antiproteinuric effect of ACE-inhibitors may be their effect on prostaglandin synthesis. It is well known that NSAIDs exert a similar antiproteinuric effect as ACE-inhibitors (18). The antiproteinuric effect of NSAIDs appears to be related to the inhibition of prostaglandin synthesis (8). Since changes in angiotensin-II levels are associated with changes in prostaglandin levels, it may be that the antiproteinuric effect of ACE-inhibitors is the result of a change in the balance between the RAAS and the prostaglandin system. We recently studied the effect of addition of NSAIDs to ACE inhibitor therapy on proteinuria. This resulted in a further fall of the proteinuria (58). A similar observation was made by Allon et al (21) in an acute study. This additive antiproteinuric effect suggest that both drugs act via different mechanism, which makes a prostaglandin-mediated antiproteinuric effect of ACE-inhibitors rather unlikely.

Thus, although there is evidence that the antiproteinuric effect of ACE-inhibition is predominantly mediated by changes in angiotensin-II synthesis, a role for other hormone systems, specifically the kinins, can as yet not be excluded.

THERAPEUTIC APPLICATIONS

As stated above, the antiproteinuric effect of ACE-inhibitors may have several therapeutic applications, such as symptomatic treatment of the proteinuria and maybe even more importantly, halting or slowing the natural progression of renal function loss. Since proteinuria and renal function loss may be related, these seemingly separate treatment goals may in the future converge to one goal that is renal protection.

As far as the symptomatic treatment of proteinuria is concerned, ACE-inhibitors may be of use to lower proteinuria in patients with the nephrotic syndrome, who do not respond to glucocorticoids and immunosuppressive agents. The need for such a treatment in these patients is to stabilize or alleviate the nephrotic condition. We have recently demonstrated that an ACE-inhibitor, in combination with a diuretic, lowers proteinuria in nephrotic patients from a mean of 10.5 ± 1.8 to 4.3 ± 4.3 g/day (59). Serum albumin rose from 28.2 ± 2.2 to 33 ± 1.6 g/l. An interesting option to even further lower protein excretion in certain patients is to combine ACE-inhibitor therapy with NSAID therapy. Indeed, we found in the above study that the combination of lisinopril and indomethacin further reduced proteinuria to 2.4 ± 0.8 g/day (59). Although such a combined treatment is very effective in lowering proteinuria, side effects may occur such as hyperkalemia and a considerable fall in GFR. Both parameters should therefore be monitored carefully when applying this therapy.

Although ACE-inhibitors effectively lower urinary protein excretion in patients with asymptomatic proteinuria, the benefit of such therapy has yet to be established. However, there are at least two reasons to advocate such a treatment.

First of all, lowering of proteinuria may reflect a lowering of an increased glomerular pressure, which may protect the kidney against further damage. Several studies have demonstrated that a patient, once having experienced a renal damage through whatever cause, will progress to end-stage renal failure, even when the underlying disease-cause has long abated. The pace at which this process takes places is individually determined (60). The possible cause for this phenomenon has been extensively studied in animal models of renal disease. One of the important factors is the slow but steady destruction of the remnant healthy nephron population by the raised intraglomerular pressure in these nephrons, although other factors such as hyperlipidemia, coagulation, and growth-stimulating factors may also play a role (1-3). ACE-inhibitors have been demonstrated in these animal models to effectively lower the intraglomerular pressure and to slow the progression of renal function loss. These effects are accompanied by a less prominent rise or even a fall in proteinuria. As such the antiproteinuric effect may thus reflect the effective lowering of intraglomerular pressure.

Also in humans, the effect of ACE-inhibitors on the progression of renal function loss has been studied. Unfortunately, these studies are either non-controlled, and/or consist of rather small patient numbers, and/or are of a retrospective nature, thus not allowing any definitive conclusions. However, the data gathered to date show that ACE-inhibitors appear also protective in the human situation, both in diabetics (29, 61, 62) and in non-diabetic renal disease (63-65).

A second reason why lowering of proteinuria may by itself protect the kidney from further damage, is supported by the hypothesis that proteinuria is not only a marker of glomerular disease, but also affects nephron function. As stated above, animal data suggest that an increased passage of proteins across the glomerular filtration barrier affects the function of mesangial and glomerular as well as tubular epithelial cells (6). By lowering the urinary protein loss with ACE-inhibitors, the kidney may be protected against further loss of nephrons.

It will be hard to dissociate the putative beneficial effects of lowering of intraglomerular pressure from that of lowering proteinuria, since the two are likely to be closely related. Moreover, other factors may also be involved in the protective effect of ACE-inhibitors, such as a lowering of systemic blood pressure (66), decreasing the mitogenic effect of angiotensin-II (67, 68), and an indirectly induced alteration in lipid metabolism and/or coagulation (69-71). The complexity of this problem is illustrated by the numerous therapeutical options, besides ACE-inhibitors, which have been advocated to have renal protective properties, such as dietary protein restriction (72), NSAID therapy (8), lipid lowering agents (69) and anticoagulant therapy (70, 71). However, it is intriguing that each of these therapies has also been proven to lower urinary protein excretion, suggesting that the reduction of proteinuria may indeed be of importance in the renal protective effects of these therapies.

Is there a special place for ACE-inhibitors in the treatment of arresting progressive renal function loss in patients with renal disease? There are several arguments pro and con. The fact that ACE-inhibitors lower systemic blood pressure, have weak but significant diuretic properties, lower angiotensin-II synthesis, lower intraglomerular pressure, and lower proteinuria, all are in favor of the use of ACE-inhibitors in patients with renal disease. None of the above therapies affects so many of the putative risk factors for progressive renal function loss. However, ACE-inhibitor therapy may be accompanied by unwanted renal side effects such as a "dramatic" fall in GFR, symptomatic hypotension, and/or hyperkalemia. Although the side effects all are reversible, they may in some patients warrant discontinuation of ACE-inhibitor therapy.

FUTURE PERSPECTIVES

The most important issue that will determine the future use of ACE-inhibitors as antiproteinuric and renal protective agents, is completion of well-designed clinical studies that prove these drugs to preserve renal function in patients with renal disease. However, even if the on-going studies render positive answers in this respect, an even greater scientific challenge will remain. It has become clear from other studies that although a large group of patients may benefit from a renal protective treatment, individual responses show great variations. Before subjecting the patient to life-long treatment with ACE-inhibitors, we would like to know whether the treatment would be of any use. The data presented above have demonstrated that the antiproteinuric response to an ACE-inhibitor depends on the dose of the drug, the pretreatment activation of the RAAS, and possibly other as yet undetermined factors. These may be of extreme importance in attaining a renal protective effect in an individual patient. Are there any factors, in particular short-term responses to the treatment, that may predict the eventual long-term protective effect? It could well be that the short-term antiproteinuric response and/or the short-term renal hemodynamic response (fall in filtration fraction) can foretell us what the individual patient's long-term response will be like. Future studies should address this issue. Furthermore, we should establish at what time intervention with ACE-inhibitors will be most beneficial. Would it not be preferable to intervene at the time that the patient has still minimal renal damage and minimal loss of GFR? However, to prove a protective effect of ACE-inhibition in such patients may take very large study populations and extremely long follow-up times. In addition, one could question whether we should treat patients with ACE-inhibitors at the time that they are (still) normotensive. Finally, we have as yet to determine whether a patient's response can be optimized by trying alternative renoprotective regimens, or a combination of different regimens. A great task lies before us to investigate all these issues, and the future will tell us whether we can get answers to these important questions

REFERENCES

1. Keane WF, Anderson S, Aurell M, de Zeeuw D, Narins RG, Povar G: Angiotensin converting enzyme inhibitors and progressive renal insufficiency. Ann Int Med, 111: 503-516, 1989.
2. Anderson S, Brenner BM: Role of intraglomerular hypertension in initiation and progression of renal disease. In: "The kidney in hypertension. Perspectives in hypertension" (Eds Kaplan N, Brenner BM, Laragh JH), Raven Press, New York, 1987, pp 67-76.
3. Klahr S, Schreiner G, Ichikawa I: The progression of renal disease. N Engl J Med, 25: 1657-1666, 1988.
4. Yoshioka T, Shigara H, Yoshida Y, Fogo A, Glick AD, Dew WM, Hoyer JR, Ichikawa I: "Intact nephrons" as the primary origin of proteinuria in chronic renal disease. J Clin Invest, 82: 1614-1623, 1988.
5. Hostetter TH, Troy JL, Brenner BM: Glomerular hemodynamics in experimental diabetes mellitus. Kidney Int, 19: 410-415, 1981.
6. Remuzzi G, Bertani T: Is glomerulosclerosis a consequence of altered glomerular permeability to macromolecules? Kidney Int, 38: 384-394, 1990.
7. Williams PS, Fass G, Bone JM: Renal pathology and proteinuria determine progression in untreated mild/moderate chronic renal failure. Q J Med, 252: 343-354, 1988.
8. Vriesendorp R, Donker AJM, de Zeeuw D, de Jong PE, van der Hem GK, Brentjens JRH: Effects of non-steroidal antiiinflammatory drugs on proteinuria. Am J Med, 81: S84-S94, 1986.
9. Heeg JE, de Jong PE, van der Hem GK, de Zeeuw D: Reduction of proteinuria by angiotensin converting enzyme inhibition. Kidney Int, 32: 78-83, 1987.
10. Taguma Y, Kitamoto Y, Futaki G, Ueda H, Monma H, Ishazaki M, Takahashi H, Sekino H, Sasaki Y: Effect of captopril on heavy proteinuria in azotemic diabetes. N Engl J Med, 313: 1617-1620, 1984.

11. Herlitz H, Edeno C, Mulec H, Westberg G, Aurell M: Captopril treatment of hypertension and renal failure in systemic lupus erythematosus. Nephron, 38: 253-256, 1984.
12. Hommel E, Parving HH, Mathiesen E, Edsberg B, Damkjaer Nielsen M, Giese J: Effect of captopril on kidney function in insulin-dependent diabetic patients with nephropathy. Br Med J, 293: 467-470, 1986.
13. Lagrue G, Robeva R, Laurent J: Antiproteinuric effect of captopril in primary glomerular disease. Nephron, 46: 99-100, 1987.
14. Marre M, Leblanc H, Suarez L, Guyenne TT, Menard J, Passa P: Converting enzyme inhibition and kidney function in normotensive diabetic patients with persistent albuminuria. Br Med J, 294: 1448-1452, 1987.
15. Trachtman H, Gauthier B: Effect of angiotensin-converting enzyme inhibitor therapy on proteinuria in children with renal disease. J Pediatr, 112: 295-298, 1988.
16. Hay U, Ludvik B, Gisinger Ch, Schernthaner G: Fehlender effekt der ACE-inhibition auf die makroproteinurie bei diabetischer nephropathie - eine langzeitstudie uber 6 monate. Schweiz Med Wschr, 188: 165-169, 1988.
17. Stornello M, Valvo EV, Puglia N, Scapellato L: Angiotensin converting enzyme inhibition with a low dose of enalapril in normotensive diabetics with persistent proteinuria. J Hypertens, 6: S464-S466, 1988.
18. Heeg JE, de Jong PE, van der Hem GK, de Zeeuw D: Efficacy and variability of the antiproteinuric effect of ACE-inhibition by lisinopril. Kidney Int, 36: 272-279, 1989.
19. Bjorck S, Mulec H, Johnson SA, Nyberg G, Aurell M: Contrasting effects of enalapril and metoprolol on proteinuria in diabetic nephropathy. Br Med J, 300: 904-907, 1990.
20. Slomowitz LA, Bergamo R, Grosvenor M, Kopple JD: Enalapril reduces albumin excretion in patients with low levels of microalbuminuria. Am J Nephrol, 10: 457-462, 1990.
21. Allon M, Pasque CB, Rodriguez M: Acute effects of captopril and ibuprofen on proteinuria in patients with nephrosis. J Lab Clin Med, 116: 462-468, 1990.
22. Cook J, Daneman D, Spino M, Sochett E, Perlman K, Williamson Balfe J: Angiotensin converting enzyme inhibitor therapy to decrease microalbuminuria in normotensive children with insulin-dependent diabetes mellitus. J Pediatr, 117: 39-45, 1990.
23. Bedogna V, Valvo E, Casagrande P, Braggio P, Fontanarosa C, Dal Santo F, Alberti D, Maschio G: Effects of ACE inhibition in normotensive patients with glomerular disease and normal renal function. Kidney Int, 38: 101-107, 1990.
24. Bakris GL: Effects of dilatiazem or lisinopril on massive proteinuria associated with diabetes mellitus. Ann Int Med, 112: 707-708, 1990.
25. Rudberg S, Aperia A, Freyschuss U, Persson B: Enalapril reduces microalbuminuria in young normotensive type1 (insulin-dependent) diabetic patients irrespective of its hypotensive effect. Diabetologica, 33: 470-476, 1990.
26. Ferder LF, Inserra F, Daccordi H, Smith RD: Enalapril improved renal function and proteinuria in chronic glomerulopathies. Nephron, 55: S90-S95, 1990.
27. Holdaas H, Hartmann A, Lien MG, Nilsen L, Jervell J, Fauchald P, Endresen L, Djoseland O, Berg KJ: Contrasting effects of lisinopril and nifedipine on albuminuria and tubular transport functions in insulin dependent diabetics with nephropathy. J Int Med, 229: 163-170, 1991
28. de Jong PE, Heeg JE, de Zeeuw D: Angiotensin-I converting enzyme inhibition and its antiproteinuric effect in renal disease. In: Proceedings XIth Int Congr Nephrol, Tokyo 1990 (in press).
29. Bjorck S, Nyberg G, Mulec H, Granerus G, Herlitz H, Aurell M: Beneficial effects of angiotensin converting enzyme inhibition on renal function in patients with diabetic nephropathy. Br Med J, 293: 471-474, 1986.
30. Ferguson RK, Irvin JD, Swanson BN, Lee RB: A comparative pilot study of enalapril, a new angiotensin converting enzyme inhibitor and hydrochlorothiazide in essential hypertension. J Clin Pharmacol, 22: 281-289, 1982.
31. Navis GJ, de Jong PE, Donker AJM, van der Hem GK, de Zeeuw D: Moderate sodium restriction in hypertensive patients, renal effects of ACE-inhibition. Kidney Int, 31: 815-819, 1987.
32. Mogensen CE: Long term antihypertensive treatment inhibiting progression of diabetic nephropathy. Br Med J, 285: 685-688, 1982.
33. Parving HH, Andersen AE, Smidt UM, Hommel E, Mathiesen ER, Svendsen PA: Effect of antihypertensive treatment on kidney function in diabetic nephropathy. Br Med J, 294: 1443-1447, 1987.

111

34. Apperloo AJ, de Zeeuw D, Sluiter HE, de Jong PE: Enalapril improves protein leakage in renal disease more than atenolol. Br Med J (in press).

35. Hollenberg NK, Meggs LG, Williams GH, Katz J, Garnic JD, Harrington: Sodium intake and renal responses to captopril in normal man and in essential hypertension. Kidney Int, 20: 240-245, 1981.

36. Bauer JH, Reams G, Gaddy P: Renal function and hemodynamics during treatment with enalapril in primary hypertension. Nephron, 44: S83-S86, 1986.

37. Hall JE, Coleman TG, Guyton AC, Kastner PR, Granger JP: Control of glomerular filtration rate by circulating angiotensin II. Am J Physiol, 241: R190-R197, 1981.

38. Navis GJ, de Jong PE, Donker AJM, van der Hem GK, de Zeeuw D: Effects of enalaprilic acid on sodium excretion and renal hemodynamics in essential hypertension. J Clin Hypertens, 3: 228-238, 1985.

39. Reams GP, Bauer JH: Effect of enalapril in subjects with hypertension associated with moderate to severe renal dysfunction. Arch Intern Med, 146: 2145-2148, 1986.

40. Heeg JE, de Zeeuw D, de Jong PE: The effects of lisinopril on renal hemodynamics in patients with renal disease. Current Opinion in Cardiol, 4: S29-S34, 1989.

41. Pelayo JC, Quan AH, Shanley PF: Angiotensin II control of the renal microcirculation in rats with reduced renal mass. Am J Physiol, 258: F414-F422, 1987.

42. Morelli E, Loon N, Meyer T, Peters W, Myers BD: Effects of converting enzyme inhibition on barrier function in diabetic nephropathy. Diabetes, 39: 76-82, 1990.

43. de Zeeuw D, Heeg JE, Stelwagen T, de Jong R, de Jong PE: The mechanism of the antiproteinuric effect of angiotensin converting enzyme inhibition. Contr Nephrol, 83: 160-165, 1990.

44. Remuzzi A, Percicucci E, Ruggenenti P, Mosconi L, Remuzzi G: Enalapril improves glomerular size-selective function in IgA nephropathy. J Am Soc Nephrol, 1: A313, 1990.

45. Heeg JE, de Jong PE, van der Hem GK, de Zeeuw D: Angiotensin II does not reverse the reduction of proteinuria by ACE-inhibition in man. Kidney Int (in press).

46. Eisenbach GM, van Liew JB, Boylan JW: Effect of angiotensin on the filtration of protein in the rat kidney: a micropuncture study. Kidney Int, 8: 80-87, 1975.

47. Bohrer MP, Deen WM, Robertson CR, Brenner BM: Mechanism of angiotensin II-induced proteinuria in the rat. Am J Physiol, 233: F13-F21, 1977.

48. Bauman JW: On the mechanism of angiotensin-induced proteinuria. I. Studies in aminonucleoside nephrotic rats and in saralasin blockade. Nephron, 27: 47-50, 1981.

49. Olivetti G, Kithier K, Giacomelli F, Wiener J: Characterization of glomerular permeability and proteinuria in acute hypertension in the rat. Kidney Int, 25: 599-607, 1984.

50. Yoshioka T, Rennke HG, Salant DJ, Deen WM, Ichikawa I: Role of abnormally high transmural pressure in the permselectivity defect of the glomerular capillary wall: a study in early passive Heymann nephritis. Circ Res, 61: 531-538, 1987.

51. Yoshioka T, Mitarai T, Kon V, Deen WM, Rennke HG, Ichikawa I: Role for angiotensin II in an overt functional proteinuria. Kidney Int, 30: 538-545, 1986.

52. Montoliu J, Botey A, Torras A, Darnell A, Revert L: Renin-induced massive proteinuria in man. Clin Nephrol, 2: 267-271, 1979.

53. Eiser AR, Moriber Katz S, Swartz C: Reversible nephrotic range proteinuria with renal artery stenosis: a clinical example of renin-associated proteinuria. Nephron, 30: 374-377, 1982.

54. Holman ND, Donker AJM, van der Meer J: Disappearance of renin-induced proteinuria by an ACE-inhibitor: a case report. Clin Nephrol, 34: 70-71, 1990.

55. Loon N, Shemesh O, Morelli E, Myers BD: Effect of angiotensin II infusion on the human glomerular filtration barrier. Am J Physiol, 257: F608-F614, 1989.

56. Yoshida Y, Kawamura T, Ikoma M, Fogo A, Ichikawa I: Effects of antihypertensive drugs on glomerular morphology. Kidney Int, 36: 626-635, 1989.

57. Hutchison FN, Martin VI: Effects of modulation of renal kallikrein-kinin system in the nephrotic syndrome. Am J Physiol, 258: F1237-F1244, 1990.

58. Heeg JE, de Jong PE, de Zeeuw D: Additive antiproteinuric effect of ACE inhibition and NSAID therapy: a clue to the mechanism of action. Clin Sci (in press).

59. Heeg JE, de Jong PE, Vriesendorp R, de Zeeuw D: Additive effect of the NSAID indomethacin and the ACE-inhibitor lisinopril. Am J Nephrol, 10: S94-S97, 1990.

60. Mitch WE, Walser M, Buffington GA, Lemann J: A simple method of estimating progression of chronic renal failure. Lancet, II: 1326-1328, 1976.

61. Parving HH, Hommel E, Schmidt UM: Protection of kidney function and decrease in albuminuria by captopril in insulin dependent diabetics with nephropathy. Br Med J, 297: 1086-1091, 1988.

62. Parving HH, Hommel E, Nielsen MD, Giese J: Effect of captopril on blood pressure and kidney function in normotensive insulin dependent diabetics with nephropathy. Br Med J, 299: 533-536, 1989.

63. Bauer JH, Reams GP, Lal SM: Renal protective effect of strict blood pressure control with enalapril therapy. Arch Int Med, 147: 1397-1400, 1987.

64. Mann JFE, Reisch C, Ritz E: Use of angiotensin-converting enzyme inhibitors for the preservation of kidney function: a retrospective study. Nephron, 55: 38-42, 1990.

65. Rodicio JL, Alcazar JM, Ruilope LM: Influence of converting enzyme inhibition on glomerular filtration rate and proteinuria. Kidney Int, 38: 590-594, 1990.

66. Brazy PC, Stead WW, Fitzwilliam JF: Progression of renal insufficiency: role of blood pressure. Kidney Int, 35: 670-674, 1989.

67. Fogo A, Hawkins EP, Berry PL, Glick AD, Chiang ML, MacDonnel RC, Ichikawa I: Glomerular hypertrophy in minimal change disease predicts subsequent progression to focal glomerular sclerosis. Kidney Int, 38: 115-123, 1990.

68. Yoshida Y, Fogo A, Ichikawa I: Glomerular hemodynamic changes vs hypertrophy in experimental glomerular sclerosis. Kidney Int, 35: 654-660, 1989.

69. Keane WF, Kasiske BL, O'Donnell MP: Hyperlipidemia and the progression of chronic renal disease. Am J Clin Nutr, 47: 157-160, 1988.

70. Purkerson ML, Joist JH, Yates J, Valdes A, Morrison A, Klahr S: Inhibition of thromboxane synthesis ameliorates the progressive kidney disease of rats with subtotal renal ablation. Proc Natl Acad Sci USA, 82: 193-197, 1985.

71. Purkerson ML, Tollefson DM, Klahr S: N-desulfated/acetylated heparin ameliorates the progression of renal disease in rats with subtotal renal ablation. J Clin Invest, 81: 69-74, 1988.

72. Rosman JB, ter Wee PM, Piers-Brecht TPM, Sluiter WJ, Meijer S, Donker AJM: Prospective randomised trial of early dietary protein restriction in chronic renal failure. Lancet, II: 1291-1296, 1984.

HYPERTENSION

Chapter 5

INSULIN RESISTANCE IN ESSENTIAL HYPERTENSION

WILLA A. HSUEH

Division of Diabetes, Hypertension and Nutrition, Department of Medicine, University of Southern California Medical Center, Los Angeles, CA, 90033, USA

An impressive correlation exists between body weight and blood pressure in all age groups. Sixteen percent of the normotensive population is obese, while 44% of the hypertensive population is obese (1-3). Eighty percent of patients with non-insulin dependent diabetes mellitus (NIDDM) are obese; thus, the prevalence of hypertension is twice as common in obesity or NIDDM compared to the nondiabetic, nonobese population (4). Accordingly, the concept emerges that obesity and diabetes are important determinants of blood pressure. However, little is understood of the basic mechanisms by which the metabolic derangements associated with these states interact to alter target organ structure and function (blood vessel contractility, renal sodium and metabolic balance, cardiac performance and hypertrophy, and sympathetic nervous system responses). Understanding these interactions not only has pathophysiologic relevance, but will provide a rational basis for antihypertensive treatment in the setting of obesity and NIDDM.

THE INSULIN RESISTANCE OF HYPERTENSION

A defect in insulin action on glucose utilization is an intrinsic metabolic characteristic of both obesity and NIDDM (5, 6). In obesity, insulin resistance induces hyperinsulinemia in order to maintain normoglycemia. NIDDM results when a faltering pancreas cannot secrete enough insulin to overcome the insulin resistance, although hyperinsulinemia is generally present in the prediabetic state and early in the development of the disease (7, 8). In obese populations, a highly significant correlation exists between fasting plasma insulin levels and blood pressure (9, 10).

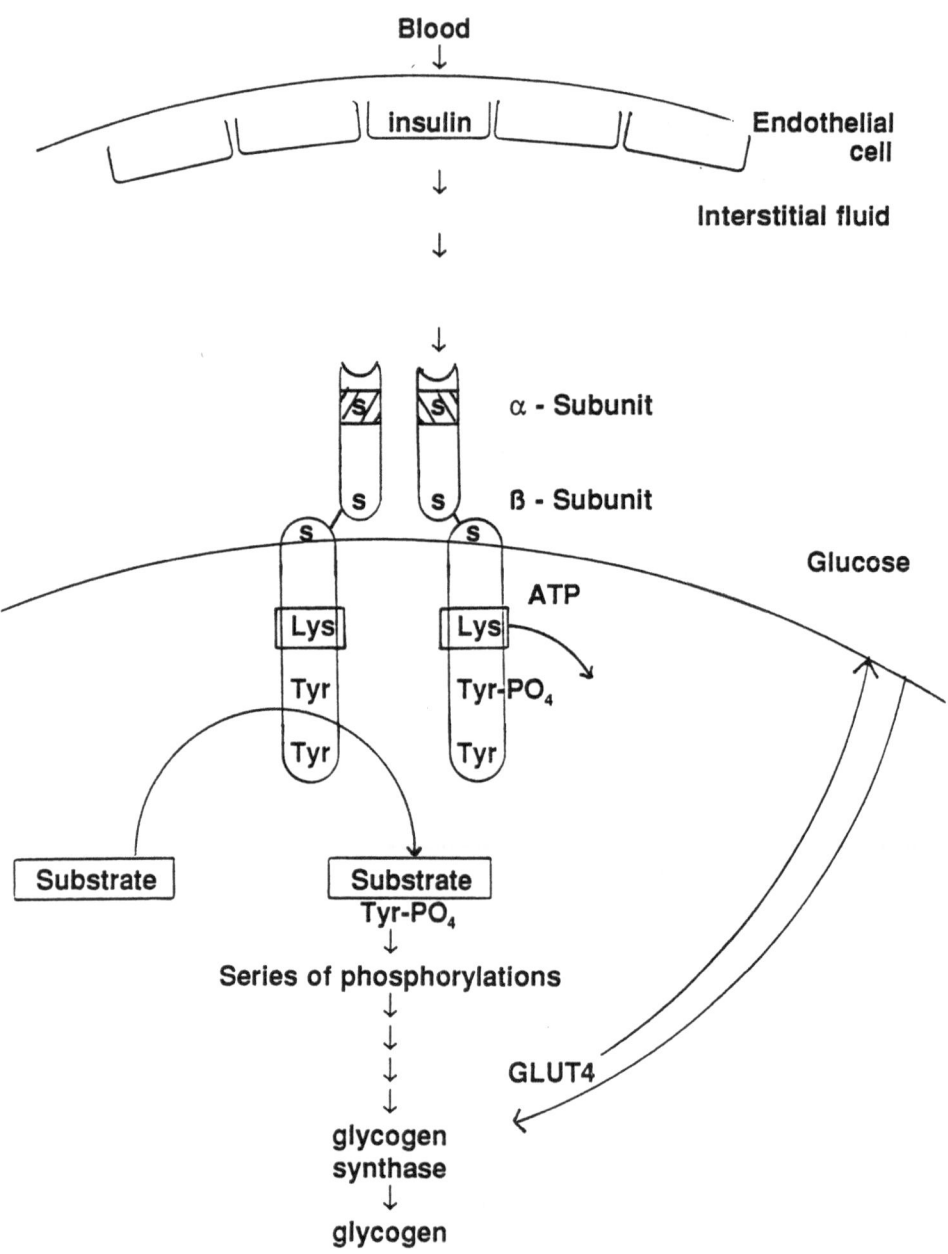

Figure 1.   Model of insulin action in muscle (see text for details)

In obese subjects, the fall in blood pressure associated with exercise training programs seems to be limited to patients who were initially hyperinsulinemic and subsequently had the greatest decrease in plasma insulin levels during training (11, 12). Other interventions such as weight loss and low fat, high fiber diets, also improve insulin sensitivity as well as lower blood pressure (13, 14). The resulting drop in plasma insulin levels directly correlates with the drop in blood pressure.

Hypertension itself, in the absence of obesity and NIDDM, is now recognized as a state of insulin resistance (15-17). Hypertensive subjects have higher basal and stimulated plasma insulin levels compared to age and weight matched controls. Results of euglycemic clamp studies in lean, nondiabetic caucasian hypertensive populations confirm that hypertensive subjects are more insulin resistant than comparable normotensive subjects; Ferranini and colleagues (15) found a 40% reduction in insulin-stimulated glucose utilization in a hypertensive compared to a normotensive group. In fact, Pollare et al (16) demonstrated that the level of insulin resistance directly correlates with the severity of hypertension. The associations between blood pressure and insulin resistance or circulating insulin levels has also been observed in blacks and Chinese and a weaker relationship has been found in Mexican-Americans (17-20). Even in the normotensive caucasian population, Saad et al (21) found a correlation between blood pressure and fasting plasma insulin levels. Thus, even in the absence of obesity, insulin directly impacts on blood pressure or blood pressure impacts on insulin action or there are common factors which are determinants of both.

In order to elucidate the etiology of the defect in insulin action in hypertension, the mechanisms of insulin action must be understood. Insulin resistance can potentially arise at several steps; however, many of the factors which determine or participate in insulin action are unknown at this time (Figure 1). Insulin must first traverse the capillary endothelial cell; this appears to be associated with vasodilation and increased blood flow (22). Upon reaching its target tissue (primarily striated muscle and adipocytes), insulin binds to a cell surface receptor and is internalized (23, 24). This turns on an extensive series of signal transduction events which begins with phosphorylation of an insulin receptor-linked tyrosine kinase (24) and then a recently described protein kinase (25), which, itself, has been shown to control the activity of glycogen synthase and hence, glycogen synthesis. Ultimately, an insulin-sensitive glucose transporter, GLUT 4, in adipose tissue and striated muscle is both transcribed and mobilized to the cell membrane to increase glucose transport into the cell (26-28). GLUT 4 is a member of a family of glucose transporters of which 5 have been described; its translocation from cytoplasmic vesicles to the plasma membrane is the most sensitive of the GLUT members to insulin (29). Skeletal muscle appears to be quantitatively the most important tissue which takes up glucose in response to insulin (30), total skeletal muscle mass accounts for approximately 70% of whole body glucose use (31). Glucose taken up by skeletal muscle is metabolized to lactate and glycogen by the "nonoxidative" pathway. Nuclear magnetic resonance spectroscopy studies suggest muscle glycogen synthesis is the principal pathway of glucose disposal in normal subjects (32). The enzyme, glycogen synthase, regulates glycogen formation; its activity in muscle correlates with muscle glycogen content (33).

In obesity and NIDDM, a post receptor defect in insulin action in the skeletal muscle plays a predominant pathophysiologic role in the insulin resistance associated with these states. Defects in insulin-induced vasodilation, insulin receptor tyrosine kinase activity, muscle glycogen synthase activity and decreased muscle glycogen content have all been described in patients with obesity and NIDDM (22, 32, 33). Bogardus and colleagues (34) found that insulin activation of glycogen synthase phosphatase, which dephosphorylates and activates glycogen synthase, is reduced in humans with insulin resistance. In addition, decreased GLUT 4 mRNA content and activity has been found in adipose tissue of humans with NIDDM and obesity (35). However, in skeletal muscle measurements of GLUT 4 gene expression appear more complicated. In biopsy samples of the *vastus lateralis* muscle, there were no significant differences in GLUT 4 mRNA or protein content in groups of lean, obese and NIDDM patients (36). In contrast, in *rectus abdominus* muscle obtained at surgery, NIDDM patients had decreased GLUT 4 mRNA compared to lean and obese controls and decreased GLUT 4 protein compared to lean controls (37). GLUT 4 protein was similarly decreased in obese controls. Thus, fiber type may affect gene expression and protein content of GLUT 4 in muscle.

In nonobese, nondiabetic subjects with essential hypertension, insulin resistance is also associated with defects in nonoxidative glucose disposal (15). Forearm studies by Ferrannini and colleagues (38), suggest that skeletal muscle is the primary site of insulin resistance in essential hypertension and that there is likely a defect in glycogen synthesis. Glucose extraction by the forearm directly correlated with diastolic blood pressure. Other effects of insulin action, such as cellular potassium uptake and inhibition of lipolysis, were not different in hypertensive and control normotensive groups (15). In contrast, obesity and NIDDM have been associated with abnormalities in these other actions of insulin (15). Nevertheless, all three states of insulin resistance appear to be accompanied by a defect in skeletal muscle glycogen synthesis. In obesity and NIDDM, this appears to be due to decreased glycogen synthase activity (30), which has not been assessed in essential hypertension. Whether other post receptor steps in insulin action such as receptor tyrosine-kinase phosphorylation or GLUT 4 gene expression and concentration are abnormal in essential hypertension also require further assessment. It is possible that the defect in insulin action in the skeletal muscle in each of these disorders begins with a defect in a different step in the cascade of events mediating insulin action and that abnormal glycogen synthesis is the final result. Decreased glucose transport into the cell itself can decrease glycogen synthase activity. Kelly and Mandarino (39) maintained hyperglycemia during insulin clamps in NIDDM subjects and found similar activity of glycogen synthase in NIDDM and normal controls. However, Henry and colleagues (40) demonstrated decreased glycogen synthase activity in NIDDM despite normalization of glucose transport, suggesting an intrinsic defect in glycogen synthase activity exists in NIDDM.

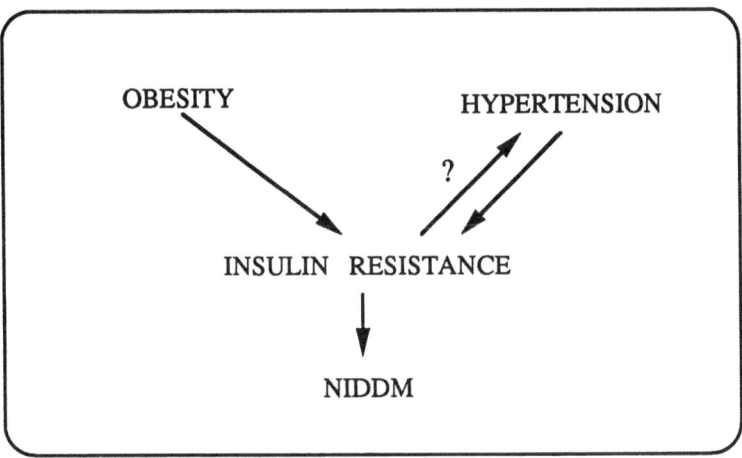

Figure 2.   Obesity leads to insulin resistance. Insulin resistance plays a pathophysiologic role in NIDDM. The relationship between hypertension and insulin resistance remains to be determined. In all of these states skeletal muscle is the major site of insulin resistance.

THE SPECTRUM OF INSULIN RESISTANCE

Since a defect in skeletal muscle glycogen synthesis in response to insulin is a key metabolic abnormality in obesity, NIDDM and hypertension, all of these diseases may represent different degrees in the spectrum of insulin resistance, such that hypertension is associated with the mildest levels of insulin resistance progressing to obesity and then NIDDM. Lean hypertensives have a 40% reduction in insulin-stimulated glucose utilization (15). Obese subjects have an 80% or greater reduction compared to lean normals, while NIDDM subjects have an 80% or more reduction combined with a pancreatic defect in insulin production (5). Each of these states, however, has a different relationship to insulin resistance, since insulin resistance plays a different role in the pathophysiology of these diseases (Figure 2).

121

Obesity induces insulin resistance. The progression from a lean to obese state decreases insulin sensitivity and induces hyperinsulinemia. Weight loss improves insulin sensitivity and decreases insulin levels, although in obesity the weight loss can be modest without necessitating return to the lean state. Thus, weight itself or food intake is a major determinant of insulin action. Therefore, in obesity, derangements in insulin action may result from genetic defects, but are primarily induced by environmental influences on insulin target cells such as increased caloric intake, dietary composition, and physical inactivity (41). Early studies postulated that the insulin resistance and hyperinsulinemia of obesity are the direct result of overeating, particularly carbohydrates (42). Ingestion of excess calories stimulates pancreatic insulin secretion; the resulting chronic hyperinsulinemia down-regulates insulin receptors and decreases insulin binding to target cells (43). However, more recent studies suggest that the insulin resistance of obesity is not due to a decrease in insulin receptors, but due to a post receptor defect (44). It is also possible that alterations in other metabolites, such as increased lipolysis and excess free fatty acids, may induce insulin resistance in obesity. Free fatty acids decrease insulin uptake into skeletal muscle (45).

In lean or obese NIDDM, insulin resistance plays an integral role in the development of the disease. Several longitudinal studies have demonstrated that insulin resistance and hyperinsulinemia occur in the prediabetic state (7, 8). In addition, non-diabetic subjects with a parental history of diabetes have higher plasma insulin levels than nondiabetics without such a parental history (7, 8). Obesity likely contributes to the insulin resistance of NIDDM, since 80% of NIDDM subjects are obese. However, lean NIDDM subjects are also insulin resistant. Since adipocytes from obese individuals display decreased insulin action on both glucose transport and antilipolysis, while adipocytes from NIDDM patients display only abnormalities in glucose transport, Bogardus et al (46) have suggested that the post receptor defect in insulin action is different in obesity compared to NIDDM and obesity. As discussed above, skeletal muscle is a primary tissue, resistant to insulin in NIDDM. However, modeling studies by Bergman (47) and other observations (48) suggest insulin resistance is not the sole defect in NIDDM. Liver production of glucose is inappropriate in NIDDM (49). A defect in pancreatic insulin production to overcome the insulin resistance also plays a prominent role in the development of diabetes (50). In addition, insulin-independent uptake of glucose is also abnormal in NIDDM (47).

The complex relationship between insulin resistance and hypertension is not yet unraveled. A strong correlation exists in certain races, particularly caucasians, but which one precedes the other is the subject of intense interest. A scenario either for insulin resistance causing hypertension or hypertension aggravating insulin resistance could be postulated. In human studies, Haffner and colleagues (20) present compelling evidence that insulin resistance precedes hypertension. In prehypertensive subjects from the San Antonio Heart Study which was composed of Mexican-Americans and non-Hispanic whites, plasma insulin concentrations were 30% higher than in subjects who remained normotensive. However, after adjustment for obesity and body fat distribution, this difference was only of border line statistical significance. Nevertheless, in lean subjects hyperinsulinemia had a predictive value in hypertension, suggesting that insulin may have played a pathophysiologic role in the development of high blood pressure. Ferrari et al (51) recently reported that young lean normotensive offspring of essential hypertensives in Switzerland had higher fasting plasma insulin and lower insulin sensitivity than comparable offspring from normotensive parents. In the Tecumseh study, Julio and coworkers (52) found that borderline hypertensive subjects had higher insulin and triglyceride levels, lower HDL cholesterol levels, but were more overweight than normotensive subjects. In adolescent black males with borderline hypertension, plasma insulin levels and insulin resistance were higher than normotensive controls (53); however, hypertensive subjects were taller with more muscle mass than the normotensives. Thus, a defect in insulin action may be an antecedent to elevated blood pressure. In contrast, no definitive evidence exists that hypertension, *per se*, impacts on insulin action. Longitudinal studies of insulin sensitivity in prehypertensives and hypertensives classified by race, salt sensitivity (54), responses to angiotensin II (55), etc. will be important to further address this issue.

Table 1. Contribution of insulin to the development of elevated blood pressure.

Hyperinsulinemia increases blood pressure by:

1. Enhanced sympathetic nervous system activity
2. Increased renal sodium reabsorption
3. Growth effects on vascular and cardiac smooth muscle
4. Atherogenic effects
5. Ionic effects
    Increased intracellular calcium
    Decreased intracellular magnesium

BLOOD PRESSURE REGULATION AND INSULIN

Insulin has been implicated to contribute to the development and maintenance of elevated blood pressure, since it impacts on a number of systems which ultimately contribute to determination of mean arterial pressure (Table 1). Acute infusion of insulin causes vasodilation *in vivo* or when added to hanging vessels *in vitro* (56). This response may be important for insulin action (22). During insulin clamp studies which maintain physiologic hyperinsulinemia, normal subjects consistently develop sodium retention and enhanced sympathetic nervous system activity (57, 58). Resnick et al (59) suggest hyperinsulinemia may be associated with increased intracellular calcium and decreased intracellular magnesium; both would contribute to increased vascular reactivity as well as enhanced angiotensin II responses. Acute hyperinsulinemia effected by a euglycemic clamp has generally not been associated with increased blood pressure, although Rowe et al (58) reported an increase in blood pressure in normal subjects in this setting. In addition, when angiotensin II (AII) was administered before and during a euglycemic insulin infusion to normal subjects, we observed no difference in the pressor response to AII (T. Buchanan, W. Hsueh unpublished observations). Thus, acute hyperinsulinemia in the physiological range does not appear to increase blood pressure or sensitivity to pressors in normal subjects.

Whether chronic hyperinsulinemia increases blood pressure and thereby contributes to the increased incidence of hypertension in obesity and early NIDDM is currently under investigation. In addition to its other effects on mechanisms which regulate blood pressure, chronic exposure to insulin may also contribute to growth of vascular smooth muscle (60) and may potentiate the development of atherosclerosis (61). Both of these effects could alter vascular reactivity such that normal vasodilatory responses are impaired. Animal studies have demonstrated an inconsistent effect of insulin on blood pressure. Hall et al (62) infused insulin into normal and uremic dogs for 7 days while maintaining euglycemia and found no blood pressure rise in either group, despite salt loading or concomitant norepinephrine infusion. In contrast, 2 rat models (Table 2) have been developed in which hyperinsulinemia precedes a rise in blood pressure. When rats are given 66% fructose in their diet, they develop hepatic insulin resistance and hyperinsulinemia (63). Within 3 weeks on this diet there is a significant rise in blood pressure compared to animals fed a normal diet. Clonidine administration lowered the blood pressure but not the hyperinsulinemia, suggesting a role for the sympathetic nervous system in the development of hypertension but not insulin resistance in this model (64). Exercise (by improving tissue insulin resistance) and somatostatin (by suppressing insulin release) prevented both the hyperinsulinemia and the hypertension (65, 66). Therefore, altering insulin responses impacted on hypertension, suggesting insulin can participate in the development of hypertension. In the hearts of the fructose fed animals the α_2 subunit of sodium-potassium ATP'ase is decreased (67); this also occurs when norepinephrine is added to cultured rat cardiocytes, suggesting there is enhanced adrenergic activity in the fructose-fed model (68). The renal α and β sodium-potassium ATP'ase subunits appeared normal. Thus, in the fructose-fed rat model the sympathetic nervous system plays a prominent role in mediating the hyperinsulinemic-induced rise in blood pressure.

Table 2. Animal models of insulin resistance and hypertension.

RAT MODEL	OBESITY	INSULIN RESISTANT	HYPERTENSION
Fructose-fed	-	+++	++
Insulin infused	-	? probably	+
Zucker	++	+++	+
2 Kidney, 1-clip renovascular	-	-	+++
SHR	-	probably not	+++

In another model, when insulin is administered via osmotic minipump to normal rats in doses which cause physiologic increases in insulin and they are also given 4% glucose and 2% sodium chloride *ad lib* in their drinking water, blood pressure increases compared to saline-infused control animals (69). The blood pressure rises by day 3-4 of the infusion and remains elevated during 10 days of infusion. When the pump is removed, blood pressure falls gradually (10-14 days) to that of control animals. The insulin-infused and saline-infused animals maintained similar body weight throughout the experiments. Blood pressure was measured continuously by an interarterial telemetry device. Preliminary studies suggest the high salt diet plays a role in the development of elevated blood pressure in this model. When insulin was chronically infused intraarterially into a normal rat which was also given large doses of intravenous glucose, Hall et al (70) demonstrated a 10 mm Hg rise in blood pressure which was statistically significant. Although the mechanism of the insulin-induced rise in blood pressure remains to be determined, these models also suggest chronic physiologic hyperinsulinemia can increase blood pressure. In both models, significant hypoglycemia was not present and blood pressure was measured in the conscious, minimally restrained state.

The Zucker rat is a model of genetic obesity which develops Type 2 diabetes mellitus and ultimately glomerulosclerosis (71, 72). This model is hyperinsulinemic and has insulin resistance primarily in peripheral tissues such as skeletal muscles. The Zucker rat has been reported to be hypertensive compared to lean Zucker controls (determined in the unanesthetized state) prior to the development of diabetes (73), although other investigators have not identified an elevated blood pressure in this model (74). Chan and Tuck (T. Chan and M. Tuck, unpublished observations) observed enhanced pressor responses in large and medium size vessels of Zucker animals *in vitro* and found decreased insulin receptor tyrosine kinase activity in vascular smooth muscle of obese animals compared to their lean controls. Insulin resistance to glucose uptake appears to be associated with a decreased vasodilatory response to insulin in obese man (22). It is possible that insulin resistance in the vessels of obese Zucker rats relates to the abnormal vessel response to insulin.

Rocchini and colleagues (14, 75) have demonstrated in humans that insulin enhances renal sodium reabsorption as a mechanism to increase blood pressure in obesity. They found that a high salt diet increased blood pressure in obese caucasian adolescents, but weight loss normalized their pressure natriuresis curves. The drop in blood pressure with weight loss correlated with baseline plasma norepinephrine and plasma aldosterone levels, suggesting these hormones played a role in salt sensitivity in these subjects. These investigators also demonstrated that obese hyperinsulinemic adolescents retain more salt during an oral glucose load compared to nonobese adolescents (14), and that the rise in blood pressure associated with weight gain in the dog is salt-dependent (76). Faulkner et al (53) also reported that adolescent black males with borderline hypertension were hyperinsulinemic, insulin resistant, and salt sensitive. These patients were also reported to have a lower sodium-potassium-chloride cotransport which correlated with sodium sensitivity and a higher intracellular sodium concentration. Thus, a primary effect of insulin on blood pressure may be through its effect on the kidney and cellular ion transport. The sympathetic system may also play a role since obese hypertensive subjects have been reported to have enhanced sympathetic nervous system activity (77) and increased sympathetic activity in the kidney increases sodium reabsorption (78). Humans with insulinoma were reported to be normotensive with no drop in blood pressure after surgery, despite normalization of blood glucose and insulin levels (79). However, patients were significantly hypoglycemic and whether this affected vasoregulatory mechanisms is unknown. Hypoglycemia in the chronic insulin infused rat prevents the rise in blood pressure (Meehan P, Hsueh W, unpublished observations).

Not all obese populations are characterized by hypertension. Pima Indians are generally obese, insulin resistant and have a high incidence of NIDDM, but a relatively low incidence of hypertension compared to caucasian populations (80). In normotensive or hypertensive Pimas, there was no relationship of plasma insulin levels to blood pressure (80). Mexican-Americans also have a higher incidence of insulin resistance and NIDDM, but a lower incidence of hypertension (81). Thus, certain ethnic groups may have activated other mechanisms to overcome the effect of hyperinsulinemia on blood pressure. In support of this possibility is the observation that Mexican-Americans have a lower incidence of salt-sensitivity (82).

DOES HYPERTENSION IMPACT ON INSULIN ACTION?

Hypertension, *per se*, does not appear to directly affect insulin action. In caucasian populations, only 40% of hypertensives manifest insulin resistance and hyperinsulinemia (15). This may be due to the large overlap of these measurements in hypertensive vs normotensive groups, despite matching for age, sex and race. Measurements of plasma insulin are a relatively crude indicator of insulin sensitivity. However, when circulating insulin was measured hourly throughout a 24h period, the hypertensive group had a significantly greater area under their plasma insulin curve than did matched normotensives (9). Using the more sensitive euglycemic clamp technique, there is a 20% coefficient of variation in insulin sensitivity in normals (83), so that small differences in insulin sensitivity may be difficult to detect between hypertensives and normals. In addition, because of its complexity to perform, the clamp approach is impossible to apply to large populations of hypertensives and normotensives. The simpler "minimal model" technique of Bergman (47) will be useful to assess insulin sensitivity in large populations.

Animal models of hypertension also provide some evidence that elevated blood pressure does not affect insulin sensitivity. In the rat 2-kidney, 1-clip Goldblatt model of hypertension, Buchanan et al (84) did not demonstrate insulin resistance in hypertensive compared to normotensive sham-operated animals, using either the euglycemic clamp or the minimal model. Animals were studied at 1 and 3 months of age while awake and free to move. In the hypertensive group, there was also no relationship between blood pressure and the integrated insulin response to injected glucose. Surprisingly, these investigators found a significant direct relationship between blood pressure and plasma insulin levels in the normotensive control group of animals, which is similar to the relationship between blood pressure and plasma insulin in normotensive caucasians. These data suggest that in normal animals there are factors which relate blood pressure and insulin action. However, the induction of secondary hypertension due to activation of the renin-angiotensin system did not detectably reduce insulin sensitivity, suggesting that not all models of hypertension are associated with insulin resistance.

The spontaneously hypertensive rat (SHR) is considered to be a model of human essential hypertension (85). A hyperactive sympathetic nervous system may mediate the hypertension (86), although many other abnormalities in vasoregulatory systems have been identified in the SHR (87). These animals are hyperinsulinemic, largely due to a hyperresponsive pancreatic β cell (88). These animals have been reported to be insulin resistant when studied in the anesthetized state (89). However, when SHR were studied in the conscious, mobile state, results of glucose clamps, performed during somatostatin infusion to suppress endogenous insulin release, demonstrated no difference in glucose clearance or hepatic glucose output between SHR and Wistar Kyoto (WKY) controls (88). Thus, in the face of hypertension in this model insulin's action on glucose metabolism does not appear to be impaired.

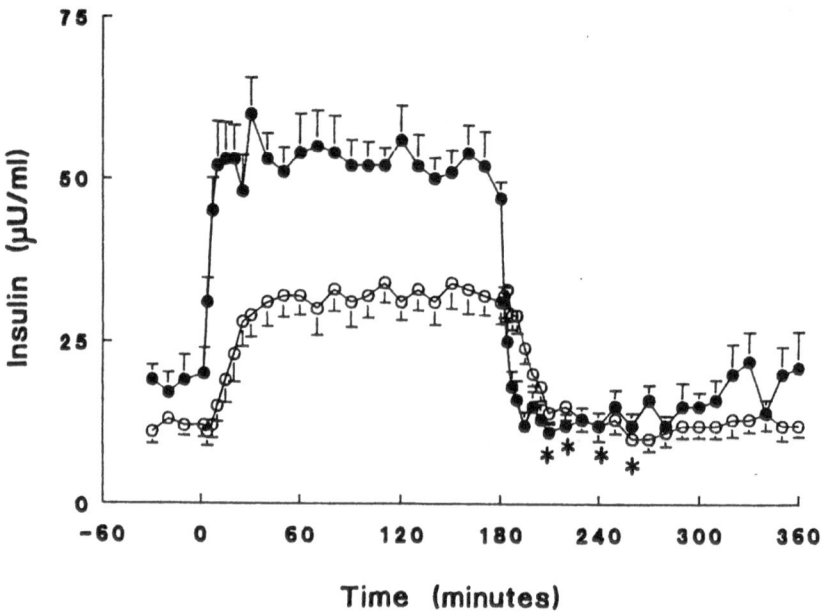

Time (minutes)

Figure 3. Gradient between plasma (closed circles) and lymph (open circles) insulin levels during an insulin infusion. Lymph insulin levels only reach 60% of those in plasma suggesting capillary endothelial cell insulin transport is rate limiting. [Reproduced from Yang JY, Hope ID, Ader M, Bergman RN: Insulin transport across capillaries is rate limiting for insulin action in dogs. J Clin Invest, 84: 1620-1628, 1989, by copyright permission of the American Society of Clinical Investigation].

Although hypertension does not directly affect insulin action, it is possible that chronic elevation of blood pressure may indirectly affect insulin sensitivity.

The first step in insulin action requires that it traverse the capillary endothelium from the plasma to reach insulin sensitive tissues. The endothelium is a major target organ of damage resulting from hypertension (90), so that endothelial cell damage may impair insulin transport. Insulin binds to a receptor on endothelial cells and is internalized, whereupon it can be shuttled to two possible pathways (91). One is to the lysosome which is associated with degradation. The other pathway involves transport of insulin through endothelial cells by plasmalemmal vesicles and release into subendothelial tissue as biologically intact insulin. The majority of insulin is shunted to the latter pathway (probably >90%), although endothelial cells from different vascular beds shunt to the two pathways differently. Capillary endothelial cells degrade less insulin and transport more insulin than large vessel endothelial cells (92).

Bergman and colleagues (93) demonstrated a gradient between plasma and lymph insulin levels in the dog, such that lymph insulin levels rose slower than plasma levels during an insulin infusion and peaked at only 60% of the levels reached in plasma (Figure 3). These data suggest endothelial insulin transport may regulate levels of insulin ultimately seen by target tissue. A plasma-lymph gradient of insulin has also been demonstrated in the rat (94).

Insulin has vasodilatory activity and its action on glucose transport has been linked to its vasodilatory response. Obese subjects were demonstrated to have decreased leg glucose uptake in response to insulin, which correlated with a diminished increase in leg blood flow (22). Based on theoretical calculations, leg blood flow contributed up to 40% of leg glucose uptake in high physiologic concentrations in normal individuals. These data suggest that the inability of insulin to increase blood flow in insulin-sensitive tissues in obese subjects contributes to their decreased insulin sensitivity (95).

In forearm studies in normal subjects, certain vasodilators enhanced both blood flow and glucose uptake in the absence of administration of exogenous insulin (96). Thus, vasodilators such as insulin, kinins and prostaglandins may be opening up previously underperfused capillaries exposing more muscle cells to insulin and glucose, thereby leading to increased glucose uptake by muscle cells. Whether the action of these vasodilators requires intact endothelial cells is a critical issue. Endothelial cells release a family of "endothelial-derived relaxing factors" (EDRF) which are nitrovasodilators (97). Substances such as acetylcholine, which antagonize the vasoconstrictive effect of norepinephrine, do so only in vessels with intact endothelium (98). Acetylcholine and other vasodilators such as bradykinin, serotonin, histamine, etc. act by stimulating EDRF release from endothelium. Endothelial cell damage by hypertension could also potentially impair EDRF vasodilatory responses (90). In addition, in the presence of hypertension endothelial cell morphology changes, permeability increases and there is deposition of connective tissue matrix with intimal thickening (90).

Whether damage or dysfunction of endothelial cells impairs insulin transport to subendothelial tissues or prevents normal vasodilatory responses leading to insulin resistance remains to be investigated.

HYPERTENSION, HYPERINSULINEMIA AND THE RISK OF ATHEROSCLEROSIS

Hypertension is a well defined risk factor for atherosclerosis (100). Endothelial damage resulting from hypertension is likely a contributing factor to the development of atherosclerosis in the vascular wall. Damage or dysfunction of the endothelium has been implicated to causally participate in the formation of the atherosclerotic plaque (101). In high-fat, low-cholesterol fed monkeys, the first morphologic change detected in the vasculature was the adherence of LDL laden monocytes to the endothelial surface (102). These monocytes continued to accumulate between endothelial cells and in subendothelial areas to form fatty streaks to which smooth muscle cells gradually migrate. In some areas the endothelial cells were denuded, exposing the fatty streaks to the circulation and providing sites for platelet adherence, aggregation, and thrombosis. These streaks advanced to plaques containing a proliferation of smooth muscle cells and collagen (103). Endothelial cells produce a host of vasoactive substances and growth factors that regulate vascular smooth muscle cell activity in a paracrine fashion (97). Loss of normal production of these factors combined with frank loss of the mechanical barrier the endothelium provides from the circulation, leads to intimal accumulation of smooth muscle cells, which in addition to endothelial damage is critical in the development of atherosclerosis (104). Hypertension accelerates this entire process (105).

Insulin impacts on a number of steps in the pathogenesis of atherosclerosis, such that Stout and coworkers (61) suggest that chronic physiologic elevations of insulin are atherogenic. Long-term insulin administration increases intimal lipid deposition in some animals (106) and inhibits regression of diet-induced atherosclerosis (107). *In vitro*, insulin stimulates cholesterol synthesis and LDL binding in vascular smooth muscle cells and in monocyte macrophages (108). Perfusion studies suggest insulin stimulates the uptake of labeled glucose into aortic lipids (109). Insulin is also a potent mitogen to stimulate proliferation of vascular smooth muscle cells (110). This effect is largely mediated through insulin-like growth factor 1 (IGF1) receptors, which are different from the insulin receptors mediating glucose transport (111, 112). Thus, in states of insulin resistance associated with receptor or post receptor defects, proliferative effects in response to insulin may still occur. In addition to proliferation, insulin has effects on migration of smooth muscle cells. These cells migrate from media to intima in the process of atherosclerosis formation (101). Insulin does not itself stimulate vascular smooth muscle cell migration, but augments 12-HETE, though not PDGF-induced migration (113).

Epidemiologic studies have demonstrated an independent association between hyperinsulinemia and ischemic heart disease. Five population studies found higher insulin responses to oral glucose in subjects at greater risk of cardiovascular disease (114-119). Three prospective studies suggest that hyperinsulinemia precedes a coronary artery disease event (116-119). In caucasian male government workers followed for 5-10 years, the incidence of coronary artery disease was significantly greater in subjects who had either higher fasting or 2h glucose-stimulated insulin levels (116). In another study which included caucasian men and women, 1h glucose-stimulated insulin levels were significantly related to the 6 year incidence of and 12 year mortality from coronary artery disease in men, but not in women (119). Zavaroni, et al (120) performed a meta-analysis of these prospective studies and found that the hyperinsulinemic groups tended to have other risk factors for atherosclerosis which included high triglycerides, lower HDL-cholesterol, higher total cholesterol, more obesity (particularly upper body), more glucose intolerance and a greater incidence of hypertension. Insulin stimulates hepatic VLDL triglyceride production and secretion, but whether it contributes to development of these other risk factors for atherosclerotic heart disease remains to be investigated. Williams and colleagues (121) found that these risk factors co-cluster in 12% of the hypertensive population and in some hypertensive families. Thus, clinical and epidemiologic evidence support animal and tissue studies suggesting hyperinsulinemia may contribute to the development of atherosclerosis.

THERAPEUTIC IMPLICATIONS

The treatments of hypertension and NIDDM are clearly impacted by these studies. Weight loss and physical training is the best approach to both, since these activities lower blood pressure and improve insulin resistance. However, compliance may be a problem. If pharmacologic agents must be employed, their effects on carbohydrate and lipid metabolism and risk factors for atherosclerosis must be carefully considered.

Measurement of circulating insulin or assessment of insulin resistance is not clinically applicable at this time in each isolated case of essential hypertension. However, a complete assessment of risk factors for atherosclerosis is warranted with the consideration that hyperinsulinemia will likely be present in hypertensive subjects with obesity or NIDDM and may be more prevalent in caucasian and oriental hypertensives compared to hypertensives of other ethnic origins. Thus, in high-risk patients, the choice of anti-hypertensive therapy should favorably impact on insulin action and lipid profiles rather than worsen these parameters.

Thiazide diuretics and β-blockers, previously integral components of the antihypertensive regime, have unfavorable effects on both carbohydrate and lipid metabolism. Thiazide diuretics worsen peripheral insulin sensitivity and impair pancreatic insulin release; these effects may be due, in part, to potassium and magnesium depletion (122, 123). Thiazides also increase VLDL triglyceride and LDL cholesterol levels without changing HDL cholesterol (124). Beta-blockers, both cardioselective and non-selective, decrease insulin sensitivity, decrease nutrient stimulated insulin levels and reduce HDL cholesterol (124, 125). Both the thiazide and β-blocker class of antihypertensives increase the tendency to glucose intolerance in patients with essential hypertension; patients on the combination have a 12-fold increase incidence of developing diabetes mellitus (126).

Calcium channel blockers, in general, have no detectable effect on insulin action or plasma lipids. Essential hypertensive patients studied before and after 24 weeks of diltiazem demonstrated no change in insulin sensitivity when they were studied using a euglycemic, hyperinsulinemic clamp (125). Lipid profiles also remained unaltered during this study. Verapamil and nifedipine have been reported to have no effect on plasma lipids (124). Because the various calcium channel blockers have differing mechanisms of action, each specific agent needs to be studied for its effects on insulin sensitivity.

Two agents, captopril and prazosin, have been demonstrated with the euglycemic clamp to improve insulin sensitivity in patients with essential hypertension (127, 128). Using the euglycemic clamp, Pollare, et al (127) found a 12% improvement in insulin sensitivity in hypertensive subjects given chronic captopril for 4 months; this was associated with a slight reduction in circulating insulin levels and no change in lipid profiles. In hypertensive patients with NIDDM, Rett et al (129) demonstrated a 40% increase in glucose utilization during a euglycemic, hyperinsulinemic clamp study after a single oral dose of 25 mg captopril. In normal subjects, these investigators also demonstrated that captopril caused an increase in forearm glucose uptake which correlated with an increase in forearm blood flow (129). Captopril stimulates tissue kinins and vasodilatory prostaglandins (130), which may contribute to its effect on insulin action. When bradykinin or PGE_2 are administered to normal subjects, both increase forearm blood flow as well as glucose uptake (96). Whether other angiotensin converting enzyme (ACE) inhibitors have a similar effect on insulin action remains to be determined. As a class ACE inhibitors do not alter lipid profiles in hypertensive or hypertensive diabetic subjects (127, 131), although one study reported improved levels of total cholesterol, HDL cholesterol, and triglycerides with long-term captopril administration (132). Captopril may also have a positive local vascular effect since it inhibits myointimal proliferation (133), which is a major vascular structural change in hypertension and atherosclerosis.

Prazosin, the α_1 adrenoreceptor blocking drug, improved insulin sensitivity in obese hypertensive men as demonstrated by the euglycemic clamp and improved glucose uptake by 14% (128). In another group of patients with mild hypertension prazosin decreased insulin responses measured every 2 hours throughout the day and significantly decreased fasting plasma triglyceride and total cholesterol concentrations, increased HDL cholesterol, and decreased apolipoprotein B levels by 25% (134). This impressive effect on lipid profiles is consistent with what has been demonstrated for blockade of the alpha adrenergic system. Alpha blockade has been shown to cause increased serum lipoprotein lipase activity, increased hydrolysis of triglyceride rich lipoproteins, increased receptor-mediated clearance of LDL cholesterol and inhibition of hepatic cholesterol and triglyceride synthesis. The exact role of the sympathetic nervous system in these functions are unknown. However, these observations on ACE inhibitors and alpha blockades provide rational approaches to lowering blood pressure while improving carbohydrate and lipid metabolism and vascular cell biology.

REFERENCES

1. Kannel WB, Npahtali B, Skinner JJ, et al: The relation of adiposity to blood pressure and development of hypertension: The Framingham Study. Ann Int Med, 67: 48-59, 1967.
2. Stamer R, Stamler J, Reidinger WF, Algera G, Roberts RH: Weight and blood pressure findings in hypertension screening of one million Americans. JAMA, 240: 1607-1610, 1978.
3. National Heart Blood & Lung Institute. Hypertension Statistics, 1989.
4. Sowers JR, Levy J, Zemel MB: Hypertension and Diabetes. The Medical Clinics of North America, 72: 1399-1414, 1988.
5. Kolterman IG, Insel J, Saekow M, Olefsky JM: Mechanisms of insulin resistance in human obesity. J Clin Invest, 65: 1273, 1980.
6. Hollenbeck CB, Chen Y-DI, Reaven GM: A comparison of the relative effects of obesity and insulin-dependent diabetes mellitus on *in vivo* insulin stimulated glucose utilization. Diabetes, 33: 622-626, 1984.
7. Eriksson J, Franssila-Kallunki A, Ekstrand A, et al: Early metabolic defects in persons at risk for non-insulin dependent diabetes mellitus. N Engl J Med, 321: 337-343, 1989.
8. Saad MF, Knowler WC, Pettitt DJ, Nelson RG, Mott DM, Bennett PH: Sequential changes in serum insulin concentration during development of non-insulin-dependent diabetes. Lancet, I: 1356-1359, 1989.
9. Swislocki ALM, Hoffman BB, Reaven GM: Insulin resistance, glucose intolerance and hyperinsulinemia in patients with hypertension. Amer Jour Hyper, 2: 419-423, 1989.
10. Manicardi V, Camellini L, Bellodi G, Coscelli C, Ferrannini E: Evidence for an association of high blood pressure and hyperinsulinemia in obese man. J Clin Endocrinol Metab, 62: 1302-1304, 1986.
11. Krotkiewski M, Mandroukas K, Sjostrom L, Sullivan L, Wetterqvist H, Bjorntorp P: Effects of long-term physical training on body fat, metabolism and blood pressure. Metabolism, 28: 650-658, 1979.
12. Bjorntorp P, de Jonge K, Sullivan L: The effect of physical training on insulin production in obesity. Metabolism, 19: 631-638, 1970.

13. Reisin E, Abel R, Modan M, Silverberg DS, Eliahou HE, Modan B: Effect of weight loss without salt restriction in the reduction of blood pressure in overweight hypertensive patients. N Engl J Med, 298: 1-6, 1978.
14. Rocchini AP, Key J, Bondie D, Chico R, Moorehead C, Katch V, Martin M: The effect of weight loss on sensitivity of blood pressure to sodium in obese adolescents. N Engl J Med, 321: 580-585, 1989.
15. Ferrannini E, Buzzigoli G, Bonadonna R, Giorico MA, Oleggini M, Graziadei L, Pedrinelli R, Brandi L, Bevilacqua S: Insulin resistance in essential hypertension. N Engl J Med, 317: 350-357, 1987.
16. Pollare T, Lithell H, Berne C: Insulin resistance is a characteristic feature of primary hypertension independent of obesity. Metabolism, 39: 167-174, 1990.
17. Reaven GM, Hoffman BB: A role for insulin in the aetiology and course of hypertension? Lancet, II: 435-437, 1987.
18. Falkner B: Differences in blacks and whites with essential hypertension: biochemistry and endocrine, Hypertension, 15: 681-686, 1990.
19. Shen D-C, Shieh S-M, Fuh MM-T, Wu D-A, Chen Y-DI, Reaven GM: Resistance to insulin-stimulated-glucose uptake in patients with hypertension. J Clin Endocrinol Metab, 66: 580-583, 1988.
20. Haffner SM, Ferrannini E, Hazuda HP, Stern MP: Clustering of cardiovascular risk factors in confirmed prehypertensive individuals: The San Antonio heart study, 1991 (submitted for publication).
21. Saad MF, Lillioja S, Nyomba BL, Castillo C, Ferraro R, Gregorio MD, Ravussin E, Knowler WC, Bennett PH, Howard BV and Bogardus C: Racial differences in the relation between blood pressure and insulin resistance. N Engl J Med, 324: 733-739, 1991.
22. Laakso M, Edelman SV, Brechtel G, Baron AD: Decreased effect of insulin to stimulate skeletal muscle blood flow in obese man. J Clin Invest, 85: 1844-1852, 1990.
23. Kolterman OG, Gray RS, Griffin PB, Insel J, Scarlett JA, Olefsky JM: Receptor and postreceptor defects contribute to the insulin resistance in non-insulin-dependent diabetes mellitus. J Clin Invest, 68: 957-969, 1981.
24. Kahn CR, White MF: The insulin receptor and the molecular mechanisms of insulin action. J Clin Invest, 83: 1151-1156, 1988.
25. Gottesman MM, Pastan I: The multidrug transporter, a double edged sword. J Biol Chem, 263: 12163-12166, 1988.
26. Thorens B, Sarkar HK, Kaback HR, Lodish HF: Cloning and functional expression in bacteria of a novel glucose transporter present in liver, intestine, kidney and pancreatic islets. Cell, 55: 281-290, 1988.
27. Bell GI, Kayano T, Buse JB, Burant CF, Takeda J, Lin D, Fukumoto H, Seino S: Molecular biology of mammalian glucose transporters. Diabetes Care, 13: 198-208, 1990.
28. Thorens B, Charron MJ, Lodish HF: Molecular Physiology of Glucose Transporters. Diabetes Care, 13: 209-218, 1990.
29. Klip A, Paquet MR: Glucose transport and glucose transporters in muscle and their metabolic regulation. Diabetes Care, 13: 228-243, 1990.
30. Bogardus C: Perspective: does insulin resistance primarily affect skeletal muscle? Diabetes/Metabolism Reviews, 5: 527-528, 1989.
31. Kida Y, Esposito-Del Puente A, Bogardus C, Mott DM: Insulin resistance is associated with reduced fasting and insulin-stimulated glycogen synthase phosphatase activity in human skeletal muscle. J Clin Invest, 85: 476-481, 1990.
32. Shulman GI, Rothman DL, Jue T, Stein P, Defronzo RA, Shulman RG: Quantitation of muscle glycogen synthesis in normal subjects and subjects with non-insulin-dependent diabetes by ^{13}C nuclear magnetic resonance spectroscopy. N Engl J Med, 322: 223-228, 1990.
33. Bogardus C, Lillioja S, Stone K, Mott D: Correlation between muscle glycogen synthase activity and in vivo insulin action in man. J Clin Invest, 73: 1185-1190, 1984.
34. Freymond D, Bogardus C, Okubo M, Stone K, Mott D: Impaired insulin-stimulated muscle glycogen synthase activation in vivo in man is related to low fasting glycogen synthase phosphatase activity. J Clin Invest, 82: 1503-1509, 1988.
35. Garvey WT, Maianu L, Huecksteadt TP, Birnbaum MJ, Molina JM, Ciaraldi TP. GLUT4 Transporter Gene expression in NIDDM. J Clin Invest, 1991 (in press).

36. Pederson O, Bak JF, Andersen PH, Lund S, Moller DE, Flier JS, Kahn BB: Evidence against altered expression of GLUT 1 or GLUT 4 in skeletal muscle of patients with obesity of NIDDM. Diabetes, 39: 865-870, 1988.

37. Elton CW, Roy L, Moller DE, Pilch PF, Pories WJ, Atkinson SM, Dohm GL: Decreased expression of an insulin-sensitive glucose transporter in muscle from insulin-resistant obese and diabetic patients. Diabetes, 39 (suppl. 1): 120A, 1990.

38. Natali A, Santora D, Palombo C, Cerri M, Ghione S, Ferrannini E: Impaired insulin action on skeletal muscle metabolism in essential hypertension. Hypertension, 17: 170-178, 1991.

39. Kelley D, Mandarino LJ: Hyperglycemia normalizes insulin-stimulated skeletal muscle glucose oxidation and storage in noninsulin-dependent diabetes mellitus. J Clin Invest, 86: 1999-2007, 1990.

40. Thorburn AW, Gumbiner B, Bulacan F, Brechtel G, Henry RR: Multiple defects in muscle glycogen synthase activity contribute to reduced glycogen synthesis in non-insulin dependent diabetes mellitus. J Clin Invest, 87: 489-495, 1991.

41. Salans LB: The Obesities. In: "Endocrinology and Metabolism" (Eds P Felig, JD Baxter, AE Broadus, LA Frohman), McGraw-Hill, New York, 1987.

42. Grey N, Kipnis DM: Effect of diet composition on hyperinsulinemia of obesity. N Engl J Med, 285: 837, 1975.

43. Roth J, Kahn CR, Lesniask MA, Gorden P, De Meyts P, Megyesi K, Meville DM, Gavin JR, Soll AH, Freychet P, Goldine I, Barr Rs, Archer JA: Receptors for insulin NSILA-S and growth hormone. Recent Prog Horm Res, 31: 95, 1975.

44. Olefsky J, Kolterman O: Mechanisms of insulin resistance in obesity and noninsulin-dependent (type II) diabetes. Am J Med, 70: 151, 1981.

45. Reaven GM: The role of insulin resistance in the pathogenesis and treatment of noninsulin dependent diabetes mellitus. Am J Med, 74: 1, 1983.

46. Bogardus C: Perspective: Does insulin resistance primarily affect skeletal muscle? Diabetes Met Rev, 5: 527-528, 1989.

47. Bergman RN: Toward physiological understanding of glucose tolerance. Minimal-model approach. Diabetes, 38: 1512-1527, 1989.

48. DeFronzo RA: The triumvirate: ß-cell, muscle, liver   A collusion responsible for NIDDM. Diabetes, 37: 667-687, 1988.

49. DeFronzo RA, Simonson D, Ferrannini E: Hepatic and peripheral insulin resistance: a common feature in non-insulin dependent and insulin dependent diabetes. Diabetologia, 23: 313-319, 1982.

50. Unger RH: Diabetic hyperglycemia: link to impaired glucose transport in pancreatic ß cells. Science, 251: 1200-1205, 1991.

51. Ferrari P, Weidmann P, Shaw S, Giachino D, Riesen W, Allemann Y, Heynen G: Altered insulin sensitivity, hyperinsulinemia, and dyslipidemia in hypertension prone humans. Clin Res, 39: 353A, 1991.

52. Julius S, Jamerson K, Mejia A, Krause L, Schork N, Jones K: The association of borderline hypertension with target organ changes and higher coronary risk. Techumseh Blood Pressure Study. JAMA, 264: 354-358, 1990.

53. Falkner B, Hulman S, Tannenbaum, et al: Insulin resistance and blood pressure in young black males. Hypertension, 12: 352, 1988.

54. Campese VM, Ramoff MS, Levitan D: Abnormal relationship between sodium intake and sympathetic nervous activity in salt sensitive patients with essential hypertension. Kidney Int, 21: 371-378, 1982.

55. Hollenberg NK, Moor T, Shoback D, Redgrave J, Rabinowe S, Williams GH: Abnormal renal sodium handling in essential hypertension. Relation to failure of renal and adrenal modulation of responses to angiotensin II. Am J Med, 81: 412-418, 1986.

56. Yagi S, Takata S, Kiyokawa H, Yamamoto M, Noto Y, Ikeda T, Hattori N: Effects of insulin on vasoconstrictive responses to norepinephrine and angiotensin II in rabbit femoral artery and vein. Diabetes, 37: 1064-1067, 1988.

57. DeFronzo RA: The effect of renal sodium motabolism. Diabetologia, 21: 165-171, 1981.

58. Rowe JW, Young JB, Minaker KL, Stevens AL, Patotta J, Landsberg L: Effect of insulin and glucose infusions on sympathetic nervous system activity in normal man. Diabetes, 30: 219, 1981.

59. Resnick LM, Gupta RK, Gruenspan H, Alderman MH, Laragh JH: Hypertension and peripheral insulin resistance. Possible mediating role of intracellular free magnesium. Am J Hyper, 3: 373-379, 1990.

60. Stout RW, Bierman EL, Ross R: Effect of insulin on the proliferation of cultured primate arterial smooth muscle cells. Circ Res, 36: 319-327, 1980.
61. Stout RW: Insulin and atheroma 20-yr perspective. Diabetes, 13: 631-654, 1990.
62. Hall JE, Coleman TG, Mizelle HL, Smith MJ Jr: Chronic hyperinsulinemia and blood pressure regulation. Am J Physiol, 258: F722-F731, 1990.
63. Young JB, Landsberg L: Effect of oral sucrose on blood pressure in the spontaneously hyperactive rat. Metabolism, 30: 421-424, 1981.
64. Hwang IS, Ho H, Hoffman BB, Reaven GM: Fructose induced insulin resistance and hypertension in rats. Hypertension, 10: 512-516, 1987.
65. Reaven G, Ho H, Hoffman BB: Attenuation of fructose-induced hypertension in rats by exercise training. Hypertension, 12: 129-132, 1988.
66. Reaven G, Ho H, Hoffman BB: Somatostatin inhibition of fructose-induced hypertension. Hypertension, 14: 117-120, 1989.
67. Crnkovic-Markovic R, Putnam D, McDonough AA: Differential expression of Na,K-ATPase subunits in Sprague-Dawley rats with fructose induced hypertension and hyperinsulinemia. Circulation, 82: III-87, 1990.
68. Hensley CB, Ming JT, Azuma KK, McDonough AA: Thyroid hormone alters the ration of Na, K-ATPase α_1, and α_2 proteins in myocardial cells *in vivo*. Circulation, 82: III-350, 1990.
69. Meehan WP, Buchanan TA, Shargill NS, Hsueh WA: High blood pressure research: insulin, obesity, and metabolic abnormalities of hypertension. Circulation, 82: III-86, 1990.
70. Brands MW, Hildebrandt DA, Mizelle HL, Hall JE: Sustained hyperinsulinemia increases arterial pressure in conscious rats. Am J Physiol, 260: R764-R768, 1991.
71. Bray GA: The Zucker family rat. A review. Fed Proc, 36: 148-153, 1977.
72. O'Donnell MP, Kasiske BL, Cleary MP, Keane WF: Effects of genetic obesity on renal structure and function in the Zucker rat. J Lab Clin Med, 106 (5): 598-604, 1985.
73. Kurtz TW, Morris RC, Pershadsingh HA: The Zucker fatty rat as a genetic model of obesity and hypertension. Hypertension, 13: 896-901, 1989.
74. Barringer DL, Bunag RD: Uneven blunting of chronotropic baroreflexes in obese Zucker rats. Am J Physiol, 256: H417-H421, 1989.
75. Rocchini AP, Katch V, Kveselis D, Moorhead C, Martin M, Lampman R, Gregory M: Insulin and renal sodium retention in obese adolescents. Hypertension, 14: 367-374, 1989.
76. Rocchini AP, Moorehead C, London M: Salt is critical for the development of weight gain induced hypertension. Circulation 82: III-87, 1990.
77. Tuck ML, Sowers J, Dornfeld L, Kledzik G, Maxwell M: The effect of weight reduction on blood pressure, plasma renin activity and plasma aldosterone levels in obese patients. N Engl J Med, 304: 930-933, 1981.
78. Campese VM, Ramoff MS, Levitan D, Saglikes Y, Fiedler RM, Massry SG: Abnormal relationship between sodium intake and sympathetic nervous activity in salt sensitive patients with essential hypertension. Kidney Int, 21: 371-378, 1982.
79. Nobutaka T, Nunoi K, Kodama T, Nomiyama R, Iwase M, Jujishima M: Lack of association between blood pressure and insulin in patients with insulinoma. J Hypertension, 8: 479-482, 1990.
80. Saad M, Knowler W, Pettitt DJ, Nelson RG, Mott DM, Bennett PH: Insulin and hypertension relationship to obesity and glucose intolerance in Pima Indians. Diabetes, 39: 1430-1435, 1990.
81. Haffner S, Fong D, Hazadu HP, Pugh JA, Patterson JK: Hyperinsulinemia, upper body adiposity, and cardiovascular risk factors in non-diabetics. Metabolism, 37: 338-345, 1988.
82. Weinberger MH, Miller JZ, Luft FC, Grim CE, Fineberg NS: Definitions and characteristics of sodium sensitivity and blood pressure resistance. Hypertension, 8: 127-134, 1986.
83. Foley JE, Chen YD, Lardinois CK, Hollenbeck CB, Liu GC, Reaven GM: Estimates of *in vivo* insulin action in humans: comparison of the insulin clamp and the minimal model techniques. Horm Metab Res, 17: 406-409, 1985.
84. Buchanan TA, Sipos GF, Gadalah S, Yip K-P, Marsh DJ, Hsueh WA: Glucose tolerance, insulin responses to glucose and insulin sensitivity in rats with renovascular hypertension. 1991 (submitted for publication).
85. Yamori Y, Ooshima A, Okamoto K: Genetic factors involved in spontaneous hypertension in rats: an analysis of F2 segregate generation. Jpn Circ J, 36: 561-568, 1972.
86. Saavedra JM, Grobecker H, Axelrod J: Changes in centra catecholaminergic neurons in the spontaneously (genetic) hypertensive rat. Circ Res, 42: 529-534, 1978.

87. Bianchi G, Ferrari P, Barber BR: Lessons from experimental genetic hypertension. In: "Hypertension: pathophysiology, diagnosis and management" (Eds JH Laragh and BM Brenner) Raven Press Ltd, New York, 1990.

88. Buchanan TA, Sipos G, Liu C, Campese V: Hyperinsulinemia in spontaneously hypertensive rats. Clinical Research, 38: 109A, 1990.

89. Mondon CE, Reaven GM: Evidence of abnormalities of insulin metabolism in rats with spontaneous hypertension. Metabolism, 37: 303-305, 1988.

90. Chobanian AV: Adaptive and maladaptive responses of the arterial wall to hypertension. Hypertension, 15: 666-674, 1990.

91. Hachiya HL, Halban PA, King GL: Intracellular pathways of insulin transport across vascular endothelial cells. Am J Physiol, 255: C459-C464, 1988.

92. King GL, Buzney S, Kahn CR, Hetu N, Buchwald S, McDonald S, Rand LI: Differential responsiveness to insulin of endothelial and support cells from micro- and macrovessels. J Clin Invest, 71: 974-979, 1983.

93. Yang JY, Hope ID, Ader M, Bergman RN: Insulin transport across capillaries is rate limiting for insulin action in dogs. J Clin Invest, 84: 1620-1628, 1989.

94. Bryer-Ash M, Hodges N: Intravascular and interstitial compartmentalization of insulin in normal and diabetic rats. Clin Res, 39: 38A, 1991.

95. Lasko MS, Edelman SV, Olefsky JM, Brechtel G, Wallace P, Baron AD: Kinetics of in vivo muscle insulin-mediated glucose uptake in human obesity. Diabetes, 39: 965-974, 1990.

96. Dietze GJ, Rett K, Wicklmayer M, Mehnert H: ACE-inhibitors and glucose metabolism. Wein Med Wochenschr, 140: 35-39, 1990.

97. Brenner BM, Troy JL, Ballerman BJ: Endothelium-dependent vascular reponses, mediators and mechanisms. J Clin Invest, 84: 1373-1378, 1989.

98. Furchgott RF, Zawadski JV: The obligatory role of endothelial cells in the relaxation of arterial smooth muscle by acetylcholine. Nature, 288: 373-376, 1987.

99. Kannel WB: Hypertension and the risk of cardiovascular disease. In: "Hypertension: pathophysiology, diagnosis and management" (Eds JH Laragh and BM Brenner) Raven Press Ltd, New York, 1990.

100. Smith WM: Epidemiology of hypertension. Med Clin North Am, 61: 467-486, 1977.

101. Ross R: The pathogenesis of atherosclerosis - an update. N Engl J Med, 314: 488-500, 1986.

102. Faggiotto A, Ross R, Harker L: Studies of hypercholesterolemia in the nonhuman primate. I. Changes that lead to fatty streak formation. Arteriosclerosis, 4: 323-340, 1984.

103. Faggiotto A, Ross R: Studies of hypercholesterolemia in the nonhuman primate. II. Fatty streak conversion in fibrous plaque. Arteriosclerosis, 4: 341-356, 1984.

104. Ross R, Glomset JA: Atherosclerosis and the arterial smooth muscle cell. Proliferation of smooth muscle is a key event in the genesis of the lesions of atherosclerosis. Science, 180: 1332-1339, 1973.

105. Chobanian A: Overview: hypertension and atherosclerosis. Am Heart J, 116: 319-322, 1988.

106. Duff GL, Brechin DJH, Findelstein WE: The effect of alloxin diabetes on experimental cholesterol atherosclerosis in the rabbit. IV. The effect of insulin therapy on the inhibition of atherosclerosis in the alloxan-diabetic rabbit. J Exp Med, 100: 371-380, 1954.

107. Wilson RB, Martin JM, Hartroft WS: Failure of insulin therapy to prevent cardiovascular lesions in diabetic rats fed an atherogenic diet. Diabetes, 18: 225-231, 1969.

108. Stout RW, Buchanan KD, Vallance-Owen J: Arterial lipid metabolism in relation to blood glucose and plasma insulin in rats with streptozotocin-induced diabetes. Diabetologia, 8: 398-401, 1972.

109. Capron L, Philippe M, Fiessinger JN, Housset E: Diabetes and insulin: actions and interactions upon the glucose metabolism of rat aorta. Diabete Metab, 10: 78-84, 1984.

110. Pfeifle B, Ditschuneit H: Effect of insulin on growth of cultured human arterial smooth muscle cells. Diabetologia, 20: 155-158, 1981.

111. Pfeifle B, Ditschuneit H: Two seperate receptors for insulin and insulinlike growth factors on arterial smooth muscle cells. Exp Clin Endocrinol, 81: 280-286, 1983.

112. King GL, Kahn CR, Rechler MM, Nissley SP: Direct demonstration of separate receptors for growth and metabolic activities of insulin and multiplication-stimulating activity (an insulinlike growth factor) using antibodies to the insulin receptor. J Clin Invest, 66: 130-140, 1980.

113. Nakao J, Ito H, Kanayasu T, Muroto S-I: Stimulatory effect of insulin on aortic smooth muscle cellmigraton induced by 12-L-hydroxy-5, 8, 10, 14-eicosatetraenoic acid and its modulation by elevated extracellular glucose levels. Diabetes, 34: 185-191, 1985.

114. Carlson LA, Lockerbie L, Lutz W: Risk factors for ischaemic heart-disease in normal men aged 40: Edinburgh-Stockholm study. Lancet, I: 949-955, 1978.
115. Hughes LO, Cruickshank JK, Wright J, Raftery EB: Disturbances of insulin and its action in British Asian and White male survivors of myocardial infarction. Br Med J, 299: 537-541, 1989.
116. Pyörälä K: Relationship of glucose tolerance and plasma insulin to incidence of coronary heart disease: results from two population studies in Finland. Diabetes Care, 2: 131-141, 1979.
117. Pyörälä K, Savolainen E, Kaukola S, Haapakoski J: Plasma insulin as coronary heart disease risk factor: relationship to other risk factors and predictive value during 91/2 year follow-up of the Helsinki Policemen Study population. Acta Med Scand, (Suppl) 701: 38-52, 1985.
118. Ducimentiere P, Eschwege E, Papoz L, Richard JL, Claude JR, Rosselin G: Relationship of plasma insulin levels to the incidence of myocardial infarction and coronary heart disease in a middle-aged population. Diabetologia, 19: 205-210, 1980.
119. Welborn TA, Wearne K: Coronary heart disease incidence and cardiovascular mortality in Busselton with reference to glucose and insulin concentrations. Diabetes Care, 2: 154-160, 1979.
120. Zavaroni I, Bonara E, Pagliara M, Dall'Aglio E, Luchetti L, Buonanno G, Bonati PA, Bergonzani M, Gnudi L, Passeri M, Reaven GM: Risk factors for coronary artery disease in healthy persons with hyperinsulinemia and normal glucose tolerance. N Engl J Med, 320: 702-706, 1989.
121. Williams RR, Hunt SC, Hopkins PN, Stults BM, Wu LL, Hasstedt SJ, Barlow GK, Stephenson SH, Lalouel J-M, Kuida H: Familial dyslipidemic hypertension: evidence from 58 Utah families for a syndrome present in approximately 12% of patients with essential hypertension. JAMA, 259: 3570-3586, 1988.
122. Beardwood DM, Alden JS, Graham CA, Beardwood JT, Jr., Marble A: Evidence for a peripheral action of chlorothiazide in normal man. Metabolism, 15: 88-93, 1966.
123. Fajans SS, Floyd JC, Knopf RF, Rull T, Guntsche EM, Conn JW: Benzothiadiazine suppression of insulin release from normal and abnormal islet cell tissue in man. J Clin Invest, 45: 481-493, 1966.
124. Morgan TO: Metabolic effects of various antihypertensive agents. J Cardiovasc Pharmacol, 15 (Suppl 5): S39-S-45, 1990.
125. Pollare T, Lithell H, Morlin C, Prantare H, Hvarfner A, Ljunghall S: Metabolic effects of diltiazem and atenolol: results from a randomized, double-blind study with parallel groups. J Hypertension, 7: 551-559, 1989.
126. Bengtsson C, Blohme G, Lapidus L, Lindquist O, Lundgren H, Nystroem E, Petersen K, Sigurdsson JA: Do antihypertensive drugs precipitate diabetes? Br Med J, 289: 1495-1497, 1984.
127. Pollare T. Lithell H, Berne C: A comparison of the effects of hydrochlorothizide and captopril on glucose and lipid metabolism in patients with hypertension. N Engl J Med, 321: 868-873, 1989.
128. Pollare T, Lithell H, Selinus I, Berne C: Application of prazosin is associated with an increase of insulin sensitivity in obese patients with hypertension. Diabetologia, 31: 415-420, 1988.
129. Rett K, Jauch KW, Wicklmayr M, Dietze G, Fink E, Mehnert H: Angiotensin converting enzyme inhibitors in diabetes: experimental and human experience. Postgrad Med J, 62 (Suppl 1): 59-64, 1986.
130. Zusman RM: Effects of converting-enzyme inhibitors on the renin-angiotensin-aldosterone, bradykinin, and arachidonic acid-prostaglandin systems: correlation of chemical structure and biologic activity. Am J Kidney Dis, 10: 13-23, 1987.
131. Weinberger MH: Influence of an angiotensin converting-enzyme inhibitor on diuretic-induced metabolic effects in hypertension. Hypertension, 5 (Suppl 3): 132-138, 1983.
132. Costa FV, Borghi C, Ambrosioni E: Hypolipidemic effects of long-term antihypertensive treatment with captopril. Am J Med, 84 (suppl 3): 159-161, 1983.
133. Powell JS, Clozel J-P, Müller RKM, Kuhn H, Hefti F, Hosang M, Baumgartner HR: Inhibitors of angiotensin-converting enzyme prevent myointimal proliferation after vascular injury. Science, 245: 186-188, 1989.
134. Swislocki ALM, Hoffman BB, Sheu WH-H, Chen Y-DI, Reaven GM: Effect of prazosin treatment on carbohydrate and lipoprotein metabolism in patients with hypertension. Am J Med, 86 (Suppl 1B): 14-18, 1989.

THE KIDNEY AND DIABETES

Chapter 6

RISK FACTORS AND OPTIMAL BLOOD PRESSURE LEVEL FOR INSULIN-DEPENDENT DIABETIC PATIENTS

CARL ERIK MOGENSEN

Medical Department M (Diabetes and Endocrinology), Aarhus Kommunehospital, University of Aarhus, DK-8000 Aarhus C, Denmark

Usually diabetic nephropathy with end-stage-renal disease takes about 25-30 years to develop as outlined in Table 1 and three main periods may be defined (1), each lasting more or less one decade, starting with the acute changes (*Stage I*) at diagnosis of diabetes, which also involve abnormalities in the kidney, - but the degree of these changes at diagnosis are probably not predictive of subsequent disease (1, 2). *Stage II* usually lasts 10 years, and is characterized by renal hyperfunction and hypertrophy without any clinical or laboratory signs of disease (normal albumin excretion), but structural changes in glomeruli are developing. Long-term follow-up studies have, however, shown that patients with most severe early renal involvement (hyperfiltration associated with poor metabolic control) are those most prone to development of late nephropathy (3). In the following decade (*Stage III*) a very characteristic abnormality develops, namely microalbuminuria (3, 4), which is defined as an elevated urinary albumin excretion rate, below the proteinuric range. Usually this, too, is a slow process, and the increase in albuminuria from normal to the proteinuric level may also last about 10 years, although with considerable variations in rate of progression. The third decade (*Stage IV*) is the well-known clinically apparent diabetic nephropathy, known since the thirties, with proteinuria increasing blood pressure and eventually end-stage-renal-failure (ESRF, *Stage V*) after a fairly linear fall in GFR, again lasting about 10 years. The aim of this paper is to discuss in further details the natural history, risk factors, endpoints as well as effect of antihypertensive treatment in incipient and overt nephropathy.

141

Table 1. Schematic natural history outline of diabetic nephropathy in Insulin Dependent Diabetes Mellitus (IDDM).

STAGE

	I At diagnosis, changes	II First decade (≈7-13 y)	III Second decade (≈7-25 y)	IV Third decade (or last ≈8-12 y)	V ESRF
GFR	High(*)	HF (total and single nephron)	Still HF, but declining GFR	Fall rate 12 ml/y; single-nephron-HF likely	Close to zero
UAER	High(*) or normal	Normal, but slightly increasing	Increasing microalbuminuria	Increasing proteinuria	Still P
BP or HT	BP usually normal	BP comparable with background population (HT seen in ≈5%-10%)	BP increasing 3% per year	HT increasing 7% per year	High BP
Suggested basic changes	Metabolic and hemodynamic changes, plus hyperphagia	Metabolic: Glycemia↑, AR↑, Hormones↑ — Hemodynamic: Normal BP but intrarenal HT likely — Diet: Usually high in protein	Metabolic: Glycemia↑, AR↑, Hormones↑ — Hemodynamic: Systemic and intrarenal HT — Diet: Usually high in protein	Metabolic: Glycemia↑, AR↑, Hormones↑ — Hemodynamic: Systemic and intrarenal HT — Diet: Usually high in protein — Nephron closure	Nephron closure
Other concomitant abnormality	HbA$_{1c}$↑ and many metabolic changes	Possibly hyperperfusion	Retinopathy and neuropathy, lipid changes and vascular disease in general	As III, but increasing in severity	Uremia
Main structural counterparts	Hypertrophy of nephrons	Hypertrophy of nephrons, BM thickening after ≈2 years Mesangial expansion after ≈5 years	Microalbuminuria associated with more advanced ultrastructural lesions	Advancing structural lesion especially mesangial expansion and glomerular closure	Nephron closure

ESRF = End Stage Renal Failure; HF = Hyperfiltration; UAER = Urinary Albumin Excretion Rate; P = Proteinuria; HT = Hypertension; BP = Blood Pressure;
AR = Aldose Reductase activity; BM = Basement Membrane
(*) reversible

142

GENETICS, RISK FACTORS AND INTERVENTION

Studies of the natural history of diabetic patients have revealed a number of risk factors of late diabetic nephropathy (1), possibly including genetic factors (5) although there is controversy in this latter area (6).

Table 2. Effect parameters or surrogate endpoints in diabetic nephropathy.

Parameter	Technical problems	Association to progression, possibly to ESRF	Main confounding elements	Evidence of amelioration by intervention
Hyperfiltration or GFR measurement	Constant infusion technique required	Found by one group in retrospective analysis	Poor metabolic control	Optimized insulin treatment. Somatostatin analogues. ARI (*) Low protein diet
Microalbuminuria or measurement of UAE	Due to variability are multiple collections necessary	Found in 3 independent studies	Marginal BP elevation found in microalbuminuria in addition to somewhat poorer control	Optimized insulin treatment.Low protein diet. Antihypertensive therapy (including ACE inhibitors)
Development of BP elevation	Due to observer bias blinded procedures or ambulatory 24 h procedures required	Not clearly documented to be independent from proteinuria	Associated to microalbuminuria and proteinuria	Antihypertensive treatment. Practically all agents effective on BP in diabetics
Degree of proteinuria or development of proteinuria	Multiple collection required	Clearly associated to development of ESRF	Non-diabetic renal disease	Antihypertensive treatment (including ACE inhibitors). Low protein diet
Fall rate of GFR	Exact GFR measurement necessary	Clearly associated to development of ESRF	Non-exact measures of GFR	Antihypertensive treatment (including ACE inhibitors). Low protein diet
Structural analysis of renal biopsies	No studies available on representativity/ reproducibility	Likely, but no documentation in longitudinal studies	Predictive value not known	No data available

BP = blood pressure; ESRF = End Stage Renal Failure; UAE = urinary albumin excretion
(*) Aldose reductase inhibitors

Identification of risk factors is important, but obviously it cannot be taken for granted that a risk factor is in fact involved in the pathogenetic process. However, if long-term intervention e.g. with adequate dosages of drugs, based on the risk factor idea, appears successful, it seems likely that the risk factor is actually involved in the pathogenesis of disease. On the other hand, if intervention is unsuccessful, the risk factor may not be involved in the pathogenesis, but is rather an innocent bystander.

One important point is monitoring of treatment-effect and reliable effect-parameters or endpoints are crucial (Table 2). The most sceptical or critical attitude regarding a chronic disease like diabetes would require increased longevity or postponement of end-stage-renal-failure. The fulfilment of such criteria would require extremely long-term follow-up of patients. Hence, one has to consider intermediate endpoints or surrogates for final end points. For instance, if the fall rate in GFR can be reduced on a long-term basis, it is also likely that end-stage-renal-failure can be postponed, although extrapolation over many years may not necessarily be permissible.

Reduction of microalbuminuria may be considered beneficial, because microalbuminuria is likely to be the earliest reliable parameter in the disease process (3, 7), readily detectable and reproducible by standard laboratory procedures. An even earlier abnormality is hyperfiltration, and amelioration of this physiological abnormality may also be beneficial in the long run, although this is less certain.

Thus far physiological parameters of renal functions are the main test parameters very early in the course of the disease process. Evaluation of renal biopsies have not yet been performed systematically in treatment trials (8). Quantitative evaluation of renal biopsies is not an easy procedure, and one biopsy specimen may not be representative of the integrated renal system, which is in contrast to functional studies. To rely on quantitative structural analysis of renal biopsy specimens requires not only more experience but also a considerable break-through in technology, which must be attained before the procedure can be considered as safe and practical in clinical medicine.

EFFECT PARAMETER ENDPOINTS AND INTERMEDIATE ENDPOINTS

The following effect parameters or endpoints can be considered in clinical trials as outlined in Table 2.

Hyperfiltration

Hyperfiltration is an early phenomenon in the course of diabetes. It may be associated to late nephropathy (3), but in the literature in general is not so clear an association as we see with microalbuminuria. However, new prospective studies shows that hyperfiltration in fact is a strong independent predictor of nephropathy (S. Rudberg & G. Dahlquist, in preparation). In a multiple regression analysis we also found hyperfiltration stronger correlated to subsequent renal disease than microalbuminuria (9). Therefore reduction in significant hyperfiltration may in theory be considered beneficial. Obviously this is a very early parameter, probably the earliest pathophysiologic change that can be detected.

Microalbuminuria

Microalbuminuria is defined as increased urinary albumin excretion (UAE, UAER, or AER)[*] but below the proteinuric level, and according to an international consensus (4) the range 20-200 µg/min is proposed. Obviously there may be a "grey area" in lower level as well as in the high level, also because as a considerable variability in UAER, around 40-50% (10). It should also be noted that microalbuminuria may be induced by very poor metabolic control, physical exercise and urinary tract infection or cardiac decompensation. Such causes should of course be excluded and if so the term incipient diabetic nephropathy may be employed (10).

The first assays used for measurement of albumin excretion rate in the low range was radioimmunoassays (11), but at the present time there is a large number of assays available, mainly immunochemical assays (7, 12). Although sensitivity may not be as high as radioimmunoassay there usually will suited for clinical practice and for research purposes (7, 12). If sensitive measurements are necessary e.g. measurement of albumin in diluted urine from clearance studies, radioimmunoassay may be advantageous. Microalbuminuria in Insulin Dependent Diabetes Mellitus (IDDM) patients is usually found in 10-20% of individuals in cross-sectional studies (13-17), not only in clinic based studies, but also in epidemiological studies (18). Independent studies from 3 centres (19-21) document the strong predictive power of microalbuminuria and this concept has now been widely accepted.

New studies suggest that there may be a difference between low range microalbuminuria 20-70 µg/min where the prognosis may be better than in the high range, between 70-200 µg/min (22). The lower range microalbuminuria may be easier to stabilize by fair metabolic control in contrast to the high range (22, 23). Figure 1 complies data from

---

[*] UAE = Urinary Albumin Excretion; UAER = Urinary Albumin Excretion Rate; AER = Albumin Excretion Rate

two papers (19, 20) on the predictive value of microalbuminuria and Figure 2 shows long-term follow-up data from Mogensen and Christensen (19).

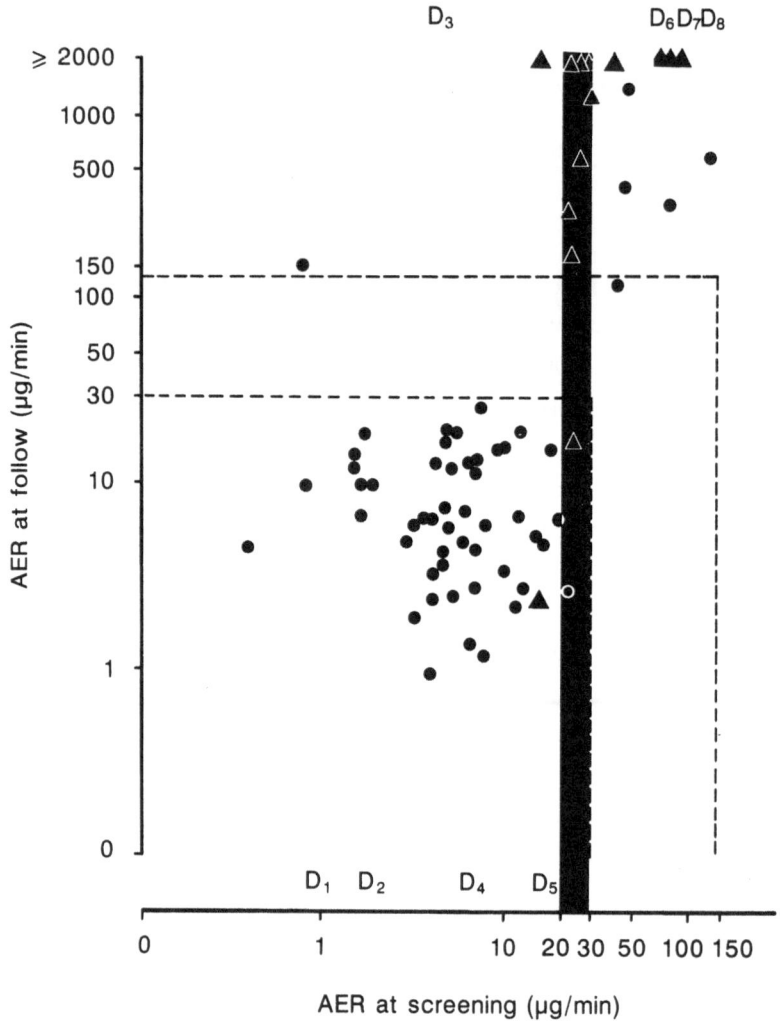

Figure 1. Urinary albumin excretion at follow-up plotted against initial urinary albumin excretion rate at screening. The figure shows data from two follow-up studies (Refs. 19, 20). A combination of the two materials suggests that a cut-off point 20 µg/min is relevant in progression of renal disease. (D = dead patient)

Finally persistent microalbuminuria cannot be considered as an epiphenomenon. It is quite likely to be an expression of the proper disease process, like proteinuria, but earlier in the course of the disease.

Important studies are now being conducted to correlate microalbuminuria with structural lesions.

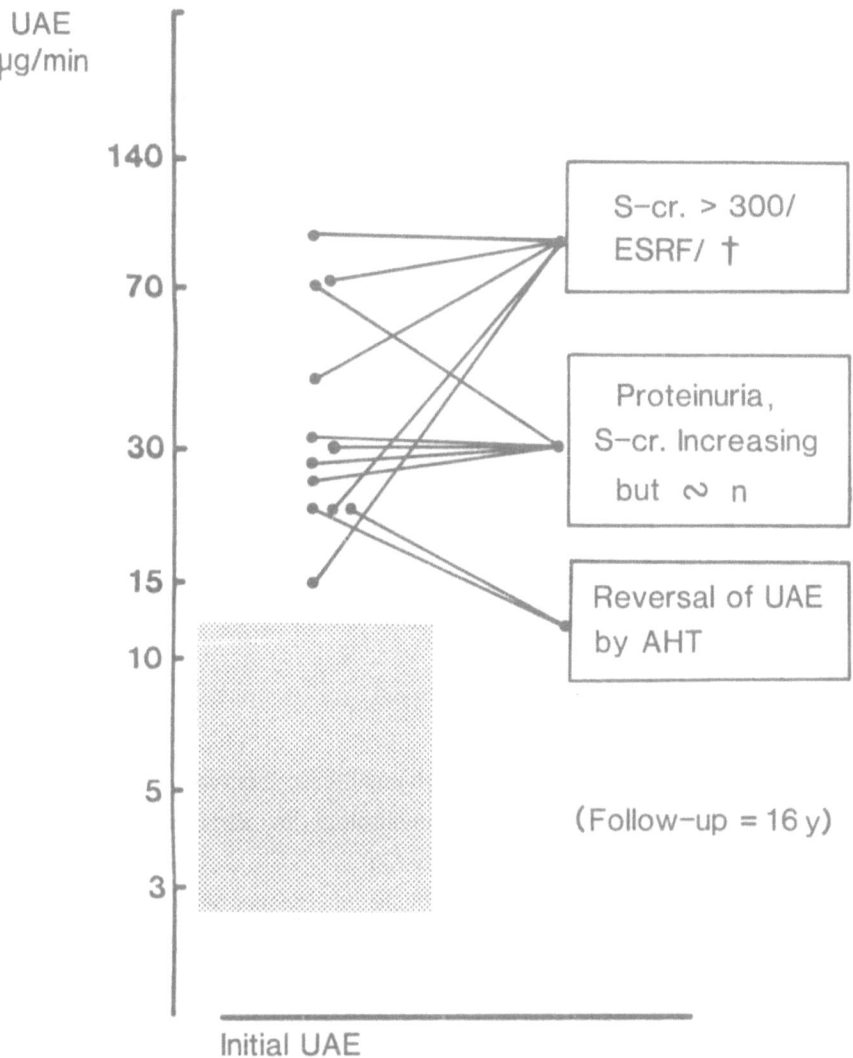

Figure 2. 16 yr follow-up of 12 of the patients shown in Figure 1, namely those progressing (Ref. 19). Five patients progressed to end-stage-renal-failure (ESRF) or death. Five patients progressed to proteinuria with increasing serum creatinine but still within the normal level (~n). Two patients were treated early with antihypertensive treatment (AHT) and reversed (UAE = Urinary Albumin Excretion) [Reprinted from Mogensen CE: Prediction of clinical diabetic nephropathy in IDDM patients. Alternatives to microalbuminuria? Diabetes, 39: 761-767, 1990, with permission. Copyright (c) 1990 by the American Diabetes Association].

So far available studies have not dealt with appropriate selection of patients with microalbuminuria (3, 24).

Degree of proteinuria or development of proteinuria

Proteinuria has long been considered the hallmark of diabetic nephropathy and it is usually defined as a 24 hr total urinary protein excretion of more than 0.5 g/day (25). It is quite clear that patients with proteinuria do have a poor prognosis and therefore it seem reasonable to use development of proteinuria (from microalbuminuria) as an important effect-parameter. However, new procedures has been introduced regarding urinary proteins, especially measurement of urinary albumin by specific procedures. Therefore the total urinary protein excretion may be replaced by albumin excretion and 0.5 g/24 h of total protein corresponds to approximately 300 mg albumin/24 h period (4, 10, 25). Obviously, a mean of values of at least 3 collections should be used. There is some variability in urinary protein excretion and this may be a weakness in this context, for instance in patients where excretion rate may fluctuate around 300 mg/24 h period. Also it seems quite clear that the situation of a patient is not very different if the excretion rate is 290 mg/24 h compared to 310 mg/24 h. However, if groups of patients are considered together the effect of this variability may be eliminated although the number of patients required for analysis may be rather high unless the treatment effect is pronounced. Based on these consideration one may prefer to use the increase rate in albumin excretion, better than a rather arbitrary limit as 300 mg/24 h or 200 µg/min.

Fall rate of GFR

Determination of progression of chronic renal disease is really a key parameter in nephrological research, not only in diabetic nephrology, but surprisingly little emphasis was placed on this issue in classical nephrology (26).

For instance in 1976 Mitch et al (27) published their paper on progression of chronic renal failure using a simple method based on estimation of inverse serum creatinine. The same year the data were published on measurement of progression in diabetic renal disease based on classical constant infusion techniques as introduced by Homer Smith (28). The former procedure has been used in many papers (26) including data based on creatinine clearance measurements, but these procedures clearly have to be abandoned (26, 29, 30). The latter procedure remains standard although the constant infusion technique in many studies has been replaced by the single shot procedure (because of the advantage that urine samples have not to be collected) using e.g. Cr-51-EDTA as filtration marker, a procedure that correlates fairly well the constant infusion technique although not all agree (B. Myers, personal communication).

Clearly it is important to calculate exactly the rate of progression expressed as fall rate of GFR (ml/min/mo) and therefore at least 3 measurements of GFR are necessary over a certain period of time e.g. at least 2 years (or better measurement twice every year). Rate of change in GFR can be estimated by ordinary least squares regression, a procedure that may be optimized by break point analysis (26, 31). Obviously, the main idea is to see if the fall rate of GFR is really changed by intervention. It is important to consider that GFR may fall acutely days or weeks after intervention (due to decreased intraglomerular pressure?), whereafter it stabilizes with a reduced fall rate.

In diabetic nephropathy a fall rate of GFR is usually very linear, although this is not always the case (32). If the linearity is accepted it seems clear that by extrapolation change in the fall rate of GFR certainly will postpone the development of end-stage-renal-failure. Therefore documentation of a reduction in the fall rate of GFR over a prolonged period of time, e.g. more than 3-4 years, really must be a key effect-parameter in the evaluation of intervention. However, it should be noted that change in fall rate of GFR is correlated to change in urinary protein excretion, and therefore it could be suggested that a reduction in proteinuria or microalbuminuria also is a clear indication of beneficial effect.

End-stage-renal-failure or death

End-stage-renal-failure may be defined as GFR values less than 5-10 ml/min. Obviously this is a very strong end-point, but since end-stage diabetic nephropathy usually takes 3 decades to develop this end-point may be difficult, although it may be used in proteinuric patients with a 10 year perspective. Without intervention the proteinuric stage usually lasts 10 years, but the advent of antihypertensive treatment seems to have prolonged this phase considerably (33-35). Therefore the use of this end-point may be quite unpractical, unless clinical trials had to go on for one to two decades. Mortality is closely related to end-stage-renal-failure because diabetic patients even on dialysis and transplantation programmes often have a rather poor prognosis.

Blood pressure elevation

Blood pressure elevation is related to development of diabetic nephropathy and elevated blood pressure is associated to progression of renal disease. However, increase in blood pressure usually cannot be used as endpoint in trials. Rather blood pressure elevation is considered a risk factor.

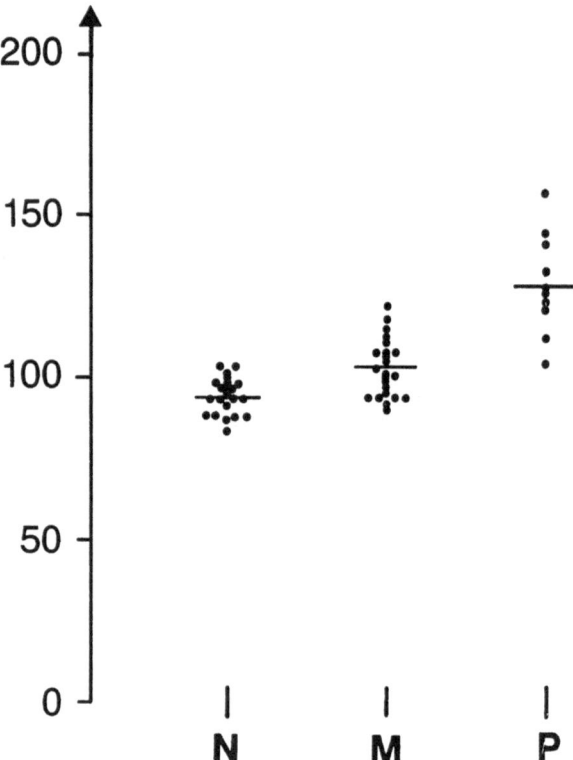

Figure 3.   Mean Blood Pressure (mm Hg) in normoalbuminuric (N), microalbuminuric (M) and proteinuric (P) Insulin Dependent Diabetes Mellitus (IDDM) patients.

Figures 3 and 4 show mean arterial pressure and GFR values in IDDM patients with various degree of renal involvement (normoalbuminuria, microalbuminuria, proteinuria or "macroalbuminuria").

Renal biopsies

Obviously, data from renal biopsies is potentially important in the evaluation of progression of renal disease and its modulation by intervention. However, in most studies it is not feasible to do repeated biopsies and also there is no experience regarding relevant parameters, although basement membrane thickening (early in the course) and mesangial expansions (some years later) are clearly important parameters (8). However, there may be problems regarding representativity of renal biopsy and so far biopsies are not considered in most clinical trials.

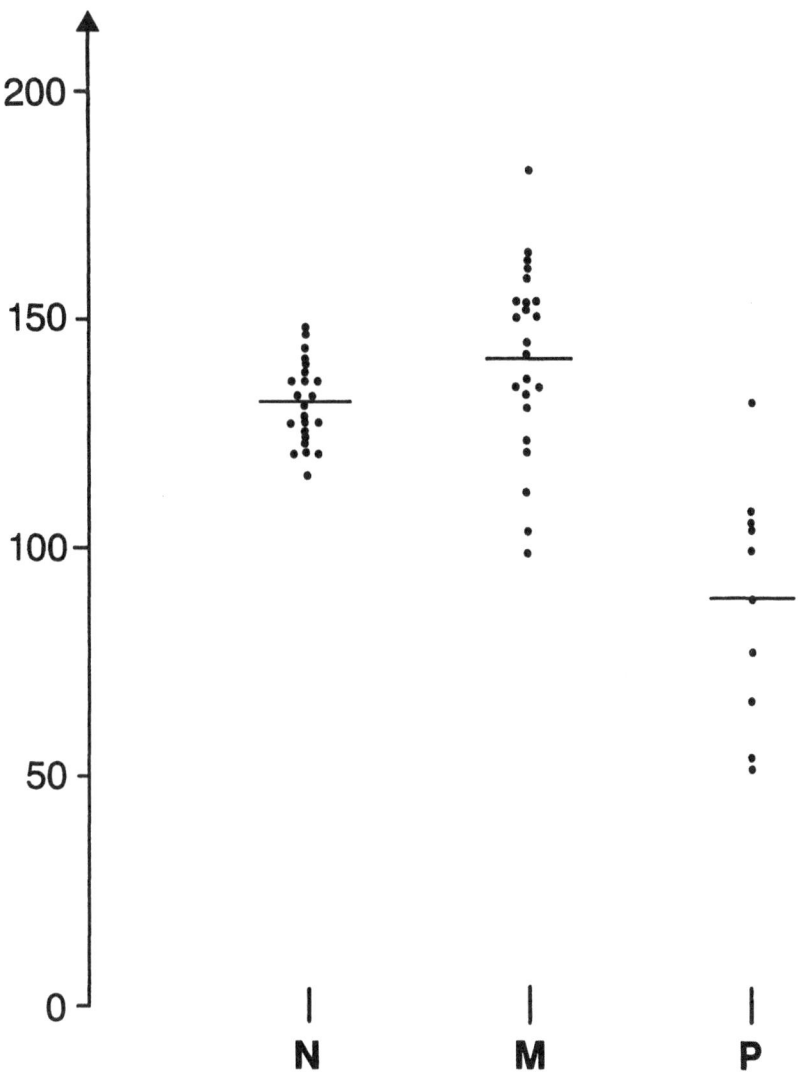

Figure 4. GFR (ml/min/1.73 m^2) in normoalbuminuric (N), microalbuminuric (M) and proteinuric (P) Insulin Dependent Diabetes Mellitus (IDDM) patients. GFR shows wide range in the microalbuminuric patients (many hyperfiltering) and reduction in proteinuric patients.

EFFECT OF INTERVENTION

Blood Pressure in microalbuminuric individuals and effect of antihypertensive treatment

A review in this area has been given previously (36). The first studies describing elevated BP in microalbuminuric individuals were published only 5-6 years ago (9, 19, 37-

40) and Table 3 also includes some further data from studies published from 1984 to 1990 (14, 15, 18, 41-46). Typically, in these studies the mean age of microalbuminuric patients is around 30 years. It appears that recorded BP is declining from 1984 to 1990, probably because many patients are now being treated with antihypertensive agents, and thus not included in the surveys. Wilson & Luetscher (45) in addition to elevated BP and poorer control also found microalbuminuria and retinopathy to be associated with increased prorenin-levels. Elevated BP in microalbuminuric individuals has recently been observed in studies using 24-hr BP-monitoring and in this study BP appeared to be normal in normoalbuminuric patients (46).

Table 3. Changing level of blood pressure in microalbuminuria.

Authors (Ref. #)	Year of publication	Mean Age (years)	Mean BP (Syst/Dia) (mm Hg)	Mean MAP (mm Hg)
Mogensen & Christensen (19)	1984	35	138/92	107
Mathiesen et al (21)	1984	31	131/85	100
Wiseman et al (39)	1984	34	136/87	103
Feldt-Rasmussen et al (40)	1985	32	135/86	102
Christensen & Mogensen (48)	1985	27	133/88	103
Berglund et al (15)	1987	33	135/77	96
Le Floch et al (42)	1990	45	133/77	96
Hansen, Mogensen et al (46)	1990	30	125/82	96
Wiegmann et al (41)	1990	21	120/81	94
Cook et al (52)	1990	14	108/64	79

BP = blood pressure; MAP = Mean Arterial blood Pressure
Korotkoff's phase 5 used in all studies in defining diastolic BP

A few longitudinal studies have been published documenting that BP rises with time in microalbuminuric in contrast to normoalbuminuric subjects (23, 37). An even steeper rise is seen in proteinuric patients (47). In addition, rise in microalbuminuria is correlated to BP-level (23, 48) (Figure 5).

Rather high BP is noted in Figure 5, all in the untreated situation also in overt nephropathy (28), and such patients would of course receive antihypertensive treatment to-day. It is not completely clarified whether some BP-elevation trickers development of microalbuminuria from the normoalbuminuric range or whether microalbuminuria (e.g. by glomerular damage) induces increase in BP. However, it is an interesting observation that BP increases in microalbuminuric patients and indeed a self-perpetuating process may prevail. By some undefined mechanism renal abnormalities responsible for microalbuminuria increases BP, and on the other hand BP-elevation increases microalbuminuria, eventuating in proteinuria and overt hypertension and after many years severe diabetic nephropathy and uremia develops.

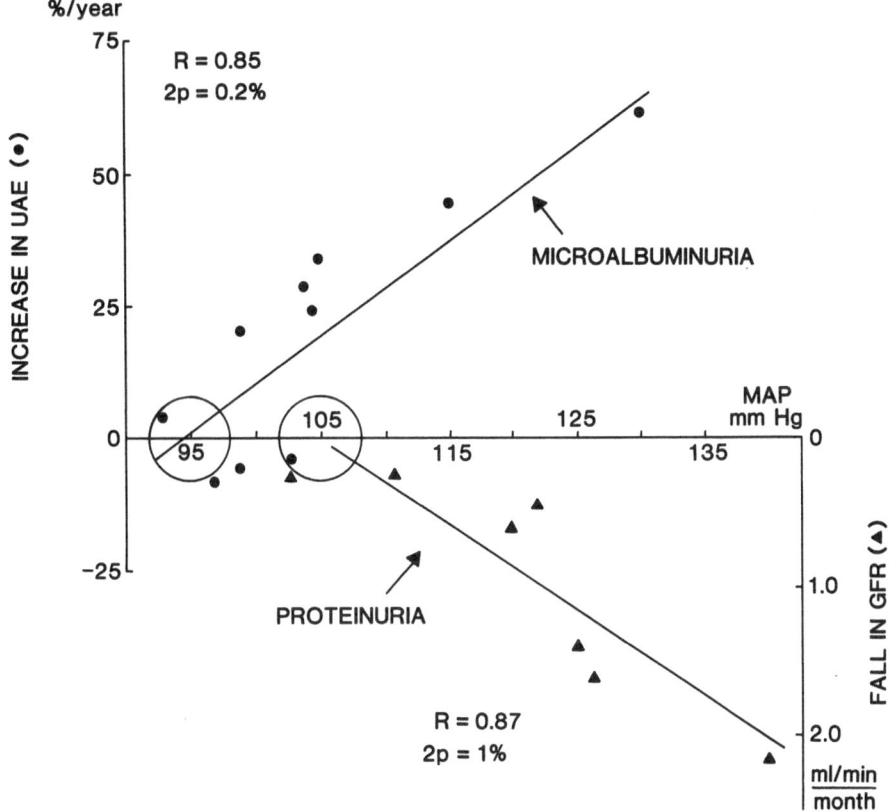

Figure 5. Threshold for progression in microalbuminuria (95 mm Hg) and fall rate of GFR (105 mm Hg) in insulin-dependent diabetes mellitus (IDDM) patients. (Modified from Refs 28 and 48). The upper part of the figure shows correlation between percentage increase in urinary albumin excretion (UAE) and mean arterial blood pressure (MAP) in the observation period of 5 years. The lower part shows correlation between fall rate in GFR and MAP at the end of the observation period of 3 years.

Within this context it is therefore not surprising that antihypertensive treatment is effective in reducing microalbuminuria after a few months of intervention (49-53) and at the same time such patients show stable GFR (54, 55). However, studies over several years also including a control group have not been able to document that GFR is better preserved than in a comparable control group (55) probably because the threshold for progression in microalbuminuria is lower than the BP-threshold for inducing fall in GFR (by glomerular destruction and closure). A rather low Mean Arterial blood Pressure (MAP) is observed in this trial (90-95 mm Hg) (55). However, the control group show clear rise in microalbuminuria and development of proteinuria in a significant number of patients. In the one-year study by Marre et al (50) BP was higher before treatment (MAP ≈100 mm Hg) and GFR was better preserved in the ACE-treated group. Table 4 shows data on MAP before and during treatment in microalbuminuric patients (49, 50, 53-56). It appears that MAP during treatment is around 90-95 mm Hg. It is therefore suggested that this level in MAP may be able to protect against significant deterioration in renal function. However, no long-term studies have been conducted and an extremely long-term follow-up period is probably needed, simply because such studies will not include patients with clear elevation of BP but only include "slow progressers" with rather low blood pressure. Antihypertensive treatment is simply considered clinically mandatory in such individuals with elevated BP and are therefore not included in trials as control subjects.

Table 4. Mean Arterial blood Pressure (MAP) before and during treatment in incipient nephropathy in Insulin Dependent Diabetes Mellitus (IDDM).

Authors (Ref. #)	Year of publication	Mean MAP (mm Hg)
Microalbuminuria reduced:		
Christensen & Mogensen (53, 54)	1985, 1987	107 → 93
Marre, Passa et al (49, 50)	1987, 1988	100 → 90
Mathiessen, Parving et al (55)	1990	96 → 93 (n.s.)
Cooper, Jerums et al (*) (ACE-I) (56)	1991	102 → 98
Cooper, Jerums et al (*) (Ca-A) (56)	1991	109 → 99

(*) some NIDDM (Non Insulin Dependent Diabetes Mellitus) included.
ACE-I = Angiotensin Converting Enzyme Inhibitor.
Ca-A = Calcium Antagonist.

Also exercise-induced-microalbuminuria can be reduced by long-term antihypertensive treatment (57) and a new study shows that the acute exercise-induced elevation in microalbuminuria is reduced by ACE-inhibition (58).

Hypertension in proteinuric IDDM patients and effect of antihypertensive treatment

It has been known for many years that diabetic patients with proteinuria often show a considerable increase in BP (28) and it also became clear that they show a dramatic rise in BP with time (47).

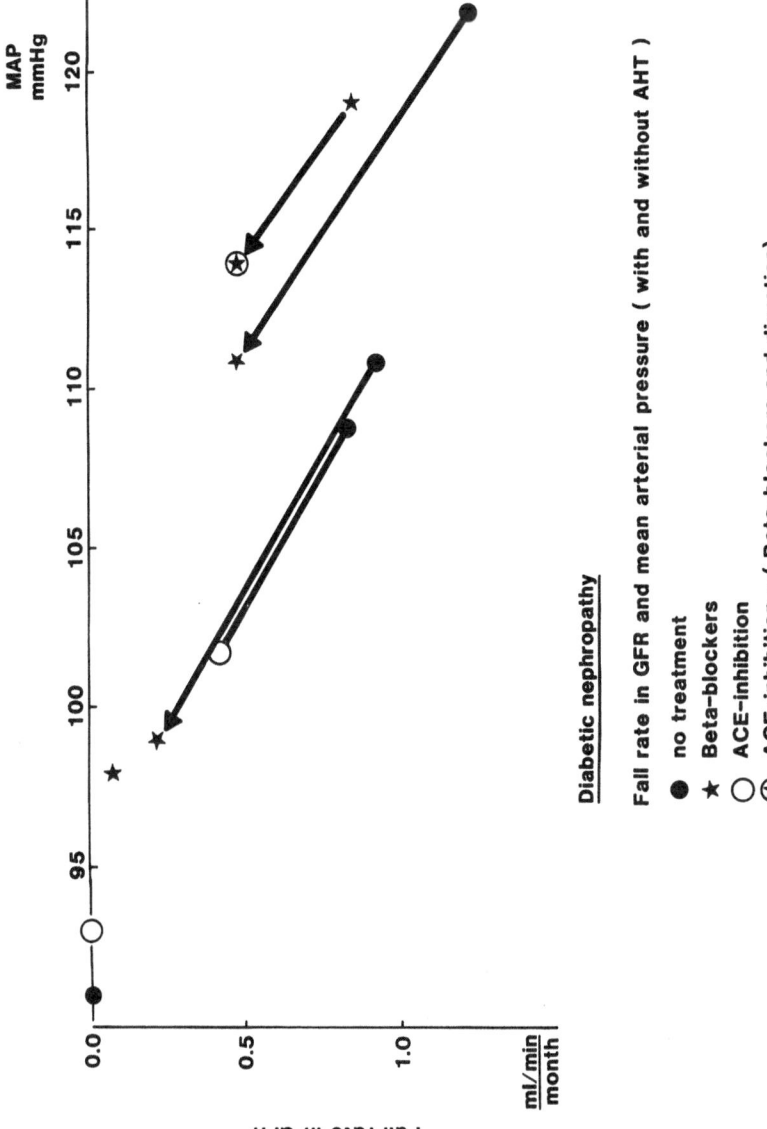

Figure 6. Fall rate in GFR plotted against mean arterial blood pressure (MAP) in trials with and without antihypertensive treatment (data from Refs 54, 55, 59-62) in groups of patients. (AHT = antihypertensive treatment).

155

Importantly, MAP in the untreated situation was shown to be correlated to the fall rate of GFR in a series of such patients published in 1976 (28) as seen in Figure 5. This observation appeared to be extremely important to therapy because it suggested that reduction in BP might also be able to reduce the fall rate in GFR and indeed subsequent studies documented that not only proteinuria was reduced (28), but also fall rate of GFR (59-62).

Figure 6 shows the correlation between fall rate in GFR and BP in a number of long-term antihypertensive trials conducted over more than two years (59-62), not only in overt nephropathy, but also in patients with incipient nephropathy (54, 55). It is not simple to extrapolate a BP to a level where renal function must be considered stable, but as seen from a level in MAP at around 100-105 mm Hg may be appropriate. In patients with incipient diabetic nephropathy a BP-level of around 95 mean arterial BP seems to be able to preserve stable albumin excretion or to reduce UAER and also without fall in GFR (Table 4). Quite often microalbuminuria is reduced with well preserved GFR, which may relate to the lower threshold for occurrence of microalbuminuria than for reduction in fall rate of GFR.

Triple-treatment with diuretics, beta-blockers and ACE-inhibitors seems to have a pathophysiologic rationale. New studies (63, 64) support this concept since a clear continuous reduction in UAER was seen, even with stable BP. Thus the addition of ACE-inhibition reduced UAER without significant BP-reduction which may suggest a specific renal effect of ACE-inhibitors, also when added to conventional treatment. These studies also show that this triple-treatment is well tolerated by patients with incipient or early nephropathy (63, 64).

Other factors determining progression in renal disease

BP-elevation is evidently a main risk factor for the initiation and progression of renal disease in diabetes, but other pathogenetic mechanisms may exist apart from elevated BP and elevated intraglomerular pressure although the latter may be a common phenomenon associated with other risk factors e.g. poor metabolic control and high dietary proteins and possibly other factors (65). One important factor is obviously quality of metabolic control and although a small intervention trial in overt nephropathy was negative (66), it is likely that poor metabolic control in IDDM patients still is a risk factor not only in the occurrence and increase rate of microalbuminuria (23, 67-70), but also for the fall rate of GFR (71). Recently much interest is focused on the role of lipids in renal disease, and in one analysis it appeared that diabetic patients who had the highest serum cholesterol during antihypertensive treatment also had the highest level of progression rate, that is fall rate of

GFR (72). Therefore abnormal lipids may play a role in producing renal injury and lipid lowering agents may be effective in protecting against progression in renal disease. So far no studies are available in this area in diabetic individuals, but this is an interesting new avenue in clinical research (73, 74). However, there is more evidence suggesting that a protein reduced diet reduces not only fall rate of GFR but also microalbuminuria and hyperfiltration (75-80) although the effect on fall rate of GFR has been questioned (81).

REFERENCES

1. Mogensen CE: Prevention and treatment of renal disease in insulin-dependent diabetes mellitus. Sem Nephrol, 10: 260-273, 1990.
2. Mogensen CE, Schmitz A, Christensen CK: Comparative renal pathophysiology relevant to IDDM and NIDDM patients. Diabetes/Metab Rev, 4: 453-483, 1988.
3. Mogensen CE: Prediction of clinical diabetic nephropathy in IDDM patients. Alternatives to microalbuminuria? Diabetes, 39: 761-767, 1990.
4. Mogensen CE, Chachati A, Christensen CK, Close CF, Deckert T, Hommel E, Kastrup J, Lefebvre P, Mathiesen ER, Feldt-Rasmussen B, Schmitz A, Viberti GC: Microalbuminuria: an early marker of renal involvement in diabetes. Uremia Invest, 9: 85-95, 1985-86.
5. Viberti GC: New insights into the genesis of diabetic kidney disease in insulin-dependent diabetic patients. In: "The Diabetes Annual/5" (Eds KGMM Alberti, LP Krall), Elsevier Science Publishers, B.V.,1990, pp 301-311.
6. Jensen JS, Mathiesen ER, Nørgaard K, Hommel E, Borch-Johnsen K, Funder J, Brahm J, Parving H-H, Deckert T: Increased blood pressure and erythrocyte sodium/lithium countertransport activity are not inherited in diabetic nephropathy. Diabetologia, 33: 619-624, 1990.
7. Rowe DJF, Dawnay A, Watts GF: Microalbuminuria in diabetes mellitus: review and recommendations for the measurement of albumin in urine. An Clin Biochem, 27: 297-312, 1990.
8. Mauer SM, Chavers BM, Steffes MW: Should there be an expanded role for kidney biopsy in the management of patients with type I diabetes? Am J Kidney Dis, 16: 96-100, 1990.
9. Mogensen CE, Christensen CK: Blood pressure changes and renal function in incipient and overt diabetic nephropathy. Hypertension, 7 (suppl II): II-64 - II-73, 1985.
10. Mogensen CE: Microalbuminuria as a predictor of clinical diabetic nephropathy. Kidney Int, 31: 673-689, 1987.
11. Keen H, Chlouverakis C: An immunoassay method for urinary albumin at low concentrations. Lancet, II: 913-914, 1963.
12. Townsend JC: Increased albumin excretion in diabetes. J Clin Path, 43: 3-8, 1990.
13. Niazy S, Feldt-Rasmussen B, Deckert T: Microalbuminuria in insulin-dependent diabetes: prevalence and practical consequences. J Diabetic Compl, 1: 76-80, 1987.
14. Parving H-H, Hommel E, Mathiesen E, Skøtt P, Edsberg B, Bahnsen M, Lauritzen M, Hougaard P, Lauritzen E: Prevalence of microalbuminuria, arterial hypertension, retinopathy and neuropathy in patients with insulin dependent diabetes. Br Med J, 296: 156-160, 1988.
15. Berglund J, Lins P, Adamson U, Lins L: Microalbuminuria in long-term insulin dependent diabetes mellitus. Acta Med Scand, 222: 333-338, 1987.
16. Mogensen CE: A complete screening of urinary albumin concentration in an unselected diabetic out-patient-clinic population (1082 patients). Diabetic Nephropathy, 2: 11-18, 1983.
17. Mathiesen ER, Saurbrey N, Hommel E, Parving H-H: Prevalence of microalbuminuria in children with type 1 (insulin-dependent) diabetes mellitus. Diabetologia, 29: 640-643, 1986.
18. Berglund J, Newberg K: Incipient diabetic nephropathy in a Swedish province - impact of past glycemic control, blood pressure and smoking habits. Diabetologia, 33 (suppl): 140A, 1990.
19. Mogensen CE, Christensen CK: Predicting diabetic nephropathy in insulin-dependent patients. N Engl J Med, 311: 89-93, 1984.
20. Viberti GC, Jarrett RJ, Mahmud U, Hill RD, Argyropoulos A, Keen H: Microalbuminuria as a predictor of clinical nephropathy in insulin-dependent diabetes mellitus. Lancet, I: 1430-1434, 1982.

21. Mathiesen ER, Oxenbøll B, Johansen K, Svendsen PA, Deckert T: Incipient nephropathy in type I (insulin-dependent) diabetes. Diabetologia, 26: 406-410, 1984.
22. Feldt-Rasmussen B: Association of poor metabolic control for five to eight years and progression of diabetic renal disease. Diabetologia, 32: 486A, 1989.
23. Feldt-Rasmussen B, Mathiesen E, Deckert T: Effect of two years of strict metabolic control on the progression of incipient nephropathy in insulin-dependent diabetes. Lancet, II: 1300-1304, 1986.
24. Chavers BM, Bilous RW, Ellis EN, Steffes MW, Mauer M: Glomerular lesions and urinary albumin excretion in type I diabetes without overt proteinuria. N Engl J Med, 320: 966-970, 1989.
25. Drury PL, Watkins PJ, Viberti GC, Walker JD: Diabetic nephropathy. Br Med Bull, 45: 127-147, 1989.
26. Walser M: Editorial Review. Progression of chronic renal failure in man. Kidney Int, 37: 1195-1210, 1990.
27. Mitch WE, Buffington G, Lemann J, Walser M: Progression of chronic renal failure: a simple method of estimation. Lancet, II: 1326-1331, 1976.
28. Mogensen CE: Progression of nephropathy in long-term diabetics with proteinuria and effect of initial anti-hypertensive treatment. Scand J Clin Lab Invest, 36: 383-388, 1976.
29. Nordén G, Björck S, Granerus G, Nyberg G: Estimation of renal function in diabetic nephropathy. Nephron, 47: 36-42, 1987.
30. Shemesh O, Golbetz H, Kriss JP, Myers BD: Limitations of creatinine as a filtration marker in glomerulopathic patients. Kidney Int, 28: 830-838, 1985.
31. Viberti GC, Walker J, Dodds R: Low protein diet and progression of renal disease in diabetic nephropathy. Lancet, 335: 550-551, 1990 (Letter).
32. Nyberg G, Nordén G, Björck S, Larsson O: Progression of diabetic nephropathy - a multifactorial process. Scand J Urol Nephrol, 108 (suppl): 35-40, 1988.
33. Mathiesen ER, Borch Johnsen K, Jensen DV, et al: Improved survival in patients with diabetic nephropathy. Diabetologia, 32: 884-886, 1989.
34. Parving H-H, Hommel E: Prognosis in diabetic nephropathy. Br Med J, 299: 230-233, 1989.
35. Hasslacher C, Borgholte G, Ritz E, Wahl P: Impact of hypertension on prognosis of IDDM. Diabete Metab, 15: 338-342, 1989.
36. Mogensen CE: Therapeutic interventions in nephropathy of IDDM. Diabetes Care, 11 (suppl 1): 10-15, 1988.
37. Christensen CK: Abnormal albuminuria and blood pressure rise in incipient diabetic nephropathy induced by exercise. Kidney Int, 25: 819-823, 1984.
38. Mathiesen ER, Oxenbøll B, Johansen K, Svendsen PA, Deckert T: Incipient nephropathy in type I (insulin-dependent) diabetes. Diabetologia, 26: 406-410, 1984.
39. Wiseman M, Viberti GC, Mackintosh D, Jarrett RJ, Keen H: Glycaemia, arterial pressure and micro-albuminuria in type 1 (insulin-dependent) diabetes mellitus. Diabetologia, 26: 401-405, 1984.
40. Feldt-Rasmussen B, Borch-Johnsen K, Mathiesen ER: Hypertension in diabetes as related to nephropathy. Early blood pressure changes. Hypertension, 7 (suppl II): II-18 - II-20, 1985.
41. Wiegmann TB, Chonko AM, Barnard MJ, MacDougall ML, Folscroft J, Stephenson J, Kyner JL, Moore WV: Comparison of albumin excretion rate obtained with different times of collection. Diabetes Care, 13: 864-871, 1990.
42. Le Floch JP, Christin S, Bertherat J, Perlemuter L, Hazard J: Blood pressure and microvascular complications in type 1 (insulin-dependent) diabetic patients without hypertension. Diabete Metab, 16: 26-29, 1990.
43. Stehouwer CDA, Fischer HRA, Hackeng WHL, den Ottolander GJH: Identifying patients with incipient diabetic nephropathy. Should 24-hour urine collections be used? Arch Intern Med, 150: 373-375, 1990.
44. Sampson MJ, Chambers J, Sprigings D, Drury PL: Intraventricular septal hypertrophy in type 1 diabetic patients with microalbuminuria or early proteinuria. Diabetic Med, 7: 126-131, 1990.
45. Wilson DM, Luetscher JA: Plasma prorenin activity and complications in children with insulin-dependent diabetes mellitus. N Engl J Med, 323: 1101-1106, 1990.
46. Hansen KW, Christensen CK, Andersen PH, Christensen JS, Mogensen CE: Ambulatory blood pressure in microalbuminuric type 1 (insulin-dependent) diabetic patients. Diabetologia, 33 (suppl): 201A, 1990.
47. Parving H-H, Andersen AR, Smidt UM, Svendsen PaA: Early aggressive antihypertensive treatment reduces rate of decline in kidney function in diabetic nephropathy. Lancet, I: 1175-1179, 1983.
48. Christensen CK, Mogensen CE: The course of incipient diabetic nephropathy: Studies of albumin excretion and blood pressure. Diabetic Med, 2: 97-102, 1985.

49.   Marre M, Leblanc H, Suarez L, Guyenne T-T, Ménard J, Passa Ph: Converting enzyme inhibition and kidney function in normotensive diabetic patients with persistent microalbuminuria. Br Med J, 294: 1448-1452, 1987.

50.   Marre M, Chatellier G, Leblanc H, Guyenne T-T, Ménard J, Passa Ph: Prevention of diabetic nephropathy with Enalapril in normotensive diabetics with microalbuminuria. Br Med J, 297: 1092-1095, 1988.

51.   Rudberg S, Aperia, Freyschuss U, Persson B: Enalapril reduces microalbuminuria in young normotensive type 1 (insulin-dependent) diabetic patients irrespective of its hypotensive effect. Diabetologia, 33: 470-476, 1990.

52.   Cook J, Daneman D, Spino M, Sochett E, Perlman K, Balfe JW: Angiotensin converting enzyme inhibitor therapy to decrease microalbuminuria in normotensive children with insulin-dependent diabetes mellitus. J Pediatr, 117: 39-45, 1990.

53.   Christensen CK, Mogensen CE: Effect of antihypertensive treatment on progression of incipient diabetic nephropathy. Hypertension, 7 (suppl II): II-109-II-113, 1985.

54.   Christensen CK, Mogensen CE: Antihypertensive treatment: long-term reversal of progression of albuminuria in incipient diabetic nephropathy. A longitudinal study of renal function. J Diabetic Compl, 1: 45-52, 1987.

55.   Mathiesen ER, Hommel E, Giese J, Parving H-H: Captopril postpones and may even prevent development of diabetic nephropathy. Diabetologia, 33 (suppl): 75A, 1990.

56.   Melbourne Diabetic Nephropathy Study Group: Comparison between perindopril and nifedipine in hypertensive and normotensive diabetic patients with microalbuminuria. Br Med J, 302: 210-216, 1991.

57.   Christensen CK, Mogensen CE: Acute and long-term effect of antihypertensive treatment on exercise-induced albuminuria in incipient diabetic nephropathy. Scand J Clin Lab Invest, 46: 553-559, 1986.

58.   Romanelli G, Giustina A, Cimino A, Valentini U, Agabiti-Rosei E, Muiesan G, Giustina G: Short term effect of captopril on microalbuminuia induced by exercise in normotensive diabetics. Br Med J, 298: 284-288, 1989.

59.   Mogensen CE: Long-term antihypertensive treatment inhibiting progression of diabetic nephropathy. Br Med J, 285: 685-689, 1982.

60.   Björck S, Nyberg G, Mulec H, Granerus G, Herlitz H, Aurell M: Beneficial effects of angiotensin converting enzyme inhibition on renal function in patients with diabetic nephropathy. Br Med J, 293: 471-474, 1986.

61.   Parving H-H, Andersen AR, Smidt UM, Hommel E, Mathiesen ER, Svendsen PAa: Effect of antihypertensive treatment on kidney function in diabetic nephropathy. Br Med J, 294: 1443-1447, 1987.

62.   Parving H-H, Hommel E, Smidt UM: Protection of kidney function and decrease in albuminuria by captopril in insulin-dependent diabetics with nephropathy. Br Med J, 297: 1086-1091, 1988.

63.   Christensen CK, Pedersen MM, Mogensen CE: Combining antihypertensive agents in early diabetic nephropathy. J Diabetic Compl, 4: 88-90, 1990.

64.   Christensen CK, Pedersen MM, Hansen KW, Schmitz A, Mogensen CE: Renal effects of ACE-inhibition in Type 1 (insulin-dependent) patients treated with betablocker and thiazide. Diabetologia, 33 (suppl): 256A, 1990.

65.   Curtis JR: Interventions in chronic renal failure. Treatment may slow progression in some cases. Br Med J, 301: 622-624, 1990.

66.   Viberti GC, Bilous RW, Mackintosh D, Bending JJ, Keen H: Long term correction of hyperglycaemia and progression of renal failure in insulin dependent diabetes. Br Med J, 286: 598-602, 1983.

67.   Mathiesen ER, Rønn B, Jensen T, Storm B, Deckert T: Relationship between blood pressure and urinary albumin excretion in the development of microalbuminuria. Diabetes, 39: 245-249, 1990.

68.   Dahl-Jørgensen K, Hanssen KF, Kierulf P, et al: Reduction of urinary albumin excretion after 4 years of continuous subcutaneous insulin infusion in insulin-dependent diabetes mellitus. Acta Endocrinol (Copenh), 117: 19-25, 1988.

69.   Bangstad H-J, Hanssen KF, Dahl-Jørgensen K, Aagenaes Ø: Microalbuminuria is associated with long term poor glycemic control in adolescent insulin dependent diabetics. Diabetes Res, 12: 71-74, 1989.

70.   Kalk WJ, Osler C, Taylor D, Panz VR: Prior long term glycaemic control and insulin therapy in insulin-dependent diabetic adolescents with microalbuminuria. Diabetes Res Clin Prac, 9: 83-88, 1990.

71. Nyberg G, Nordén G, Björck S, Larsson O: Progression of diabetic nephropathy - a multifactorial process. Scand J Urol Nephrol, 108 (suppl): 35-40, 1988.
72. Mulec H, Johnson S-A, Björck S: Relation between serum cholesterol and diabetic nephropathy. Lancet, 335: 1537-1538, 1990.
73. Moorhead JF, Chan MK, El-Nahs M, Varghese Z: Lipid nephrotoxicity in chronic progressive glomerular and tubulo-interstitial disease. Lancet, II: 1309-1311, 1982.
74. Kasiske BL, O'Donnell MP, Cowardin W, Keane WF: Lipids and the kidney. Hypertension, 15: 443-450, 1990.
75. Pedersen MM, Mogensen CE, Schønau Jørgensen F, Møller B, Lykke G, Pedersen O: Renal effects of from limitation of high dietary protein in normoalbuminuric insulin-dependent diabetic patients. Kidney Int, 36 (suppl 27): S115-S121, 1989.
76. Cohen DL, Dodds R, Viberti GC: Effect of protein restriction in insulin dependent diabetics at risk of nephropathy. Br Med J, 294: 795-798, 1987.
77. Walker JD, Dodds RA, Murrells TJ, Bending JJ, Mattock MB, Keen H, Viberti GC: Restriction of dietary protein and progression of renal failure in diabetic nephropathy. Lancet, II: 1411-1415, 1989.
78. Zeller K, Whittaker E, Sullivan L, Raskin P, Jacobson HR: Effect of restricting dietary protein on the progression of renal failure in patients with insulin-dependent diabetes mellitus. N Engl J Med, 324: 78-84, 1991.
79. Evanoff GV, Thompson C, Brown J, et al: Prolonged dietary protein restriction in diabetic nephropathy. Arch Intern Med, 149:1129-1133, 1989.
80. Anderson S: Low protein diets and diabetic nephropathy. Sem Nephrol, 10: 287-293, 1990.
81. Parving H-H: Low-protein diet and progression of renal disease in diabetic nephropathy. Lancet, 335: 411, 1990 (Letter).

THE KIDNEY IN PREGNANCY

Chapter 7

TREATMENT OF HYPERTENSION DURING PREGNANCY: DRUGS TO BE AVOIDED AND DRUGS TO BE USED

STEPHEN N STURGISS*, MARSHALL D LINDHEIMER** AND JOHN M DAVISON*

*Department of Obstetrics and Gynaecology, University of Newcastle-upon-Tyne, Princess Mary Maternity Hospital, Great North Road, Newcastle-upon-Tyne, UK, NE2 3BD and **Departments of Medicine and Obstetrics and Gynecology, University of Chicago, Chicago Lying-in Hospital, 5841 Maryland Avenue, Chicago, IL 60637, USA

This chapter focuses on hypertension during pregnancy, a common clinical problem and one of the main causes of maternal and perinatal morbidity and mortality. Drug treatment of hypertension during pregnancy is controversial not only because of our lack of understanding of cardiovascular physiology in normal pregnancy, but also because there is a clinical spectrum of hypertensive disorders in pregnancy making an aetiologic diagnosis difficult by clinical criteria alone. Therefore, before considering drugs to be avoided and drugs to be used, it is essential to briefly review the course of normal blood pressure during pregnancy, the classification of hypertensive disorders which complicate pregnancy and the pathophysiology of these disorders in pregnancy, focusing on pre-eclampsia.

BLOOD PRESSURE DURING NORMAL PREGNANCY

Blood pressure normally decreases in early pregnancy, reaching its nadir at about the stage of pregnancy at which women usually present for antenatal care. The decrease averages about 7 - 10 mm Hg for diastolic readings although in some women the decrement is more than this, such that the return of blood pressure towards nonpregnancy levels in late pregnancy might be sufficient to diagnose hypertension. Interestingly, women who are hypertensive prior to pregnancy usually have a greater decrease in blood pressure in early pregnancy than do normotensive women, so they are more likely to be erroneously diagnosed as hypertensive.

CLASSIFICATION OF HYPERTENSION DURING PREGNANCY

The most crucial factor in the classification of increased blood pressure during pregnancy is the differentiation of hypertension that precedes pregnancy from a pregnancy-specific condition, which is characterised by poor perfusion of many organs and which usually has increased blood pressure as one of its features. In the former condition, elevated blood pressure is the cardinal pathophysiological feature, while in the latter, increased blood pressure is important primarily as a sign of the underlying disorder. The impact of these two conditions on mother and fetus is quite different, as is their management. Attempts to differentiate these two classes of patients have led to confusion in terminology. In 1972 a system was proposed by the American College of Obstetricians and Gynaecologists which, although imperfect, has been in wide use for some time and has the advantage of clarity and simplicity and divides pregnant women with hypertension into 4 groups: [1] chronic hypertension, [2] pre-eclampsia/eclampsia, [3] pre-eclampsia superimposed upon chronic hypertension and [4] transient hypertension.

[1] Chronic hypertension

Chronic hypertension is defined as a blood pressure of 140/90 mm Hg or greater present prior to pregnancy or before the 20th week of pregnancy. Hypertension diagnosed for the first time during pregnancy and persisting beyond the 42nd day postpartum is also classified as chronic hypertension.

[2] Pre-eclampsia/eclampsia

Pre-eclampsia usually occurs after the 20th week of pregnancy (or earlier with trophoblastic disease) and is determined by increased blood pressure accompanied by proteinuria, edema or both. Either of the following criteria suffice for the diagnosis of hypertension in this situation: [1] systolic blood pressure increases of 30 mm Hg or more or [2] diastolic blood pressure increases of 15 mm Hg or more from early values (average values prior to 20 weeks gestation). If prior blood pressure is not known, readings of greater than or equal to 140/90 mm Hg after 20 weeks gestation are considered sufficiently elevated to satisfy the blood pressure criteria of pre-eclampsia. Of interest some pregnant women will show the blood pressure increase required for the diagnosis of pre-eclampsia without attaining 140/90 mm Hg.

Proteinuria is defined as the excretion of 0.3 g or greater in a 24-hour specimen. This will usually correlate with 30 mg/dl (1+ dipstick) or greater in a random urine sample.

164

Proteinuria usually is a late sign in the course of pre-eclampsia; although it is non-specific, its appearance greatly endorses the diagnosis of pre-eclampsia.

Edema is clinically evident swelling. Fluid retention, however, may also be apparent as a rapid increase of weight without swelling.

[3] Pre-eclampsia superimposed upon chronic hypertension

Pre-eclampsia may occur in women who have chronic hypertension and the prognosis for mother and fetus is much worse than with either condition alone. The diagnosis can be made on the basis of increases of blood pressure (30 mm Hg systolic or 15 mm Hg diastolic, or 20 mm Hg mean arterial pressure) together with the appearance of proteinuria or generalised edema.

[4] Transient hypertension

This label is used when elevated blood pressure occurs during pregnancy or in the first 24 hours postpartum without other signs of pre-eclampsia or preexisting hypertension. If any uncertainty regarding the diagnosis exists, these patients should be managed as having pre-eclampsia. It is often predictive of the eventual development of essential hypertension.

PATHOPHYSIOLOGY OF HYPERTENSION DURING PREGNANCY

A major pathophysiological feature is a marked increase in peripheral resistance. This vasospasm is due, in part, to exaggerated responsiveness to circulating angiotensin II (AII) and catecholamines and possibly an imbalance between thromboxane and prostacyclin production. Prior to therapeutic intervention, cardiac output is often decreased, pulmonary capillary wedge pressure is normal or low and intravascular volume is below that of normal pregnant women. Renal hemodynamics decrease, related in part to the characteristic morphologic lesion in the glomerulus (glomerular endotheliosis) and there may be increased vascular permeability leading to albumin loss from the intravascular space. Compromised uteroplacental perfusion often leads to fetal growth retardation.

There can be two life threatening complications. Firstly, a rapidly developing syndrome characterised by microangiopathic hemolytic anemia and marked signs of liver dysfunction as well as coagulation changes. This variant is termed HELLP - hemolysis, elevated liver enzymes, low platelets - and is an emergency necessitating termination of the pregnancy (often hemolysis is absent - hence the ELLP syndrome). Secondly, a progression to a convulsive phase, eclampsia, associated with autopsy findings of cerebral hyperemia, thrombosis and hemorrhage.

Compromised placental perfusion due to placental pathology (failure of trophoblastic invasion of spiral arteries) and vasospasm is almost certainly a major culprit in the genesis of the increased perinatal morbidity and mortality.

RATIONALE BEHIND TREATMENT OF HYPERTENSION DURING PREGNANCY

A decision to treat elevated blood pressure in pregnancy is much more controversial than in nonpregnant patients. In pregnancy the hypertension is of relatively short duration, there is the need to consider a second patient, the fetus, and the majority of clinical experience to date has been derived from nonrandomised and noncontrolled studies (often retrospective) of pregnant women with various types of hypertension.

Maternal beneficial effects

For the mother the major risks of severe hypertension are cardiac decompensation and cerebrovascular accidents. In contrast, the hazards of mild to moderate hypertension, over a period of several weeks to months, are less clear. Therefore, the rationale to treat such levels of blood pressure in nonpregnant populations (i.e. prevention of vascular pathology, which requires years to develop) cannot reasonably be applied in pregnancy.

Another question is whether or not the treatment of mild to moderate hypertension in pregnancy reduces the progression to severe hypertension and/or the need for hospitalisation?

Fetal and neonatal beneficial effects

Friedman and Neff (1), analysing data from 38,636 women, observed that fetal mortality rose abruptly when diastolic blood pressure was greater than 84 mm Hg at any stage of pregnancy. Page and Christianson (2) noted that in 14,833 single births there were increases in perinatal mortality and intrauterine growth retardation when second and third trimester mean arterial pressures exceeded 90 and 95 mm Hg, respectively. Whether or not outcome is much altered by drug therapy remains to be established. In a review of five randomised, controlled trials of drug therapy versus no treatment for hypertension during pregnancy (3) four trials failed to demonstrate a significant reduction in perinatal mortality (4-7), but the pooled relative risk of fetal or neonatal loss for all the studies showed a benefit favouring treatment. In the largest trial, in which the reduction in perinatal mortality was the greatest (8), the improved outcome was due to a reduction in the incidence of midtrimester stillbirths, leading to the suggestion that the mechanism of any potential benefit may be independent of a reduction in blood pressure *per se* (see later discussion of methyldopa therapy).

Another potential positive effect of antihypertensive therapy is the prevention of premature delivery necessitated by severe maternal hypertension. Although early studies suggested that this might be the case, gestational age at delivery in more recent trials was similar in treated and untreated subjects (4, 5).

Table 1. Food and drug administration pregnancy risk classification.

A. *Controlled studies show no risk.*Well-designed studies in humans have failed to demonstrate risk to the fetus.
B. *No evidence of risk in humans.* Either [a] animal studies demonstrate risk but human findings do not or [b] if no adequate human studies have been done, animal findings are negative.
C. *Risk cannot be ruled out.* Human studies are lacking, and animal studies are either positive for fetal risk or have not been performed. However, potential benefits may justify the potential risk.
D. *Positive evidence of risk.* Investigational or post marketing data show risk to the fetus. Nevertheless, potential benefits may outweigh the risks (e.g. for treatment of serious disease for which safer alternatives are not available).
X. *Contraindicated in pregnancy.* Studies in animals or humans (or post marketing reports) have shown fetal risk which clearly outweighs any potential benefit to the patient.

Non-beneficial effects

Any benefits must be weighed against possible adverse effects on the offspring, short and long-term. There is a paucity of data mainly because there are no standards for drug testing, either for humans or animals, which encompasses [1] effects of the agent on the ability of the fetus to withstand hypoxic stress, [2] thorough analyses of structural and functional variables in the neonate and [3] long-term assessment of intellectual and physical well-being of the offspring.

FETAL RISKS

The US Food and Drug Administration has suggested a "risk assessment classification" which theoretically assigns an individual drug according to risk posed to the fetus and/or neonate (Table 1). Most drugs have not been "risk assessed" by the manufacturers so that variable categorisation may occur between different authors. Furthermore, clinicians may be lulled into a false sense of security about drug prescribing during pregnancy because of a notation that no fetal or reproductive side effects have been described.

There have been very few studies of even crude markers of drug safety let alone any subtle effects. The teratogenicity of all antihypertensives remains virtually unknown, since drug trials of even the best-studied agents (such as methyldopa) have generally included women only when they are beyond the first trimester. Since virtually all drugs prescribed to pregnant women reach the fetus, the above considerations serve as a reminder that therapeutic agents of any kind should be prescribed to pregnant women with the utmost caution.

UTEROPLACENTAL CIRCULATORY RISKS

A major concern is that uteroplacental blood flow may be adversely affected. As the uterine spiral arteries lose their muscular media in early pregnancy and probably behave as maximally dilated passive conduits, it has been suggested that placental blood flow is not effectively autoregulated. Experiments in anaesthetised pregnant rabbits demonstrated well-maintained uteroplacental blood flow over a wide range of systemic arterial pressure (9), but studies in awake rabbits and sheep have indicated that placental perfusion is directly related to the level of systemic blood pressure (10-12). Regardless of whether placental blood flow is effectively autoregulated, it is clear that uteroplacental blood flow can be influenced by several vasoconstrictors (probably by acting on the proximal uterine vasculature) and that circulating levels of endogenous pressor hormones may be markedly augmented following excessive drug-induced decrements in maternal arterial pressure.

RECOMMENDATIONS FOR TREATMENT OF HYPERTENSION DURING PREGNANCY

Not surprisingly there are divergent recommendations regarding the treatment of hypertension during pregnancy. Some believe that drug therapy should be initiated when blood pressure is >140/90 mm Hg (13, 14), whereas others, reporting impressive fetal and maternal outcome statistics, withhold treatment until levels are 150-170/110 mm Hg (15, 16).

Our approach is an intermediate one: in the acute inpatient setting, drug therapy is initiated when diastolic blood pressure is >105 mm Hg. The goal is to lower blood pressure gradually to levels between 90 and 100 mm Hg, a point at which the risk of hypertension-induced cerebrovascular hemorrhage is extremely low.

In a chronically hypertensive woman medication is withheld as long as diastolic blood pressure is <95 mm Hg. Important exceptions to this approach are women with renal disease and/or diabetes in whom a more aggressive line is taken in order to prevent further glomerular damage.

Table 2. Drug therapy of severe hypertension in pregnancy.*

DRUG	DOSE/ROUTE°	ONSET OF ACTION	ADVERSE EFFECTS^	COMMENTS
Agent of choice				
Hydralazine	5 mg iv/im, then 5-10 mg every 20-40 mins; or constant infusion of 0.5-10 mg/hr	iv: 10 min im: 20-30 min	Headache, flushing, tachycardia, nausea, vomiting	Broad experience of safety and efficacy
Second-line agents				
Diazoxide	30-50 mg iv every 5-15 mins	2-5 min	Inhibition of labour; hyperglycaemia, fluid retention with repeated doses	Doses of 150-300 mg may cause severe hypotension
Labetalol	20 mg iv, then 20-80 mg every 20-30 min, up to 300 mg; or constant infusion of 1-2 mg/min until desired effect, then stop or reduce to 0.5 mg/min	5-10 min	Flushing, nausea, vomiting, tingling of scalp	Limited experience in pregnancy
Nifedipine	10 mg po; repeat in 30 min if necessary then 10-20 mg po every 3-6 hr	10-15 min	Flushing, headache, nausea, inhibition of labor	May adversely interact with MgSO$_4$; limited experience in pregnancy
To be avoided				
Nitroprusside	0.5-10 µg/Kg/min by constant iv infusion	Instantaneous	Cyanide toxicity, nausea, vomiting	Use only in critical care unit at low doses for briefest time feasible; may cause fetal cyanide toxicity

* Indicated for acute elevation of diastolic blood pressure to >105 mm Hg; goal is gradual reduction to 90-100 mm Hg
° Abbreviations: iv = intravenously; im = intramuscularly; po = per os (orally)
^ All agents may cause marked hypotension, especially in severe pre-eclampsia

169

In general, if pre-eclampsia or severe hypertension occurs beyond the 36th gestational week, a point at which fetal pulmonary maturity has generally occurred, delivery is the therapy of choice following control of elevated blood pressure. Delivery is also indicated regardless of gestational age if there is evidence of advanced disease or impending eclampsia, since progression is virtually inevitable unless the uterus is evacuated. Particularly worrisome symptoms and signs are: headache, blurred vision, scotomata, epigastric pain, diastolic blood pressure >110 mm Hg after 24 hrs of hospitalisation, clonus, rising serum creatinine and consumptive coagulopathy.

DRUGS TO BE USED FOR ACUTE HYPERTENSION

The ideal drug should act quickly and reliably to reduce blood pressure in a gradual manner, thereby avoiding hypotension and baroreflex-mediated sympathetic responses, both of which may reduce placental blood flow.

In addition, such a drug should act directly on the uteroplacental vasculature to reverse vasospasm induced by the hypertensive disease process and be free of adverse effects on both mother and fetus.

The ideal drug is not currently available, but several drugs used cautiously are successful in this situation (Table 2).

Hydralazine

Hydralazine is the most frequently used antihypertensive agent for control of severe hypertension and has a long record of proven effectiveness.

The effect of parenteral hydralazine on the maternal cardiovascular system has been studied using Swan Ganz catheterisation, M-mode echocardiography and radionuclide methods (17-22). In all studies, blood pressure reduction occurred in association with a reduced systemic vascular resistance and increased maternal heart rate and cardiac index. Where decreased stroke volume has been noted the rise in cardiac output was achieved from increased heart rate. Concurrently pulmonary capillary wedge pressure (PCWP) decreased, oliguria ensued and some fetuses showed cardiotocographic evidence of distress. These adverse reactions were rapidly corrected with an infusion of plasma or plasma substitute suggesting that hydralazine-induced vasodilation in pre-eclamptic women (who are known to have contraction of plasma volume) had led to relative underfilling of the circulatory volume with inability to maintain adequate venous return to the heart. Other workers, however, have shown either no change or an increase in stroke volume and in the only other study using Swan Ganz catheters, PCWP minimally increased.

It is difficult to account for the discrepancies in the findings of different workers, but numbers in each trial were small and some patients had received magnesium sulphate or anti-hypertensive treatment before investigation.

UTEROPLACENTAL CIRCULATORY RISKS

Hydralazine administration to normotensive pregnant ewes, or ewes made hypertensive with phenylephrine, resulted in decreased and increased blood flow, respectively. However, these early studies have been criticised because of the use of uterine artery flow probes, which are unable to differentiate between myometrial and placental circulation. More recently, a radioactive labeled microsphere technique has been used to assess organ blood flow during administration of hydralazine to spontaneously hypertensive rats (23). Hydralazine produced opposite effects on the myometrial and placental circulation, with a 45% reduction in myometrial vascular resistance resulting in a 57% increase in flow and a 43% increase in placental vascular resistance resulting in a 44% reduction in flow. In addition, rats with the highest blood pressure tended to have the lowest placental perfusion after drug administration. It is possible that the divergent effects on myometrial and placental hemodynamics are due to catecholamine release and reflex sympathetic activation after vasodilator therapy. There are abundant alpha-adrenergic receptors on uterine spiral arteries and in pre-eclampsia the response to circulating vasoactive agents is not completely attenuated.

The results of human studies using radionuclide methods have been similarly variable and overall hydralazine had no effect on uteroplacental blood flow (20-22). In one study there was a non-significant increment in mean intervillous blood flow (IVBF) from 92 to 76 ml/min/100 ml, but the range of percentage change was from an increment of 35% to a decrement of 69% (20). No consistent means of predicting individual response from baseline parameters was found, but there appeared to be a significant correlation between change in maternal blood pressure and change in uteroplacental blood flow index. Patients with minimal change in blood pressure experienced the largest drop in uteroplacental flow (21).

FETAL RISKS

Decrements in uteroplacental blood flow are likely to manifest clinically as fetal distress.

Several studies have shown cardiotocographic fetal distress with parenteral hydralazine. There is a report of fetal distress in 19 of 33 women who were given 12.5 mg of intravenous hydralazine to control diastolic blood pressure (DBP) of greater than or equal to 110 mm Hg (24), but the reduction of DBP to 70 - 90 mm Hg indicates the dose of hydralazine was excessive. In addition, 13 of the 19 neonates showing fetal heart rate changes were growth retarded (<10th percentile).

Another study aimed to reduce DBP to 100 mm Hg with hydralazine 5 mg intravenously at 10 minute intervals (25). Fetal distress occurred in two patients, one where 15 mg of hydralazine had lowered blood pressure from 174/113 to 164/78 mm Hg with late decelerations 90 minutes from the start of the study and another where 10 mg of hydralazine had reduced blood pressure from 182/123 to 152/89 mm Hg with fetal distress after 80 minutes.

The role of intravascular volume depletion in contributing to fetal distress has been emphasised and fetal distress usually resolves after an infusion of plasma or plasma substitute.

In one study of 23 pre-eclamptic women who were volume expanded before vasodilator therapy, there were no abnormal cardiotocograms (17).

Calcium channel blocking agents

Calcium channel blocking agents are easy to administer, rapidly and effectively lower blood pressure and have minimal side effects.

There are two groups, the dihydropyridine group (which includes nifedipine and nicardipine) and the phenylalkyline group (which includes verapamil), both having pharmacological properties theoretically useful in the treatment of pregnancy hypertension.

The dihydropyridine compounds dilate precapillary arterioles with a reduction of blood pressure proportionate to the pre-treatment level of hypertension. In addition, the renin-angiotensin-aldosterone system is not activated, renal blood flow is maintained despite the decrement in perfusion pressure, cerebral arterioles are preferentially dilated and platelet aggregation is inhibited.

Alternatively, verapamil inhibits calcium influx in sino-atrial and atrio-ventricular nodes, limiting the reflex tachycardia that can occur with the dihydropyridine drugs.

Furthermore, verapamil has a short duration of action when given intravenously, increases renal and liver perfusion (in non-pregnant subjects), causes pregnancy specific uterine artery vasodilation and inhibits platelet aggregation.

Despite these theoretical advantages calcium antagonists have not yet been widely used in obstetrics.

UTEROPLACENTAL CIRCULATORY RISKS

Administration of nifedipine to normotensive pregnant sheep and monkeys caused a reduction of blood pressure with significant decrements in uterine blood flow, fetal hypoxia and in some cases fetal acidosis (26, 27).

Normotensive animals, however, are inappropriate models to study the placental hemodynamic response to antihypertensive agents as placental vasculature is already maximally dilated and no compensatory additional vasodilation can occur in response to a reduction in perfusion pressure.

Nicardipine administered to pregnant ewes (made hypertensive with an angiotensin infusion) caused increased placental vascular resistance with reduced uterine blood flow and fetal deaths in some cases (28, 29). The maternal vascular component of the ovine placenta, however, has an anomalous response to all vasodilatators and this study is probably irrelevant to human pregnancy.

More encouragingly in spontaneously hypertensive rats (arguably a better model for hypertensive human pregnancy), placental blood flow remained constant despite reduced perfusion pressure indicating compensatory or drug-induced placental vasodilatation (30).

In hypertensive human pregnancy radionuclide methods and pulsed doppler ultrasound have been used to study the effect of nifedipine on placental vasculature. Flow velocity waveforms showed either no change or a decrease in systolic/diastolic ratio of up to 30% (31, 32).

Doppler assessment of fetal and placental vasculature during nifedipine tocolytic therapy demonstrated no significant change in pulsatility index in fetal vessels and maternal uterine arteries (33). Radionuclide methods have demonstrated constant uteroplacental blood flow despite a drop in mean arterial pressure, indicating reduction of uterine vascular resistance in proportion to the decrement in perfusion pressure (34).

In humans there is a 6-17% reduction in blood pressure after single dose (or long-term therapy) within 20 minutes, with maximum effect at 50 minutes to 2-4 hours. In patients already receiving other antihypertensive therapy nifedipine reduces blood pressure significantly within 10 minutes with the effect lasting up to 8 hours (35). In the same report side effects include hot flushes, palpitations and headache, but fetal heart rate was not altered and bleeding at delivery was not excessive. Fetal outcome was as expected in women with this severity of disease.

Nifedipine and hydralazine have been compared as acute and long-term therapy in women with severe pre-eclampsia (36). Nifedipine was more effective at controlling blood pressure, caused less fetal distress (1 vs 11 cases) and was associated with heavier infants born at a later gestational age with fewer neonatal complications. Reduction of blood pressure in the acute situation was more gradual and predictable with nifedipine, but the bolus dose of hydralazine was larger than recommended by other authors and the intervals between administration were not stated.

Diazoxide

This congener of the thiazide diuretics is a potent arteriolar vasodilator. Intravenous 300 mg boluses have been recommended, but not infrequently caused precipitous decrements in blood pressure. Current recommendations are to administer the drug in smaller doses (see Table 2) more frequently or by continuous infusion.

UTEROPLACENTAL CIRCULATORY RISKS

In normotensive and hypertensive sheep uterine blood flow is reduced, the magnitude of change being directly related to the degree of blood pressure reduction. Apparently, the adverse hemodynamic effects of bolus diazoxide administration can be markedly attenuated by a slow infusion protocol.

FETAL RISKS

As with other smooth muscle relaxants, labor may be arrested, an effect that can generally be overcome by the administration of syntocinon. Maternal and neonatal hyperglycemia can occur due to suppression of insulin release and severe degeneration of pancreatic islet cells has been reported in animals subjected to repeat administration of diazoxide. Long-term follow-up of children exposed to diazoxide in-utero is required, focusing on the incidence of diabetes or other disorders of pancreatic function.

Labetalol

The parenteral use of this adrenergic inhibitor, with combined beta and alpha-1 blocking properties, has been reported to reduce blood pressure more reliably than hydralazine (37, 38), but others have found both drugs similarly efficacious (25, 39) and well tolerated (25, 38). It seem likely that labetalol causes no change in uteroplacental, umbilical venous or fetal aortic blood flow, and, where fetal distress (39) and neonatal bradycardia (40) have occurred, it is unclear if these were drug effects or due to the underlying maternal disease.

Sodium nitroprusside

Use of this potent vasodilator has been reported in very few pregnant women, usually in an emergency situation such as pulmonary edema or life threatening hypertension unresponsive to more conventional therapy. This drug, which is metabolised to cyanide and thiocyanate, crosses the placenta, thus regarding concern regarding potential fetal toxicity. Although brief infusions of relatively low doses (<4 mg/kg b.w./min) have not been associated with maternal or fetal cyanide levels in the toxic range or with clinically evident toxicity, nitroprusside remains drug of last resort during pregnancy and should be avoided.

ANTICONVULSANT DRUGS TO BE USED IN HYPERTENSION DURING PREGNANCY

The cause of convulsions is unknown, but as approximately 20% of these women have minimally elevated blood pressure shortly before convulsing, control of blood pressure will not entirely prevent eclamptic fits.

Magnesium sulphate

In the United States magnesium sulphate has long been the drug of choice for prophylaxis and treatment of eclamptic seizures despite considerable uncertainty as to its mode of action. Proposed sites of action are within the central nervous system or peripherally at the neuromuscular junction. If magnesium does have a central effect it must do so by a mechanism that does not alter the electro-encephalogram (EEG) as abnormal EEG traces have been documented in pre-eclamptic and eclamptic women despite adequate serum magnesium levels. Furthermore, continuous EEG's recorded during magnesium therapy have shown no quantitative differences before, during or after treatment (41). There is concern that if magnesium does not act centrally then peripheral manifestation of seizures will be masked while potentially injurious changes proceed within the cerebral cortex. Evidence for peripheral neuromuscular blockade is lack of anaesthesia or sensory deficit in patients with severe hypermagnesemia and greater deposition of magnesium in peripheral tissues (compared to within the brain) following intravenous administration.

Recent evidence is more supportive of a central mode of action. Previous studies suggested that the blood brain barrier keeps central nervous system magnesium levels

175

within physiological limits, but a significant increment (19%) in cerebrospinal fluid magnesium levels are apparent four or more hours after intravenous administration (42) and furthermore, serum magnesium levels correlate with those in cerebrospinal fluid.

A substantial component of neuronal damage in prolonged seizures is associated with calcium influx through the N-methyl-D-aspartate (NMDA) subtype of glutamate channel (43). NMDA antagonists, which include magnesium, confer protection from cerebral ischemia and magnesium protects cultured hippocampal cells against anoxia or glutamate-induced injury (44, 45). Other suggested beneficial effects of magnesium include calcium channel mediated reversal of cerebral vasospasm and intracellular calcium substitution, blocking the calcium mediated feedback process that can lead to cell death. Furthermore, magnesium will enhance endothelial production of prostacyclin and modify response to vasoactive substances found in serum samples of pre-eclamptic patients.

ARGUMENTS WHY MAGNESIUM SULPHATE SHOULD BE USED

There is extensive documentation of magnesium sulphate in treating eclampsia or preventing seizures in pre-eclampsia. In a study of 245 eclamptic women who were managed with magnesium sulphate there was only one mortality, which was due to cardiorespiratory arrest following inadvertent administration of a 20 g intravenous bolus dose of magnesium (rather than the correct 4 g), illustrating the potentially fatal consequences of deviating from a standard regimen (46). Non-fatal magnesium intoxication occurred in a further three cases and in all instances this was due to deviation from the standard protocol - specifically giving more than 8 g at the outset of treatment or continuing to administer intramuscular magnesium despite lack of a patellar reflex. Perinatal outcome was impressive as of 79 fetuses alive at the time of eclampsia 71 survived to be discharged from hospital and magnesium intoxication was not diagnosed in any neonate. In a similar report of 262 eclamptic women managed with magnesium there was only one death, this occurring in a patient who suffered cardiorespiratory arrest before administration of magnesium (47). Lastly in a study of 1,870 women receiving magnesium to prevent eclampsia there were only 11 seizures (0.6%) and no serious adverse effects (48).

ARGUMENTS WHY MAGNESIUM SULPHATE SHOULD BE AVOIDED

Magnesium sulphate is not used as an anticonvulsant in any other situation and abnormal electroencephalographic activity can occur despite adequate magnesium levels. Opponents argue that magnesium sulphate is not a proven anticonvulsant, doubt the

176

excellent results in the literature and caution that profound maternal hypotension, hypothermia and cardiovascular collapse can occur as well as neonatal flaccidity, hyporeflexia and respiratory distress. Maternal osteomalacia has also been reported in association with prolonged intravenous tocolytic therapy (49).

Benzodiazepines

It has been argued that as eclamptic seizures are identical to those arising from a variety of other pathologies then drugs with proven anticonvulsant efficacy, such as benzodiazepines, should be used.

Diazepam, which rapidly controls seizures, has been used in pre-eclampsia, eclampsia and status epilepticus during pregnancy. The resultant maternal sedation, however, can interfere with neurological assessment, impair respiration and lead to increased risk of aspiration of gastric contents. Large doses of diazepam (more than 30 mg) administered during labor have been associated with reduced fetal heart rate variability, neonatal respiratory depression, hypotonia, feeding disturbance and hypothermia. It has been argued that there is little evidence that these complications occur when benzodiazepines are administered intravenously around the time of delivery.

A recent study has compared diazepam (a 10 mg intravenous bolus dose followed by an intravenous infusion) to magnesium sulphate (a 4 g bolus followed by 10 g intramuscularly) in the management of 51 women with eclampsia (50). Overall maternal morbidity (defined as recurrent convulsions, cardiopulmonary problems, coagulation failure and renal failure) was non-significantly lower in the magnesium group (29%) than in women treated with diazepam (52%). Recurrent convulsions after stabilisation (one hour of treatment) were commoner in the diazepam group (4 cases vs 1), and furthermore the patient in the magnesium group who convulsed did not receive the correct maintenance dose as stated in the protocol.

Three women in the diazepam group developed pneumonia and one patient experienced respiratory depression, whereas none treated with magnesium had respiratory complications. Diminished urine output was less common in magnesium treated women (3 cases vs 12).

Babies born to mothers receiving magnesium sulphate had significantly higher Apgar scores at one and five minutes, and required less frequent intubation, intermittent positive pressure ventilation and admission to the neonatal intensive care unit. The study, however, was undertaken in a busy obstetric unit in the developing world and the authors mentioned that patient supervision (and especially titration of intravenous diazepam) may have been less than ideal.

Phenytoin

Recent reports have advocated phenytoin as the drug of choice in pre-eclampsia or eclampsia on the basis that it is an effective anticonvulsant and does not cause maternal sedation nor effect respiratory drive. Where an intravenous infusion of phenytoin was used for seizure prophylaxis in 24 women with moderate to severe pre-eclampsia and two women with eclampsia none convulsed and the drug was well tolerated (51). One woman had a hypotensive episode (130/80 to 95/50 mm Hg) which resolved without any therapy or adjustment of the infusion rate and one neonate developed a cephalhematoma.

Phenytoin has been used alone or in combination with diazepam, frusemide and hydralazine and the main benefit of adding phenytoin was greater reduction of blood pressure and less maternal sedation (52). There are reports, however, of women having further seizures after phenytoin and in some the serum phenytoin levels were apparently in the therapeutic range (47, 53). In a comparative study of phenytoin and magnesium sulphate in the management of 22 eclamptic further convulsions occurred in four of the 11 women receiving phenytoin (compared to none in the women receiving magnesium sulphate)(54). Two of these women had low-borderline phenytoin levels (45 and 46 μmols/l), but the other two had levels of 65 and 70 μmols/l. There are other problems with phenytoin: discomfort at the infusion site, the requirement for continuous maternal heart rate monitoring and the effect of serum albumin on levels of free unbound "active" drug. The consensus is that phenytoin (at least in the range declared therapeutic in the non-pregnant population) is not an effective an anticonvulsant as magnesium sulphate.

Are anticonvulsants really necessary?

It must also be concluded that there is little evidence that anticonvulsants are required in pre-eclampsia. Most of the data reviewed refer to eclampsia - when the risk of recurrent seizures certainly warrants anticonvulsant therapy. Demonstrating the superiority of one anticonvulsant over another in this setting, however, does not justify the use of that same drug in pre-eclampsia, when the risk of a convulsion is very low, whatever the treatment. Using the occurrence of a convulsions as an end point, the size of a trial to compare anticonvulsants with each other or a control would need to be so large it is difficult to believe that such a study could ever be accomplished.

DRUGS TO BE USED FOR CHRONIC HYPERTENSION

Methyldopa

Methyldopa was one of the first drugs used in the treatment of hypertension in pregnancy (Table 3). Its clinical use has been well documented and long-term follow-up of infants exposed to the drug in-utero has been more extensive than with any other antihypertensive agent. There is no excess of congenital malformation in babies of women who received methyldopa in early pregnancy nor is there any evidence of long-term problems.

Table 3. Drug therapy of chronic hypertension in pregnancy*

DRUG	DOSE	ADVERSE EFFECTS AND COMMENTS
Agent of choice Methyldopa	500-3,000 mg in 2-4 divided doses	Safety for mother and fetus (after 1st trimester) is well documented.
Second line agents Hydralazine	50-300 mg in 2-4 divided doses	Few controlled trials but extensive experience with few serious adverse effects documented; several reports of neonatal thrombocytopenia.
Beta-adrenergic inhibitors (and the combined alpha-beta blocker, labetalol)	Dependent on specific agent used	May cause fetal bradycardia and impair fetal responses to hypoxia. Risk of intra-uterine growth retardation remains unclear
Third line agents Thiazide diuretics	Dependent on agent used	Most controlled studies in normotensive gravidas; little data in hypertensive gestation. Implicated in volume depletion, electrolyte imbalance, pancreatitis and thrombocytopenia.
Clonidine	0.1-0.8 mg in 2 divided doses	Limited data
Nifedipine	30-120 mg in 3-4 divided doses	Limited data; may inhibit labour; potential for severe hypotension in patients receiving $MgSO_4$
Prazosin	1-30 mg in 2-3 divided doses	Limited data
To be avoided Angiotensin-converting enzyme inhibitors	Dependent on agent used	High rates of fetal loss in animals. Several cases of neonatal anuric renal failure in humans.

* Note that safety during the third trimester has not been established for any antihypertensive agent

MATERNAL RISKS AND ANTIHYPERTENSIVE EFFICACY

The only maternal side effects that have occurred significantly more frequently in treated women are lethargy and drowsiness (8). There is a report of a treated patient developing a positive Coomb's test, but this was not associated with a clinical problem and the baby was unaffected (8).

Methyldopa has been assessed in controlled trials and compared to other antihypertensive agents (6, 8, 14, 55, 56). In all studies blood pressure reduction was significant, tending to be greatest in those women with higher pre-treatment hypertension. In one study there was a significant reduction in the incidence of severe hypertension and maximum blood pressure in labor (8), but this has not been confirmed and a study of women with chronic hypertension revealed no difference in requirement for additional antihypertensive medication between methyldopa treated women and controls (55). No preventative effect on the development of pre-eclampsia - usually diagnosed on the basis of biochemical indices of renal involvement - has been demonstrated.

In studies comparing methyldopa to a beta-blocking compound there was a suggestion that methyldopa was the more effective antihypertensive even though there was no significant difference between groups in level of blood pressure reduction. In one study methyldopa reduced mean predelivery blood pressure to 115/70 whereas oxprenolol reduced blood pressure to 130/82 (14). Furthermore, seven women taking methyldopa required additional antihypertensive therapy compared to 11 women receiving oxprenolol. In a similar study six of 24 women receiving oxprenolol required additional antihypertensive therapy compared to no women receiving methyldopa (56). However, this may have been because women admitted to the trial with early onset hypertension who were subsequently allocated to treatment with oxprenolol had a higher systolic blood pressure.

FETAL AND NEONATAL BENEFITS AND RISKS

Earlier studies demonstrated an improvement in the rate of pregnancy loss, but this has not been confirmed more recently. In a study of women with chronic hypertension, treatment with methyldopa produced a significant reduction in abortion and perinatal death (6). There were three abortions and two perinatal deaths in the control group compared to none in women treated with methyldopa. However, if hypertension developed *de novo* later in pregnancy treatment with methyldopa was associated with six perinatal deaths compared to four in controls. This finding was apparently confirmed in a later study in which methyldopa was associated with a significantly improved fetal outcome (8). There were nine pregnancy losses in the control group (including four mid-pregnancy abortions, three stillbirths and two neonatal deaths) compared to only one in controls (a stillbirth). Therefore, a large component of the improved fetal outcome was again due to a reduction in the incidence of mid-pregnancy abortion. Otherwise, there was an excess of perinatal deaths in the control group, but these were ascribable to a variety of causes. The authors speculated that methyldopa may have an unexpected pharmacological effect on uterine motility or cervical competence as it seemed unlikely that control of blood pressure during the second trimester prevented pregnancy loss.

Methyldopa has been shown to have a variable effect on gestation at delivery. In two controlled investigations there was significant prolongation of pregnancy, but this effect was restricted in one study to women with chronic hypertension and in the other to women recruited after 28 weeks (6, 8). It is, however, always difficult to assess whether pregnancy prolongation was a real benefit or merely artefactual due to using level of blood pressure as a guide to timing of delivery.

A variable effect on birthweight and incidence of growth retardation has also been noted. One study demonstrated higher birthweight babies (by 200-300 g) in women on methyldopa apart from those with late onset severe hypertension whose babies were on average 85 g lighter than controls (6). In another study women in a methyldopa group had lighter infants if hypertension was of early onset, but heavier infants if hypertension was late onset (8). Methyldopa was not associated with any change in birthweight in women with chronic hypertension (54). As previously mentioned the randomised comparative studies of oxprenolol and methyldopa had conflicting results. The first study demonstrated that infants of mothers taking methyldopa weighed 400 g less than neonates of women receiving oxprenolol (14). However blood pressure reduction with methyldopa was to a mean of 115/70 which is excessively low and likely to lead to uterine hypoperfusion. In a subsequent larger study there was no significant difference in birthweight between infants of mothers receiving either methyldopa or oxprenolol and in fact the methyldopa babies weighed slightly more (3,009 g vs 2,920 g) (56).

In one of the most thorough follow-up studies a cohort of infants exposed to methyldopa in-utero were examined regularly to seven years of age (57-59). At birth and at eight weeks post-delivery there was an excess of infants in the treated group with head circumference measurements below the mean value for their gestational age and lower than non-treated controls. This difference, however, was significant only in those mothers who had begun treatment at 16 to 20 weeks gestation and linear regression analysis showed no correlation between head circumference and duration or total dose of methyldopa exposure. The authors were wary of attributing too much significance to this finding as women in the non-treatment group had infants with larger than average head circumference measurements. Interestingly, however, it is known that the human brain growth spurt which is thought to be the major period of neuroblast multiplication occurs at 10-18 weeks gestation, but reassuringly there was no detectable neurological impairment at any stage up to one year. At four years boys in the methyldopa group had significantly smaller heads than in the untreated group, a difference not apparent in girls. No significant difference was found in developmental scores, but there was a tendency for the treated group to score more highly in all sectors of assessment. At seven years boys from the untreated group were heavier and taller than those from the treated group (as were their mothers) but there were no significant differences in height and weight for girls or in head circumference for either sex. No differences were found in British Ability Scales testing and mean IQs did not differ.

Hydralazine

This agent has been used successfully in the chronic setting as a second-line agent in combination with either methyldopa or a beta-blocker (14, 56, 60, 61). In a small, prospective, randomised trial hydralazine monotherapy was shown to be as effective as hydralazine plus pindolol (62), but a much higher incidence of palpitations, dizziness and headache were observed in subjects not receiving a beta-blocker. Hydralazine appears reasonably safe for the fetus, although thrombocytopenia of uncertain etiology has been reported in a few infants (63) and there are no long-term follow-up studies on children exposed to this drug in-utero.

Beta-adrenergic blockers

The use of beta-adrenoreceptor blocking agents in pregnancy has become increasingly frequent over the last decade. Propranolol was the first beta-blocker to be used in pregnancy, but has since been abandoned as case reports and uncontrolled series revealed an apparently high incidence of neonatal side effects such as bradycardia, hypoglycemia, respiratory depression and hypotension. One series demonstrated a high incidence (75%) of unsuccessful pregnancy (defined as fetal loss or intra-uterine growth retardation) in comparison to women receiving other anti-hypertensives, but the women receiving propranolol had more severe disease (64).

With the recent introduction of cardioselective beta-blocking agents such as atenolol, oxprenolol and metoprolol, fewer neonatal side effects have been reported. Labetalol, a non-selective beta-blocking agent with some alpha-1 blocking properties, decreases systemic vascular resistance with little or no change in cardiac output, making it theoretically suited for the treatment of pre-eclampsia.

UTEROPLACENTAL CIRCULATORY RISKS

There is concern that lowering blood pressure with beta-blocking agents may reduce uteroplacental blood flow unless the placental vasculature dilates and placental vascular resistance is decreased. Radionuclide assessment of uteroplacental blood flow during and after a brief labetalol infusion or an oral dose of metoprolol in women with pregnancy-induced hypertension demonstrated significant reduction of maternal blood pressure, but no significant change in indices of uteroplacental blood flow (22, 40, 65). These data should be interpreted cautiously, however, because small numbers of women were involved and there was considerable individual variation in response.

FETAL AND NEONATAL RISKS

There is concern that beta-blocking agents may cause neonatal beta-blockade with hypotension, bradycardia, hypoglycemia and hypothermia. Two case reports exist attributing neonatal circulatory collapse to maternal therapy. In one case an infant weighing 1,500 grammes at 33 weeks was born in poor condition to a mother who had received intravenous labetalol for several hours (66). Immediate resuscitation was successful, but circulatory collapse reoccurred one hour later with secondary apnoea requiring artificial ventilation, cardiac massage, adrenaline and sodium bicarbonate. The authors attributed the circulatory collapse to labetalol intoxication as the fetus was still excreting labetalol four days after delivery. In another report an infant weighing 2,680 grammes was born in good condition at 38 weeks to a mother who had received three days of oral atenolol (67). Fifteen hours after delivery the infant developed clinical signs suggestive of beta-blockade, namely bradycardia, hypotension, hypothermia, poor peripheral perfusion and oliguria, all of which responded rapidly to a plasma protein infusion. Again, the circulatory collapse was attributed to beta-blockade as the infant was still excreting atenolol several days after delivery.

Despite these isolated case reports, controlled studies of infants born to mothers who have received beta-blocking agents have shown little evidence of clinically significant neonatal beta-blockade. Blood pressure, heart rate, respiratory rate, palmar sweating, response to cold stress and blood glucose were studied in 11 infants of mothers who had received labetalol for at least one week prior to delivery, and compared to a control group of 11 neonates born to untreated normotensive women matched for gestation and mode of delivery (68). Systolic blood pressure was significantly lower (by 5 mm Hg) in the labetalol infants at two hours after delivery, but the difference gradually resolved and became non significant at 24 hours.

In a study comparing ten infants whose mothers had received acebutalol to ten neonates whose mothers had received methyldopa, systolic blood pressure and fetal heart rate were significantly lower in the acebutalol group over all three days of the study and two infants from the acebutalol group required transfusion for hypotension (69). Six babies in the acebutalol group were hypoglycemic (blood glucose less than 1.67 mmol/litre) compared to only one in the methyldopa group. Birthweight was significantly lower in the acebutalol group, but this may indicate that the group had more severe disease rather than being a primary effect of acebutalol. Lastly, this trial was not properly randomised as decision to treat and choice of drug were dependent on physician preference.

Several large series have compared obstetric and neonatal outcome in hypertensive pregnant women receiving beta-blockers, other anti-hypertensive agents or controls (4, 14, 55, 56, 70-72). Only one study demonstrated a neonatal side effect attributable to beta-blockade (4). Bradycardia (less than 120 beats per minute) was commoner in babies whose mothers had received atenolol, but on no occasion did this require treatment.

Thus, the majority of published work has shown no immediate adverse neonatal effects and, in addition, a study at one year of infants exposed to atenolol in-utero has demonstrated no ill effects (73).

BENEFICIAL MATERNAL EFFECTS

All studies have convincingly showed that maternal beta-blockade was associated with lowered systolic and diastolic blood pressure. There was a tendency for loss of blood pressure control to be less frequent in treated women and this difference was especially marked in "early onset" hypertension. In two studies of atenolol or labetalol used for pregnancy-induced hypertension where the onset was before 32 and 31 weeks, one of 20 treated women required additional therapy compared to 12 of 25 controls (4, 71). In contrast, a study of women with chronic hypertension showed no difference in need for additional antihypertensive therapy in women receiving either labetalol, methyldopa or placebo (55).

Only one study demonstrated a significant preventative effect on development of proteinuria. Among women who were nonproteinuric at entry to the study, ten of the placebo group, but only three women treated with atenolol subsequently developed proteinuria of greater than 300 mg per 24 hours (4). Atenolol did not lead to resolution of proteinuria once established. This important finding has not been replicated in other studies, suggesting that control of blood pressure does not influence rate of progression of renal involvement.

Significant prolongation of pregnancy was not seen in any trial. One study demonstrated significantly more spontaneous labours and less frequent caesarean sections in women treated with oxprenolol compared with controls, but these findings have not been confirmed (72).

BENEFICIAL NEONATAL EFFECTS

Treatment with beta-blocking compounds has not been associated with any consistent change in birthweight (Table 4). In one study babies born to mothers receiving oxprenolol were significantly heavier (400 g) than babies whose mothers received methyldopa, but this has been attributed to excessive reduction of blood pressure in the methyldopa group with the predelivery level averaging 115/70 mm Hg (14). Furthermore, in a larger study (in which blood pressure reduction associated with methyldopa was not as marked), there was no significant difference between birthweight of infants to mothers who received methyldopa or oxprenolol (56). It can be seen from Table 5 that no investigation has demonstrated a significant reduction in the incidence of intra-uterine growth retardation in association with treatment. Interestingly, in one study the frequency of growth retardation was significantly higher in labetalol treated women than controls (70). This finding would have been replicated in another study, but for removal of patients in whom growth retardation was already diagnosed at time of entry to the study (71).

Table 4. Mean birthweight in six controlled trials of beta-blocking agents to treat hypertension during pregnancy.

STUDY	MEAN BIRTHWEIGHT (grammes)				
	Atenolol	Oxprenolol	Labetalol	Placebo	Methyldopa
Rubin et al (4)	2961			3017	
Sibai et al (70)			2204	2258	
Pickles et al (71)			2948	2913	
Plouin et al (72)		3079		3023	
Sibai et al (55)			3068	3123	3056
Gallery et al (14)		3051#		2654	
Fidler et al (56)		2920		3009	

significant (p <0.05)

There was no difference in indices of neonatal behaviour in the two studies comparing oxprenolol and methyldopa, whereas in the studies comparing beta-blocking agents to control there was a tendency for infants of mothers treated with beta-blockers to have fewer problems associated with prematurity (4, 14, 56, 71, 72).

Three studies showed a reduction in incidence of respiratory distress requiring ventilation (4 vs 16 in total), although in only one of the studies was the difference significant (4, 71, 72).

This finding was not confirmed in two other series, but the incidence of respiratory distress was not specifically mentioned in either and in one patients were exclusively suffering from chronic hypertension.

Table 5. Incidence of growth retarded infants in five controlled trials of beta-blocking agents to treat hypertension during pregnancy.

STUDY	GROWTH RETARDED INFANTS				
	Atenolol	Oxprenolol	Labetalol	Placebo	Methyldopa
Rubin et al (4)	7/46			7/39	
Sibai et al (70)			18/74#	9/78	
Pickles et al (71)			1/70	1/70	
Plouin et al (72)		5/76		8/75	
Sibai et al (55)			7/86	8/90	6/88

Figures are number of growth retarded infants and number of infants in the study
significant (p <0.05)

Nifedipine

The use of oral nifedipine in this situation has not been widely reported and its safety remains uncertain.

There is a report of nifedipine being used as second line therapy in 22 women with pregnancy-induced hypertension where atenolol had failed to reduce blood pressure to 140/90 mm Hg (74).

Nifedipine was effective in controlling blood pressure in 20 patients, but three women experienced significant hypotension and treatment had to be withdrawn in one instance. Fetal outcome was poor with perinatal mortality in the index group of 130/1,000 and nine infants weighing below the third percentile. One baby was thrombocytopenic shortly after birth and subsequently developed a hemiplegia. The group as a whole, however, had very severe disease and a poor fetal outcome was to be expected.

186

Angiotensin converting enzyme (ACE) inhibitors

There are no controlled trials of ACE inhibitors in human pregnancy. There are, however, several reports of anuric renal failure in babies exposed to this category of drug in-utero and high rates of fetal wastage in animal studies (75-77). These data strongly suggest that these drugs must be avoided during pregnancy.

Alpha-adrenergic blockers

Prazosin, an alpha-1 receptor antagonist, has been used in uncontrolled studies of chronic hypertension (78-80) and pheochromocytoma (81, 82) complicating gestation. No specific untoward effects have been identified: however, given the lack of data and lack of benefit over other, better studied agents, there is little reason to use this drug for hypertension during pregnancy except for patients with a pheochromocytoma.

Diuretics

As diuretics have not yet been proved to be beneficial and can be associated with a number of side effects, we caution against their routine use in either pre-eclampsia or chronic hypertension during pregnancy. We would, however, unhesitatingly use a diuretic for women with pulmonary edema and/or left ventricular failure.

DRUGS TO BE USED TO PREVENT PRE-ECLAMPSIA

There is no good evidence supporting the use of diuretics in the prevention of pre-eclampsia. Nor does the early treatment of mild hypertension forestall the appearance of other manifestations of pre-eclampsia - not surprisingly since the placental, cerebral, renal, hepatic and coagulation abnormalities do not appear as a direct consequence of elevated blood pressure.

Dietary calcium supplementation

Dietary calcium deficiency has been suggested as underlying hypertension in both pregnant and nonpregnant populations (83). One study has described hypocalciuria in most women with pure and superimposed hypertension during pregnancy (84), while in another investigation a 600 mg daily calcium supplement enhanced pressor resistance to an infusion of angiotensin II in healthy pregnant women as compared to nonpregnant controls chosen in a randomised manner (85). Furthermore, two randomised trials have shown small blood pressure decreases in healthy pregnant women receiving 1-2 g/day of calcium; the incidence of hypertension, however, was similar to the control group (83). In a recent preliminary report it has been claimed that calcium supplementation reduces the incidence of pre-eclampsia (86).

Low-dose aspirin therapy

There is evidence to suggest that pre-eclampsia is associated with relative deficiency of endothelial-derived prostacyclin compared to platelet-derived thromboxane, such that the platelet-aggregating and vasoconstrictor effects of thromboxane predominate.

Pregnancy associated tissues such as myometrium, decidua, chorion, amnion, trophoblast, and especially umbilical vessels can all produce prostacyclin *in vitro* (87-89). 6-keto-prostaglandin $F_{1\alpha}$, a major prostacyclin metabolite, has been measured in normal pregnancy with variable results (90-94). In pre-eclampsia, a prostacyclin deficiency in maternal and fetal tissue is apparently detectable in the first trimester, well before the clinical onset of the disease (95).

EICOSANOIDS, HUMAN PREGNANCY AND ASPIRIN

Like prostacyclin, thromboxane formation has been reported to be increased, unchanged and decreased in normal pregnancy, but the differences between studies may reflect the analytical methods used, specifically platelet activation during sampling. This can be overcome by measurement of plasma and urinary thromboxane metabolites, which have shown that maternal thromboxane levels increase during early pregnancy and remain elevated thereafter (96). Thromboxane synthesis is further increased in pregnancy-induced hypertension and, furthermore, the degree of increased synthesis correlates with disease severity (97). Placental production of thromboxane A_2 is increased in hypertensive pregnancy, but at least in normal pregnancy it has been claimed that thromboxane mainly originates from platelets (96). Recovery of aspirin-induced inhibition of thromboxane synthesis takes several days, coinciding with the rate of new platelet generation. Aspirin irreversibly binds to cyclo-oxygenase and if tissue enzyme was crucial to biosynthesis, recovery of thromboxane excretion would take place much more quickly as new tissue enzyme was created.

The long delay between reduced prostacyclin synthesis and the clinical onset of pre-eclampsia indicates that prostacyclin deficiency alone is not responsible for development of hypertension. However, it may be that hypertension occurs when the ratio of thromboxane to prostacyclin reaches a certain level and this does not develop until later in pregnancy.

Alternatively, prostacyclin may be responsible for modulating vascular response to various vasoactive compounds, such as angiotensin, and the development of clinical disease may depend on interaction between the various vasoactive agents.

Low dose aspirin could have a prophylactic effect on pre-eclampsia by inhibiting platelet cyclo-oxygenase, but sparing endothelial cyclo-oxygenase. The abnormal thromboxane predominance in pre-eclampsia will then be shifted back towards prostacyclin. Certainly in normotensive term pregnancy, low dose aspirin (60 or 80 mg/day) significantly reduced platelet thromboxane production in response to ADP or collagen stimulation and also impaired platelet aggregation while not affecting maternal serum 6-keto-prostaglandin $F_{1\alpha}$ (98). Similarly, in placentas taken from normotensive term women, aspirin at concentrations equivalent to those produced by low dose therapy reduced thromboxane production by whole villi without effecting synthesis of prostacyclin (99).

In pregnant women thought to be at risk of developing pregnancy-induced hypertension (because of a positive rollover test - a dubious test it must be admitted), treatment with aspirin reduced thromboxane concentration by almost a half (100). A slight reduction in prostacyclin concentration in women receiving either aspirin or placebo resulted in the ratio of thromboxane to prostacyclin decreasing by a third in the aspirin group, compared to controls where it increased by 51%. In the aspirin group, the mean ratio reduction was less in women who later became hypertensive.

When low dose aspirin was administered to women with a poor obstetric history or chronic hypertension, platelet generation of thromboxane (at 24 weeks and term) was reduced by over 80% (101). Urinary excretion of a prostacyclin metabolite was not modified by aspirin. Interestingly, urinary excretion of thromboxane metabolites thought to originate purely from platelets were reduced by more than metabolites reflecting more generalised production. Thus, low dose aspirin may be inhibiting platelet thromboxane to a greater degree than other thromboxane synthesis.

FETAL, NEONATAL AND MATERNAL RISKS

Low dose aspirin could affect neonatal hemostasis and lead to an increased incidence of fetal hemorrhagic complications. Other suggested neonatal side effects are an increased risk of certain cardiac malformations and/or delayed closure of the ductus arteriosus, leading to postnatal pulmonary hypertension and severe neonatal hypoxemia.

Evidence for aspirin causing neonatal bleeding problems stems from a study showing that in women who had ingested aspirin within 5 days of delivery, there was a

90% incidence of bleeding tendency in their neonates (102). The bleeding problems included profusion (>50) of petechiae over the presenting part, a cephalhematoma, a sub-conjunctival hemorrhage, bleeding from circumcision site and microscopic hematuria. These types of bleeding disturbance are characteristic of a platelet or capillary disturbance and interestingly they did not occur in infants whose mothers had taken aspirin at between 6 and 10 days pre-delivery. This suggests a site of action in neonatal platelets as recovery of full hemostatic function coincided with formation of new unaffected platelets. Abnormal bleeding occurred with much greater frequency in neonates than in their mothers and several sensitive tests of neonatal platelet function have revealed impaired adhesiveness and aggregation compared to maternal platelets. A superimposed aspirin-induced abnormality may impair hemostasis still further resulting in a clinically apparent bleeding diathesis.

The majority of these reports have involved mothers who had taken 150 - 300 mg/day of aspirin, a dose far in excess of that used in the prophylaxis of pre-eclampsia. Furthermore, several controlled studies of the use of low dose aspirin in pregnancy have revealed no clinical evidence of a bleeding diathesis in the neonate (98, 100, 101, 103, 105, 106). In particular, ultrasound examination of neonates showed no evidence of intracranial hemorrhage and several infants have undergone minor surgery without any problems (98, 101).

The suggestion that maternal aspirin ingestion may cause neonatal cardiac defects arose from a study in which there was a two to three fold increase in the incidence of four specific abnormalities: aortic stenosis, co-arctation of the aorta, hypoplasia of the left ventricle and transposition of the great arteries (107). Data from the Collaborative Perinatal Project supported the finding of increased risk for aortic stenosis, coarctation of the aorta and great vessel transposition. However a large case control study of 8,613 infants with congenital malformations found the prevalence of maternal first trimester aspirin ingestion was 26% for mothers whose infants had congenital cardiac defects and 27% for controls (108). There was no suggestion that aspirin use during the early months of pregnancy was associated with any of the previously mentioned cardiac defects.

No controlled study has shown delayed closure of the ductus arteriosus and fetal echocardiography showed no difference in several parameters of right ventricular function in infants exposed to aspirin (98). However, these were all term infants to normotensive mothers and the authors pointed out that premature babies may respond differently.

Blood loss at vaginal delivery or caesarean section has not been significantly different between aspirin treated mothers and controls. Six intra-uterine deaths have occurred, but one was due to a cord accident in labor, another was due to asphyxia with no evidence of fetal hemorrhage or abruptio placentae (104, 105). In the other study where intra-uterine deaths were recorded, all occurred before 30 weeks gestation and were associated with severe growth retardation (106).

ARGUMENTS WHY ASPIRIN SHOULD BE USED

Five randomised trials have assessed the effect of varying doses of low dose aspirin on pregnancy outcome in selected populations of women thought to be at high risk of developing pre-eclampsia or intra-uterine growth retardation (100, 101, 103-106). Table 6 summarises the number of women developing hypertension in each of these studies.

Table 6. Incidence of hypertension (+/- proteinuria) during pregnancy in six controlled trials of low-dose aspirin.

STUDY	HYPERTENSION		PRE-ECLAMPSIA	
	Aspirin	*Placebo*	*Aspirin*	*Placebo*
Beaufils et al (103)	19/48	22/45	0/48#	6/48
Wallenburg et al (104)	2/21	4/23	0/21#	7/23
Schiff et al (100)	3/34	4/31	1/34	7/31
Benigni et al (101)	0/17	3/16	-	-
McParland et al (105)	6/48	13/52	1/48	10/52
Uzan et al (106)	35/156	25/73	5/156	8/73
ALL	65/324	71/240	7/307	38/227

Figures are numbers of women developing hypertension or pre-eclampsia during pregnancy and number of patients in the study.
= significant (p <0.05)

The results are strikingly similar despite different methods of patient selection, dose of aspirin (60 - 150 mg) and duration of treatment (12 - 28 weeks until term). Methods of identifying an at risk population have included previous obstetric history, presence of chronic hypertension, the roll-over test, angiotensin sensitivity and doppler uteroplacental flow velocity waveforms, implying that all studies are likely to have included a heterogeneous population.

The incidence of pre-eclampsia was only marginally reduced, but proteinuria was almost completely abolished, indicating that aspirin prevents the severe form of the disease, which is more closely associated with morbidity and mortality in mother and infant.

In all studies, birthweight and gestational age were greater in aspirin treated women than controls (see Table 7). However, in only three of the studies were both parameters significantly greater than controls and in one other investigation gestation alone was significantly longer (101, 103, 106). Interestingly, the two studies in which a significant effect was seen on both birthweight and gestational age were those in which treatment was started in the first trimester on the basis of a poor previous obstetric history.

Table 7. Mean birthweight and gestation at delivery in five controlled trials of low-dose aspirin.

STUDY	BIRTHWEIGHT (grammes)		GESTATION AT DELIVERY (weeks)	
	Aspirin	Placebo	Aspirin	Placebo
Beaufils et al (103)	3172#	2625	38.6#	36.5
Wallenburg et al (104)	3190	3040	40	39
Schiff et al (100)	3037	2706	38.9#	37.3
Benigni et al (101)	2922#	2264	39#	35
McParland et al (105)	3068	2954	39.5	38.7
Uzan et al (106)	2751	2526	37.7	36.9

Other beneficial effects of aspirin treatment have included reduced incidence of fetal and neonatal loss, intra-uterine growth retardation, premature delivery and caesarean sections. In one study platelet count and plasma volume were higher throughout pregnancy in aspirin treated women (103).

REFERENCES

1. Friedman EA, Neff RK: Pregnancy hypertension: a systematic evaluation of clinical diagnostic criteria. PSG Publishing Company, Littleton MA, 1977.
2. Page EW, Christianson R: The impact of mean arterial pressure in the middle trimester upon the outcome of pregnancy. Am J Obstet Gynecol, 125: 740-746, 1976.
3. Fletcher AE, Bulpitt CJ: A review of clinical trials in pregnancy hypertension. In: "Hypertension in pregnancy" (Ed PC Rubin), Elsevier, New York, 1988, pp 186-201.
4. Rubin PC, Butters L, Clark DM, Reynolds B, Sumner DJ, Steedman D, Low RA, Reid JL: Placebo-controlled trial of atenolol in treatment of pregnancy-associated hypertension. Lancet, I: 431-434, 1983.
5. Whichman K, Ryden G, Karlberg G: A placebo controlled trial of metoprolol in the treatment of hypertension during pregnancy. Scand J Clin Lab Invest, 44 (Suppl 169): 90-95, 1984.
6. Leather HM, Humphreys DM, Baker P, Chadd MA: A controlled trial of hypertensive agents in hypertension of pregnancy. Lancet, II: 488-490, 1968.
7. Walker JJ, Crooks A, Erwin L, Calder AA: Labetalol in pregnancy-induced hypertension: fetal and maternal effects. In: "The investigation labetalol in the management of hypertension in pregnancy" (Eds A Riley, EM Symonds), Excerpta Medica, Amsterdam, 1982, pp 148-160.

8. Redman CWG, Beilin LJ, Bonnar J: Treatment of hypertension in pregnancy with methyldopa: blood pressure control and side effects. Br J Obstet Gynecol, 84: 419-426, 1977.

9. Venuto RC, Cox JW, Stein JH, Ferris TF: The effect of changes in perfusion pressure on uteroplacental blood flow in the pregnant rabbit. J Clin Invest, 57: 938-941, 1976.

10. Ladner C, Brinkman CR III, Weston P, Assali NS: Dynamics of uterine circulation in pregnant and nonpregnant sheep. Am J Physiol, 218: 257-263, 1970.

11. De Swiet M, Hoffbrand BI: Effect of bethanidine on placental blood flow in conscious rabbits. Am J Obstet Gynecol, 111: 374-378, 1971.

12. Greiss FC Jr: Uterine pressure flow relationships. In: "Uterine and placental blood flow" (Eds AH Moawad, MD Lindheimer), Masson, New York, 1982, pp 67-71.

13. Ferris TF: Toxaemia and hypertension. In: "Medical complications during pregnancy" (Eds GN Burrow, TF Ferris), 3rd Edition, WB Saunders, Philadelphia, 1988, pp 1-33.

14. Gallery EDM, Saunders DM, Hunyor SM, Gyory AZ: Randomised comparison of methyldopa and oxprenolol for treatment of hypertension in pregnancy. Br Med J, I: 1591-1594, 1979.

15. Sibai BM, Ardella TM, Anderson GD: Pregnancy outcome in 21 patients with mild chronic hypertension. Obstet Gynecol, 61: 571-576, 1983.

16. Pritchard JA, MacDonald PC, Gant NF: Williiams Obstetrics, 17th edition, Appleton Century Crofts, Norwalk CT, 1985.

17. Wallenburg HCS: Hemodynamics in hypertensive pregnancy. In: "Hypertension in pregnancy" (Ed PC Rubin), Elsevier, New York, 1988, pp 66-101.

18. Kuzniar J, Skret A, Piela A, Szmiegel Z, Zaczek T: Hemodynamic effects of intravenous hydralazine in pregnant women with severe hypertension. Obstet Gynecol, 66: 453-458, 1985.

19. Belfort M, Uys P, Dommisse J, Davey DA: Hemodynamic changes in gestational proteinuric hypertension: the effects of rapid volume expansion and vasodilator therapy. Br J Obstet Gynecol, 96: 634-641, 1989.

20. Jouppila P, Kirkinen P, Koivula A, Ylikorkala O: Effects of dihydralazine infusion on the fetoplacental blood flow and maternal prostanoids. Obstet Gynecol, 65: 115-118, 1985.

21. Nylund L, Lunell NO: Dihydralazine and the uteroplacental blood flow. Am J Obstet Gynecol, 158: 440-441, 1988 (Letter).

22. Suonio S, Saarikoski S, Tahvanainen K, Paakkonen A, Olkkonen H: Acute effects of dihydralazine mesylate, furosemide, and metoprolol on maternal hemodynamics in pregnancy-induced hypertension. Am J Obstet Gynecol, 155: 122-125, 1895.

23. Lipshitz J, Ahokas AR, Reynolds SL: The effect of hydralzine on placental perfusion in the spontaneously hypertensive rat. Am J Obstet Gynecol, 156: 356-359, 1987.

24. Vink GJ, Moodley J, Philpott RH: Effect of dihydralazine on the fetus in the treatment of maternal hypertension. Obstet Gynecol, 55: 519-522, 1980.

25. Mabie WC, Gonzalez AR, Sibai BM, Amon E: A comparative trial of labetalol and hydralazine in the acute management of severe hypertension complicating pregnancy. Obstet Gynecol, 70: 328-333, 1987.

26. Harake B, Gilbert RD, Ashwal S, Power GG: Nifedipine: effects on fetal and maternal hemodynamics in pregnant sheep. Am J Obstet Gynecol, 157: 1003-1008, 1987.

27. Dusay CA, Cook MJ, Veille JC: Cardiorespiratory effects of calcium channel blocker tocolysis in pregnant rhesus monkeys. In: "The physiological development of the fetus and newborn" (Eds CT Jones, PW Nathanielsz), Academic Press, London, 1985, pp 423-428.

28. Parisi VM, Salinas J, Stockmar EJ: Fetal vascular responses to maternal nicardipine administration in the hypertensive ewe. Am J Obstet Gynecol, 161: 1035-1039, 1989.

29. Parisi VM, Salinas J, Stockmar EJ: Placental vascular responses to nicardipine in the hypertensive ewe. Am J Obstet Gynecol, 161: 1039-1043, 1989.

30. Ahokas RA, Sibai BM, Anderson GD: Nifedipine does not adversely affect uteroplacental blood flow in the hypertensive term-pregnant rat. Am J Obstet Gynecol, 159: 1440-1445, 1988.

31. Pirhonen JP, Erkkola RU, Ekblad U: Uterine and fetal flow velocity waveforms in hypertensive pregnancy: the effect of a single dose of nifedipine. Obstet Gynecol, 76: 37-41, 1990.

32. Hanretty KP, Whittle MJ, Howie CA, Rubin PC: Effect of nifedipine on doppler flow velocity waveforms in severe pre-eclampsia. Br Med J, 299: 1205-1206, 1989.

33. Mari G, Kirshon B, Moise KJ, Lee W, Cotton DB: Doppler assessment of the fetal and uteroplacental circulation during nifedipine therapy for preterm labor. Am J Obstet Gynecol, 161: 1514-1518, 1989.

34. Lindow SW, Davies N, Davey DA, Smith JA: The effect of sublingual nifedipine on uteroplacental blood flow in hypertensive pregnancy. Br J Obstet Gynecol, 95: 1276-1281, 1988.

35. Walters BNJ, Redman CWG: Treatment of severe pregnancy- associated hypertension with the calcium antagonist nifedipine. Br J Obstet Gynecol, 91: 330-336, 1984.

36. Fenakel K, Fenakel G, Appelman Z, Lurie S, Katz Z, Shoham Z: Nifedipine in the treatment of severe pre-eclampsia. Obstet Gynecol, 77: 331-337, 1991.

37. Walker JJ, Greer I, Calder AA: Treatment of acute pregnancy-related hypertension: labetalol and hydralazine compared. Postgrad Med J, 52: 390-394, 1983.

38. Davey DA, Dommisse J, Garden A: Intravenous labetalol and intravenous dihydralazine in severe hypertension in pregnancy. In: "The investigation of labetalol in the management of hypertension in pregnancy" (Eds A Riley, EM Symonds), Excerpta Medica, Amsterdam, 1982, pp 51-61.

39. Ashe RG, Moodley J, Richards AM, Philpott RH: Comparison of labetalol and dihydralazine in hypertensive emergencies of pregnancy. S Afr Med J, 71: 354-356, 1987.

40. Lunell NO, Nylund L, Lewander R, Sarby B: Acute effect of an antihypertensive drug, labetalol, on uteroplacental blood flow. Br J Obstet Gynecol, 89: 640-644, 1982.

41. Sibai BM, Spinnato JA, Watson DL, Lewis JA, Anderson GD: Effect of magnesium sulphate on electroencephalographic findings in preeclampsia-eclampsia. Obstet Gynecol, 64: 261-266, 1984.

42. Thurnau GR, Kemp DB, Jarvis A: Cerebrospinal fluid levels of magnesium in patients with preeclampsia after treatment with intravenous magnesium sulphate: a preliminary report. Am J Obstet Gynecol, 157: 1435-1438, 1987.

43. Rothman SM, Olney JW: Excitotoxicity and the NMDA receptor. Trends Neurol Sci, 10: 299-302, 1987.

44. Rothman SM: Synaptic activity mediates death of hypoxic neurones. Science, 220: 536-537, 1984.

45. Finkbeiner S, Stevens CF: Application of quantitative measurements for assessing neurotoxicity. Proc Natl Acad Sci USA, 85: 4071-4074, 1988.

46. Pritchard JA, Cunningham FG, Pritchard SA: The Parkland Memorial Hospital protocol for treatment of eclampsia: Evaluation of 245 cases. Am J Obstet Gynecol, 148: 951-963, 1984.

47. Sibai BM: Magnesium sulphate is the ideal anticonvulsant in preeclampsia-eclampsia. Am J Obstet Gynecol, 162: 1141-1145, 1990.

48. Sibai BM, Lipshitz J, Anderson GD, Dilts PV Jr: Reassessment of intravenous MgSO4 therapy in preeclampsia-eclampsia. Obstet Gynecol, 51: 199-202, 1981.

49. Lamm CI, Norton KI, Murphy RJC, Wilkins IA, Rabinowitz JG: Congenital rickets associated with magnesium sulfate infusion for tocolysis. J Pediatr, 113: 1078-1082, 1988.

50. Crowther C: Magnesium sulphate versus diazepam in the management of eclampsia: a randomised controlled trial. Br J Obstet Gynecol, 97: 110-117, 1990.

51. Slater RM, Wilcox FL, Smith WD, Donnai P, Patrick J, Richardson T, Mawer GE, D'Souza SW, Anderton JM: Phenytoin infusion in severe pre-eclampsia. Lancet, I: 1417-1420, 1987.

52. Moosa SM, El Zayat SG: Phenytoin infusion in severe pre-eclampsia. Lancet, II: 1147-1148, 1987.

53. Tuffnell D, O'Donovan P, Lilford RJ, Prys-Davies A, Thornton JG: Phenytoin in pre-eclampsia. Lancet, I: 273-274, 1989.

54. Dommisse J: Phenytoin sodium and magnesium sulphate in the management of eclampsia. Br J Obstet Gynecol, 97: 104-109, 1990.

55. Sibai BM, Mabie WC, Shamsa F, Villar MA, Anderson GD: A comparison of no medication versus methyldopa or labetalol in chronic hypertension during pregnancy. Am J Obstet Gynecol, 162: 960-967, 1990.

56. Fidler J, Smith V, Fayers P, De Swiet M: Randomised controlled comparative study of methyldopa and oxprenolol in treatment of hypertension in pregnancy. Br Med J, 286: 1927-1930, 1983.

57. Moar VA, Jefferies MA, Mutch LMM: Neonatal head circumference and the treatment of maternal hypertension. Br J Obstet Gynecol, 85: 933-937, 1978.

58. Ounsted MK, Moar VA, Good FJ, Redman CWG: Hypertension during pregnancy with and without specific treatment; the development of the children at the age of four years. Br J Obstet Gynecol, 87: 19-24, 1980.

59. Cockburn J, Moar VA, Ounsted M, Redman CWG: Final report of study on hypertension during pregnancy: the effects of specific treatment on the growth and development of the children. Lancet, I: 647-649, 1982.

60. Hogstedt S, Lindeberg S, Axelsson O et al: A prospective controlled trial of metoprolol-hydralazine treatment in hypertension during pregnancy. Acta Obstet Gynecol Scand, 64: 505-510, 1985.

61. Bott-Kanner G, Schweitzr A, Reisner SH, Joel-Cohen SJ, Rosenfeld JB. Propranolol and hydralazine in the management of essential hypertension in pregnancy. Br J Obstet Gynecol, 87: 110-114, 1980.

62. Rosenfeld J, Bott-Kanner G, Boner G et al: Treatment of hypertension during pregnancy with hydralazine monotherapy or with combined therapy with hydralazine and pindolol. Eur J Obstet Gynecol Reprod Biol, 22: 197-204, 1986.

63. Widerlov E, Karlman I, Storsater J: Hydralazine-induced neonatal thrombocytopenia. N Engl J Med, 303: 1235-1237, 1980.

64. Lieberman BA, Stirrat GM, Dohen SL, Beard RW, Pinker GD, Belsey E: The possible adverse effect of propranolol on the fetus in pregnancies complicated by severe hypertension. Br J Obstet Gynecol, 85: 678-683, 1978.

65. Jouppila P, Kirkinen P, Koivula A, Ylikorkala O: Labetalol does not alter the placental and fetal blood flow or maternal prostanoids in pre-eclampsia. Br J Obstet Gynecol, 93: 543-547, 1986.

66. Haraldsson A, Geven W: Serious adverse effects of maternal labetalol in a premature infant. Acta Pediatr Scand, 78: 956-958, 1989.

67. Woods DL, Morrell DF: Atenolol: side effects in a newborn infant. Br Med J, 285: 691-692, 1982.

68. Macpherson M, Broughton Pipkin F, Rutter N: The effect of maternal labetalol on the newborn infant. Br J Obstet Gynecol, 93: 539-542, 1986.

69. Dumez Y, Tchobroutsky, Hornych H, Amiel-Tsion C: Neonatal effects of maternal administration of acebutolol. Br Med J, 283: 1077-1079, 1981.

70. Sibai BM, Gonzalez AR, Mabie WC, Moretti M: A comparison of labetalol plus hospitalization versus hospitalization alone in the management of preeclampsia remote from term. Obstet Gynecol, 70: 323-327, 1987.

71. Pickles CJ, Symonds EM, Broughton Pipkin F: The fetal outcome in a randomized double-blind controlled trial of labetalol versus placebo in pregnancy-induced hypertension. Br J Obstet Gynecol, 96: 38-43, 1989.

72. Plouin PF, Breart G, Llado J, Dalle M, Keller ME, Goujon H, Berchel C: A randomised comparison or early with conservative use of antihypertensive drugs in the management of pregnancy-induced hypertension. Br J Obstet Gynecol, 97: 134-141, 1990.

73. Reynolds B, Butters L, Evans J, Adams T, Rubin PC: First year of life after the use of atenolol in pregnancy associated hypertension. Arch Dis Child, 59: 1061-1063, 1984.

74. Constantine G, Beevers DG, Reynolds AL, Luesley DM: Nifedipine as a second line antihypertensive drug in pregnancy. Br J Obstet Gynecol, 94: 1136-1142, 1987.

75. Schubiger G, Flury G, Nussberger J: Enalapril for pregnancy-induced hypertension: acute renal failure in a neonate. Ann Intern Med, 108: 215-216, 1988.

76. Broughton Pipkin F, Symonds EM, Turner SR: The effect of captopril (SQ14225) upon mother and fetus in the chronically cannulated ewe and in the pregnant rabbit. J Physiol, 323: 415-422, 1982.

77. Ferris TF, Weir EK: Effect of captopril on uterine blood flow and prostaglandin synthesis in the pregnant rabbit. J Clin Invest, 71: 809-815, 1983.

78. Lubbe WF, Hodge JV: Combined alpha and beta-adrenceptor antagonism with prazosin and oxprenolol in control of severe hypertension in pregnancy. NZ Med J, 94: 169-172, 1981.

79. Dommisse J, Davey DA, Roos PJ: Prazosin and oxprenolol therapy in pregnancy hypertension. S Afr Med J, 64: 231-233, 1983.

80. Rubin PC, Butters L, Low RA, Reid JL. Clinical pharmacological studies with prazosin during pregnancy complicated by hypertension. Br J Clin Pharmacol, 16: 543-547, 1983.

81. Devoe LD, O'Dell BE, Castillo RA, Hadi HA, Saerle N: Metastatic phaeochromocytoma in pregnancy and fetal biophysical assessment after maternal administration of alpha-adrenergic, beta-adrenergic and dopamine antagonists. Obstet Gynecol, 68 (Suppl): 15S-18S, 1986.

82. Venuto R, Burstein P, Schneider R: Phaeochromocytoma: antepartum diagnosis and management with tumor resection in the puerperium. Am J Obstet Gynecol, 150: 431-432, 1984.

83. Belizan JM, Villar J, Repke J: The relationship between calcium intake and pregnancy-induced hypertension: up-to-date evidence. Am J Obstet Gynecol, 158: 898-902, 1988.

84. Taufield PA, Ales KL, Resnick LM, Druzin ML, Gertner JM, Laragh JH: Hypocalciuria in preeclampsia. N Engl J Med, 316: 715-718, 1987.

85. Kawasaki N, Matsui K Ito M et al: Effect of calcium supplementation on the vascular sensitivity to angiotensin II in pregnant women. Am J Obstet Gynecol, 153: 576-582, 1985.

86. Montanaro D, Bascutti G, Antonucci F, et al: Prevention of pregnancy-induced hypertension (PIH) and preeclampsia (PE) by oral calcium supplementation. 10th Int Congress Nephrol: 291, 1987, (Abstract).

87. Bamford DS, Jogee M, Williams KI: Prostacyclin formation by pregnant human myometrium. Br J Obstet Gynecol, 87: 215, 1980.

88. Mitchell MD, Bibby JB, Hicks BR, Turnbull AC: Possible role for prostacyclin in human parturition. Prostaglandins, 16: 931, 1978.

89. Rakoczi I, Tihanyi K, Falkay G, Rosza I, Demaler J, Gati I: Prostacyclin production in trophoblast. In: "Prostacyclin and pregnancy" (Eds PJ Lewis, S Moncada, J O'Grady), Raven Press, New York, 1983, pp 15-23.

90. Spitz B, Deckmyn H, van Assche FA, Vermylen J: Prostacyclin production in whole blood throughout normal pregnancy. In: "Clinical and experimental hypertension. Part B. Hypertension in pregnancy" (Eds FP Zuspan, EM Symonds), Marcel Dekker, New York, 1983, pp 191-202.

91. Mitchell MD: Prostacyclin during human pregnancy and parturition. In: "Clinical pharmacology of prostacyclin" (Eds PJ Lewis, J O'Grady), Raven Press, New York, 1981, pp 121-129.

92. Ylikorkola O, Viinikka L: Maternal plasma levels of 6-keto-prostaglandin F1-alpha during pregnancy and puerperium. Prostaglandins Leukotrienes Med, 7: 95, 1981.

93. Koullapis EN, Nicolaides KH, Collins WP, Rodeck CH, Campbell S: Plasma prostanoids in pregnacy-induced hypertension. Br J Obstet Gynecol, 89: 617, 1982.

94. Lewis PJ, Boylan P, Friedman LA, Hensby CN, Downing I: Prostacyclin in pregnancy. Br Med J, 280: 1581, 1980.

95. Fitzgerald DJ, Entman SS, Mulloy K, Fitzgerald GA: Decreased prostacyclin biosynthesis preceeding the clinical manifestation of pregnancy-induced hypertension. Circ, 5: 956-963, 1987.

96. Fitzgerald DJ, Mayo G, Catella F, Entman SS, Fitzgerald GA: Increased thromboxane biosynthesis in normal pregnancy is mainly derived from platelets. Am J Obstet Gynecol, 157: 325-330, 1987.

97. Fitzgerald DJ, Rocki W, Murray R, Mayo G, Fitzgerald GA: Thromboxane A2 synthesis in pregnancy-induced hypertension. Lancet, 335: 751-754, 1990.

98. Sibai BM, Mirro R, Chesney CM, Leffler C: Low-dose aspirin in pregnancy. Obstet Gynecol, 74: 551-556, 1989.

99. Nelson DM, Walsh SW: Aspirin differentially affects thromboxane and prostacyclin production by trophoblast and villous core compartments of human placental villi. Am J Obstet Gynecol, 161: 1593-1598, 1989.

100. Schiff E, Peleg E, Goldenberg M, Rosenthal T, Ruppin E, Tamarkin M, Barkai G, Ben-Baruch G, Yahal I, Blankstein J, Goldman B, Mashiach S: The use of aspirin to prevent pregnancy-induced hypertension and lower the ratio of thromboxane A2 to prostacyclin in relatively high risk pregnancies. N Engl J Med, 321: 351-356, 1989.

101. Benigni A, Gregorina G, Frusca T, Chiabrando C, Ballerini S, Valcamonico A, Orisio s, Piccinelli A, Pinciroli V, Fanelli R, Gastaldi A, Remuzzi G: Effect of low-dose aspirin on fetal and maternal generation of thromboxane by platelets in women at risk for pregnancy-induced hypertension. N Engl J Med, 321: 357-362, 1989.

102. Stuart MJ, Gross SJ, Elrad H, Graeber JE: Effects of acetylsalicylic-acid on maternal and neonatal hemostasis. N Engl J Med, 307: 909-912, 1982.

103. Beaufils M, Uzan S, Donsimoni R, Colau JC: Prevention of pre-eclampsia by early antiplatelet therapy. Lancet, I: 840-842, 1985.

104. Wallenburg HCS, Dekker GA, Makovitz JW, Rotmans P: Low-dose aspirin prevents pregnancy-induced hypertension and pre-eclampsia in angiotensin-sensitive primigravidae. Lancet, I: 1-3, 1986.

105. McParland P, Pearce JM, Chamberlain GVP: Doppler ultrasound and aspirin in recognition and prevention of pregnancy-induced hypertension. Lancet, 335: 1552-1555, 1990.

106. Uzan S, Beaufils M, Breart G, Bazin B, Capitant C, Paris J: Prevention of fetal growth retardation with low-dose aspirin: findings of the EPREDA trial. Lancet, 337: 1427-1431, 1991.

107. Zierler S, Rothman KJ: Congenital heart disese in relation to maternal use of Bendectin and other drugs in early pregnancy. N Engl J Med, 313: 347-352, 1985.

108. Werler MM, Mitchell AA, Shapiro S: The relation of aspirin use during the first trimester of pregnancy to congenital cardiac defects. N Engl J Med, 321: 1639-1642, 1989.

HEREDITARY RENAL DISEASES

Chapter 8

PREDICTION OF LIKELIHOOD OF POLYCYSTIC KIDNEY DISEASE IN THE FETUS WHEN A PARENT HAS AUTOSOMAL DOMINANT POLYCYSTIC KIDNEY DISEASE

PATRICIA A. GABOW* AND LOUISE WILKINS-HAUG**

*Denver General Hospital, University of Colorado Health Sciences Center, Denver, Colorado, USA
**Harvard Medical School, Department of OB/GYN, Brigham and Women's Hospital, Boston, Massachusetts, USA

As a genetic disorder, autosomal dominant polycystic kidney disease (ADPKD) is present from conception. Yet, as is often the case with such disorders, the phenotypic presentation generally only mysteriously emerges years later. Occasionally the phenotypic manifestations emerge in fetal life, permitting prenatal diagnosis with fetal imaging. In addition, gene linkage techniques now permit determination of the fetal genotype without waiting years into postnatal life for telltale clinical manifestations to occur. These possibilities for prenatal diagnosis require the clinician to understand not only the methods and issues in prenatal diagnosis, but also the outcome of an affected fetus in order to adequately counsel such families.

GENETICS OF ADPKD

ADPKD is transmitted on an autosome, not a sex chromosome, and is a dominant disease. As such, every offspring, both male and female, of an affected parent has a 50/50 chance of inheriting the gene and hence the disease; there are no skipped generations and only a person carrying the gene can transmit the disease. In 1985 Reeders et al (1) utilized DNA probes for known chromosomes and found that the culprit gene was inherited frequently with a DNA probe for the hypervariable region (3'HVR) of the alpha globin locus, placing the ADPKD gene on the short arm of chromosome 16. It is this discovery which has made asymptomatic carrier and fetal gene testing for ADPKD possible.

Table 1. Fetal diagnosis of ADPKD with ultrasonography (US) and outcome of offspring

AUTHOR	YR	PT #	RENAL FINDINGS	OUTCOME AND COMMENT
Zerres (9)	1982	Fetus	33 week US enlarged kidneys	Alive with normal renal function at 1 year - affected mother
Garel (*)	1983	Fetus 1	28 week US enlarged, echogenic kidneys cysts	Outcome unknown - affected mother
Main (10)	1983	Fetus 1	21 week US normal sized kidneys; 36 week US multiple cysts in both kidneys	Age 2 months normal renal function and blood pressure - affected mother
		Fetus 2	16 week US normal kidneys; 22 week US normal kidneys; 30 week US large kidneys	6 months clinically normal - affected mother
Zerres (11)	1985	Fetus 1	32 week US enlarged, echogenic kidneys hydrops fetalis	Fetal death; autopsy confirmed diagnosis; sibling and cousin died of "Potter Syndrome" - affected father
Fryns (12)	1986	Fetus 1	16 week US enlarged, echogenic kidneys; oligohydramnios	Therapeutic abortion; autopsy confirmed diagnosis; sibling died at birth with ADPKD - affected father
Kaariainen (13) and Gal (16)	1987	Family 2 -Fetus 1	24 week US enlarged kidneys	Alive age 8; - affected mother
		Family 2 -Fetus 2	24 week US enlarged kidneys	Alive age 2; sibling of Fetus 1 - affected mother
Sedman (14)	1987	Fetus 3	36 week US enlarged, echogenic kidneys; 1 cyst	Alive age 9 yrs, mild decrease in renal size, mild hypertension - affected mother
		Fetus 4	23 1/2 week US enlarged, echogenic kidneys; oligohydramnios	Therapeutic abortion; sibling of Fetus 3 - affected mother
Pretorius (15)	1987	Fetus 5	31 week US enlarged, echogenic kidneys; decreased amniotic fluid	Age 8 months normal renal function - affected father
Gagnadoux (*)	1988	Fetus 1	?? week US enlarged, echogenic kidneys	Alive and well at 2 yrs
Gal (16)	1989	Family 1 -Fetus 1	32 week US enlarged, echogenic kidneys; oligohydramnios	Stillbirth, sibling and cousin died at birth with ADPKD; autopsy confirmed diagnosis - affected father
		Family 5 -Fetus 1	32 week US; enlarged kidneys	Alive and well at 2 yrs with cystic kidneys - affected mother
Ceccerini (17)	1989	Fetus 1	29 week US enlarged,echogenic kidneys; bilateral cysts; oligohydramnios; lung hypoplasia	Spontaneous labor at 33 weeks Caesarean section; newborn death at 1 day - affected mother
		Fetus 2	14 week US enlarged, echogenic kidneys; several cysts	Gene linkage 11 weeks 95% chance ADPKD pregnancy terminated; autopsy confirmed diagnosis; sibling of Fetus 1 - affected mother
Journel (18)	1989	Fetus 1	35 week US enlarged, echogenic kidneys	1 yr normal renal function enlarged kidneys, bilateral cysts at birth - affected father
		Fetus 2	24 week US hyperechogenic kidneys; 35 week US increased size, hyperechogenic kidneys	7 months alive and well - affected mother
		Fetus 3	21 week US normal kidneys; 28 week US enlarged, hyperechogenic kidneys	Pregnancy terminated (thought to be ARPKD); autopsy showed microscopic cysts only affected father (diagnosed 1 yr later)
Novelli (19)	1989	Fetus 1	19 week US slightly enlarged, but normal appearance kidneys	Gene linkage 10 weeks 95% chance ADPKD pregnancy terminated; autopsy revealed several cysts - affected father

(*) = Data from Journel (18)

ADPKD has considerable phenotypic variability between members of the same family and between families. This is not uncommon in autosomal dominant disorders. However, in ADPKD some of the interfamily variability may reflect the fact that the disease which we have labelled ADPKD can, in fact, result from at least two different genetic mutations (2). That is, not all ADPKD is caused by a defective gene on chromosome 16. A number of families have now been described whose gene is not linked to the probes for chromosome 16 (2-6). The location of this other gene (or genes) is not known. This second gene, PKD2 or non-PKD1, appears to have several important differences from the chromosome 16 PKD1 gene. Families with the PKD2 gene appear to have later onset of renal cysts and later onset of renal insufficiency than families with the PKD1 gene (7). Thus, differences in causative gene could explain at least some of the interfamily variability seen with ADPKD. Since the location of the PKD2 gene is unknown, gene linkage analysis is not available for families with this ADPKD gene.

PHENOTYPIC PRESENTATION OF ADPKD IN FETAL LIFE

Ultrasonographic imaging techniques have become extremely sensitive in identifying even very small renal cysts (8) and the technology permits identification of abnormalities in tissue echogenicity. Imaging techniques permit the detection not only of fetal kidneys, but also of renal cystic disease in fetuses (9-19). Although fetal kidneys can be visualized after the 16th week of gestation (20), and the diagnosis of ADPKD has been made at this point and even at 14 weeks (17), cysts or abnormalities in echogenicity may not always be detected this early. In the few instances in which sequential studies have been done in fetuses at-risk for ADPKD, the fetal kidneys were seen and considered to be normal at 16 and 21 weeks of gestation and abnormal after 28 or 30 weeks (10, 18). This detection of abnormality in at least some instances only in the third trimester has important implications for the use of ultrasonography for prenatal diagnosis of ADPKD for possible termination of pregnancy. Specifically, ADPKD is not a disorder which fulfills the guidelines for disorders in which third trimester abortion may be acceptable (21).

The abnormal fetal kidneys are frequently large and highly echogenic; they may or may not contain discrete renal cysts (Table 1). This fetal renal appearance is compatible with both autosomal recessive polycystic kidney disease (ARPKD) and ADPKD (15). These two infantile cystic disorders cannot be distinguished on the basis of imaging information alone (22). In fact, the major discriminating feature between ADPKD and ARPKD in fetal or neonatal life is the presence of ADPKD in a parent. Family history of ADPKD must be sought in this circumstance, but a negative family history does not exclude ADPKD. Only 60 to 75% of all ADPKD subjects give a positive family history, but approximately 90% will, in fact, have an affected parent if the parent undergoes the appropriate imaging studies (23). In addition, 62% of affected parents who have a neonate with clinically manifest ADPKD will be unaware that they have the disease until the child's disease prompts parental investigation (15). Therefore, parents of such a child or affected fetus should undergo imaging studies. If both parents have negative imaging studies the child either has ARPKD or the fetus is the offspring of a different father. This latter possibility should not be forgotten as there is a finite occurrence of non-paternity among married couples.

Sedman et al (14) suggested that presentation of ADPKD in fetal or neonatal life occurred more frequently with an affected father than with an affected mother; however, other studies have not demonstrated this effect of parental gender (13). Moreover, in the fetuses reported thus far with phenotypic manifestation of ADPKD on ultrasound, both parental genders appear equally represented (Table 1).

There is, however, a suggestion that early fetal and neonatal presentation of ADPKD clusters in families (Table 1). That is to say, if a family has one such early-onset affected child, other children who inherit the ADPKD gene would also present early in life. A possible explanation for this suggested clustering of early onset disease might be that such children are homozygous for the ADPKD gene, inheriting one ADPKD from each parent. However, in instances where we have examined both parents this has not occurred. It has also been suggested that these early onset children could have inherited an ADPKD gene from one parent and an ARPKD gene from the other parent (24, 25). Since the ARPKD gene requires two copies to be clinically apparent the disease would not be manifested in that parent.

However, it is postulated that the ARPKD gene in some manner might magnify the effect of the dominant ADPKD gene. Until the ARPKD gene location is identified this hypothesis cannot be tested. As yet, there are no prospective studies of fetuses at 50% risk for ADPKD to determine the frequency of abnormal fetal kidneys or to examine the hypothesis of family clustering of early disease.

The discovery of large hyperechoic or cystic kidneys in a fetus raises the question of the both short and long-term outcome for such an offspring. If the fetus is determined to have ADPKD, the outcome generally appears good for the short term. Of 20 such fetuses reported in the literature five were therapeutically aborted, three were stillborn or died at 1 day, one outcome was unknown, and the eleven others were alive and doing well at follow-up at ages two months to nine years (Table 1). Long-term follow-up is not yet available in children with fetal manifestation of ADPKD.

202

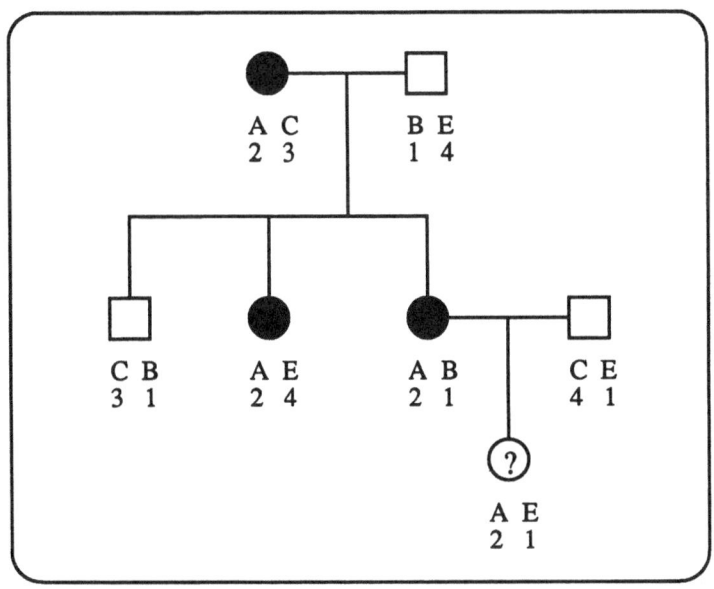

Figure 1. Pedigree of an ADPKD family with the ADPKD gene on chromosome 16 (PKD1). Two arbitrary markers for each person's two chromosomes are displayed below the symbol. In this family all affected subjects inherited the markers A and 2 with ADPKD. Therefore in this family these markers segregate with the PKD1 gene. The use of two rather than one marker, particularly if they are known to be on either side of the gene, increases accuracy of presentation. Although the family is small, there are no crossovers of markers, raising confidence that this is a PKD1 family. Thus, the fetus who has inherited the markers A and 2 on chromosome 16 has very likely (>95% chance) inherited the ADPKD gene as well.

PRENATAL GENETIC TESTING

The commercial availability of the 3'HVR probe as well as other probes on chromosome 16 on either side of the ADPKD gene permit the use of gene linkage analysis for both presymptomatic adults and fetal diagnosis (see below) (17, 19, 26). Since the method depends upon DNA located near the ADPKD gene (DNA probes) being inherited with the ADPKD gene, a certain family structure must be present to utilize the method. There must be at least two affected subjects and the affected and unaffected parent must have different probe types in order to assess which marker type is linked to the ADPKD gene in this family (Figure 1). In the family depicted two different probes were utilized to improve the accuracy of the prediction (27). The ADPKD gene is being transmitted with the probe types A and 2 since all affected individuals have inherited the chromosome with these markers from the affected grandmother. If fetal testing were done on the offspring in the third generation, she would have a greater than 95% chance of carrying the ADPKD gene since she inherited marker types A and 2 which are on the chromosome with the

ADPKD gene. The predictions made with gene linkage are never unequivocally 100 or zero percent because the gene itself is not what is identified. Hence, some possibility for error is always present. The error results from cross-over of genetic material from one chromosome to another. During meiosis, the probe on the chromosome with the ADPKD gene can exchange with the probe on the other chromosome 16 bearing the normal gene (cross-over). If that occurred and only one marker had been used it would have been concluded incorrectly from the gene linkage analysis that this subject did not have ADPKD. Using a probe closer to the ADPKD gene or using probes on either side of the gene decrease the chances of making an error due to cross-over. The use of more than one probe also increases the chances that each parent will have different probe types. Another potential source of error or, more correctly, a reason why gene linkage cannot be used in a family is that the family is a PKD2 family whose gene is not on chromosome 16. Data suggests that 90% of ADPKD in the Caucasian population is due to the PKD1 gene (28). Therefore, in a Caucasian family there is little error introduced by the infrequent presence of the PKD2 gene in the population. However, in families in which a cross-over is observed or in non-Caucasian families more family members must be tested to first verify that the family is PKD1 and hence appropriate for utilization of chromosome 16 probes.

To utilize this technique to determine the fetal genotype, fetal DNA can be obtained from fetal lymphocytes by amniocentesis or from the placenta by chorionic villus sampling. Early evaluation of the fetus is desirable if the diagnosis of ADPKD would influence the continuation of the pregnancy. Chorionic villus sampling at 9 to 12 weeks gestation affords the earliest time for procurement of fetal cells. Placental cells obtained by transcervical or transabdominal catheter require two weeks of culturing to yield a sufficient quantity of DNA for probe analysis. Approximately two additional weeks are then required to complete the probe analysis. Given the time frame of four weeks for results, chorionic villus sampling offers the advantage of obtaining fetal cells early in the gestation. This in fact has been utilized in ADPKD (17, 19, 26). Chorionic villus sampling procedures are associated with approximately a 1% inadequate sample rate, a 1% failed culture rate and a 1-2% increase in the overall fetal loss rate (29). For gestations greater than 12 weeks, amniocentesis remains an option as cells for culture can be obtained from the amniotic fluid. The constraint of 4 weeks for results should be considered, however, when offering amniocentesis in the second trimester. A diagnosis and subsequent termination of pregnancy at more than 16 weeks gestation is associated with greater maternal mortality and morbidity than a similar procedure at an earlier gestational age. For these reasons, ideally the asymptomatic but at-risk individual or the affected subject who wishes prenatal diagnosis should [1] be identified by linked marker studies early in his (her) reproductive years, [2] receive preconception or early pregnancy counselling regarding the availability of prenatal diagnosis and [3] should be offered chorionic villus sampling at 9-12 weeks to allow diagnosis early in gestation.

The physician and the family must understand the interpretation of a test which identifies the fetus as an ADPKD gene carrier. Reported odds for linkage greater than 95% implies that the fetus would be highly likely to manifest ADPKD in post-natal life but it does not provide any information regarding the age of onset of symptoms, presence of extrarenal manifestations or the likelihood of end-stage renal disease. It is well to remember the natural history of the renal defect in counselling the family. That is, 70% of all ADPKD patients are alive without end-stage renal disease at age 58 (30). Moreover, in counselling families the physician must be aware of the complexity of attitudes surrounding prenatal diagnosis of this disease.

In a recent study of 107 ADPKD kindreds, 141 ADPKD subjects were queried regarding the use of gene testing (31). Sixty-five percent of the ADPKD patients indicated that they would utilize gene linkage analysis to determine the gene status of an at-risk fetus. However, only 8% of them indicated they would terminate a pregnancy for ADPKD. In contrast, 25% would terminate the pregnancy for an unspecified "very serious medical problem" in the fetus, suggesting that in some sense individuals with ADPKD did not consider it a "very serious medical problem" for the fetus. It is also noteworthy that approximately one-third of these affected individuals were uncertain about the termination of pregnancy for ADPKD. The late onset of ADPKD and its relatively benign outcome may account for the lower anticipated use of prenatal testing and less frequent perceived willingness to terminate a pregnancy for ADPKD than has been reported for Huntington's disease (32, 33) and cystic fibrosis (34).

Moreover, there is often a difference between what patients state they will do regarding testing and what actually occurs (32). In this regard, it appears that there has been little use of prenatal testing for ADPKD. Despite the availability of the probes since 1985, only rare reports of prenatal gene testing and termination have appeared (17, 19, 26). In fact, no patient in our population has utilized prenatal testing when presented with the opportunity.

Thus, although the technology exists to determine both phenotypic and genotypic status of a fetus at risk for ADPKD, it remains to be determined if these technologies will be utilized. Nonetheless, physicians caring for ADPKD families should inform them of the availability of these technologies and they should counsel them regarding their use. Independent of any immediate clinical utilization of prenatal diagnosis, identification of phenotypically affected fetuses will expand our understanding of the natural history of the disease which will improve our counselling of families with early onset offspring.

ACKNOWLODGEMENT

This research was supported by Grant 5 P01 DK34039, Human Polycystic Kidney Disease (PKD), awarded by the Department of Health and Human Services, Public Health Service, NIDDK, and the Clinical Research Center, Grant MORR-00051 from the General Clinical Research Centers Research Program of the Division of Research Resources, National Institutes of Health.

REFERENCES

1. Reeders ST, Breuning MH, Davies KE, Nicholls RD, Jarman AP, Higgs DR, Pearson PL, Weatherall DJ: A highly polymorphic DNA marker linked to adult polycystic kidney disease on chromosome 16. Nature, 317: 542-544, 1985.
2. Kimberling WJ, Fain PR, Kenyon JB, Goldgar D, Sujansky E, Gabow PA: Linkage heterogeneity of autosomal dominant polycystic kidney disease. N Engl J Med, 319: 913-918, 1988.
3. Romeo G, Devoto M, Costa G, Roncuzzi L, Catizone L, Zucchelli P, Germino GG, Keith T, Weatherall DJ, Reeders ST: A second genetic locus for autosomal dominant polycystic kidney disease. Lancet, II: 8-10, 1988.
4. Norby S, Sorensen AWS, Boesen P: Non-allelic genetic heterogeneity of autosomal dominant polycystic kidney disease? In: "Genetics of kidney disorders" (Ed Christos S Bartsocas), Alan R. Liss Inc, New York, 1989.
5. Dawson DB, Torres VE, Charboneau JW, Thibodeau SN: Detection of a family with autosomal dominant polycystic kidney disease loosely linked to DNA markers from 16p. Kidney Int, 35: 203, 1989 (Abstract).
6. Brissenden JE, Roscoe JM, Silverman M: Linkage heterogeneity for autosomal dominant polycystic kidney disease studied by DNA and chromosomal analysis. Kidney Int, 37: 247, 1990 (Abstract).
7. Parfrey PS, Bear JC, Morgan J, Cramer BC, McManamon PJ, Gault MH, Churchill DN, Singh M, Hewitt R, Somlo S, Reeders ST: The diagnosis and prognosis of autosomal dominant polycystic kidney disease. N Engl J Med, 323: 1085-1090, 1990.
8. Levine E, Grantham JJ: The role of computed tomography in the evaluation of adult polycystic kidney disease. Am J Kidney Dis, 1: 99-105, 1981.
9. Zerres K, Weiss H, Bulla M, Roth B: Prenatal diagnosis of an early manifestation of autosomal dominant adult-type polycystic kidney disease. Lancet, II: 988, 1982 (Letter).
10. Main D, Mennuti MT, Cornfeld D, Coleman B: Prenatal diagnosis of adult polycystic kidney disease. Lancet, II: 337-338, 1983.
11. Zerres K, Hansmann M, Knopfle G, Stephan M: Prenatal diagnosis of genetically determined early manifestation of autosomal dominant polycystic kidney disease? Hum Genet, 71: 368-369, 1985.
12. Fryns JP, Vandenberghe K, Moerman F: Mid-trimester ultrasonographic diagnosis of early manifesting "adult" form of polycystic kidney disease. Hum Genet, 74: 461, 1986.
13. Kaariainen H: Polycystic kidney disease in children: a genetic and epidemiological study of 82 Finnish patients. J Med Genetics, 24: 474-481, 1987.
14. Sedman A, Bell P, Manco-Johnson M, Schrier R, Warady BA, Heard EO, Butler-Simon N, Gabow P: Autosomal dominant polycystic kidney disease in childhood: a longitudinal study. Kidney Int, 31: 1000-1005, 1987.
15. Pretorius DH, Lee ME, Manco-Johnson ML, Weingast GR, Sedman AB, Gabow PA: Diagnosis of autosomal dominant polycystic disease in utero and in the young infant. J Ultrasound Med, 6: 249-255, 1987.
16. Gal A, Wirth B, Kaariainen H, Lucotte G, Landais P, Gillessen-Kaesbach G, Muller-Wiefel DE, Zerres K: Childhood manifestations of autosomal dominant polycystic kidney disease: no evidence for genetic heterogeneity. Clinical Genetics, 35: 13-19, 1989.

17. Ceccherini I, Lituania M, Cordone MS, Perfumo F, Gusmano R, Callea F, Archidiacono N, Romeo G: Autosomal dominant polycystic kidney disease: prenatal diagnosis by DNA analysis and sonography at 14 weeks. Prenat Diagn, 9: 751-758, 1989.

18. Journel H, Guyot C, Barc RM, Belbeoch P, Quemener A, Jouan H: Unexpected ultrasonographic prenatal diagnosis of autosomal dominant polycystic kidney disease. Prenat Diagn, 9: 663-671, 1989.

19. Novelli G, Frontali M, Baldini D, Bosman C, Dallapiccola B, Pachi A, Torcia F: Prenatal diagnosis of adult polycystic kidney disease with DNA markers on chromosome 16 and the genetic heterogeneity problem. Prenat Diagn, 9: 759-767, 1989.

20. Cohen HL, Haller JO: Diagnostic sonography of the fetal genitourinary tract. Urol Radiol, 9: 88-98, 1987.

21. Chervenak FA, Farley MA, Walters LR, Hobbins JC, Mahoney MJ: When is termination of pregnancy during the third trimester morally justifiable? N Engl J Med, 310: 501-504, 1984.

22. Cole BR, Conley SB, Stapleton FB: Polycystic kidney disease in the first year of life. J Pediatr, 111: 693-699, 1987.

23. Gabow PA, Iklé DW, Holmes JH: Polycystic kidney disease: prospective analysis of nonazotemic patients and family members. Ann Intern Med, 101: 238-247, 1984.

24. Taitz LS, Brown CB, Blank CE, Steiner GM: Screening for polycystic kidney disease: importance of clinical presentation in the newborn. Arch Dis Child, 62: 45-49, 1987.

25. Zerres K, Propping P: Autosomal dominant polycystic kidney disease in children. Arch Dis Child, 62: 870-871, 1987.

26. Reeders ST, Gal A, Propping P, Waldherr R, Davies KE, Zerres K, Hogenkamp T, Schmidt W, Dolata MM, Weatherall DJ: Prenatal diagnosis of autosomal dominant polycystic kidney disease with a DNA probe. Lancet, II: 6-8, 1986.

27. Breuning MH, Reeders ST, Brunner H, Ijdo JW, Saris JJ, Verwest A, van Ommen GJB, Pearson PL: Improved early diagnosis of adult polycystic kidney disease with flanking DNA markers. Lancet, II: 1359-1361, 1987.

28. Kimberling WJ, Pieke SA, Kenyon JB, Gabow PA: An estimate of the proportion of families with autosomal dominant polycystic kidney disease unlinked to chromosome 16. Kidney Int, 37: 249, 1990 (Abstract).

29. Rhoads GG, Jackson LG, Schlesselman SE, De La Cruz FF, Desnick RJ, Golbus MS, Ledbetter DH, Lubs HA, Mahoney MJ, Pergament E, Simpson JL, Carpenter RJ, Elias S, Ginsberg NA, Goldberg JD, Hobbins JC, Lynch L, Shiono PH, Wapner RJ, Zachary JM: The safety and efficacy of chorionic villus sampling for early prenatal diagnosis of cytogenetic abnormalities. N Engl J Med, 320: 609-617, 1989.

30. Churchill DN, Bear JC, Morgan J, Payne RH, McManamon PJ, Gault MH: Prognosis of adult onset polycystic kidney disease re-evaluated. Kidney Int, 26: 190-193, 1984.

31. Sujansky E, Kreutzer SB, Johnson AM, Lezotte DC, Schrier RW, Gabow PA: Attitudes of at-risk and affected individuals regarding presymptomatic testing for autosomal dominant polycystic kidney disease. Am J Med Genet, 35: 510-515, 1990.

32. Meissen GJ, Berchek RL: Intended use of predictive testing by those at risk for Huntington disease. Am J Med Genet, 26: 283-293, 1987.

33. Kessler S, Field T, Worth L, Mosbarger H: Attitudes of persons at risk for Huntington disease toward predictive testing. Am J Med Genet, 26: 259-270, 1987.

34. Evers-Kiebooms G: Decision making in Huntington's disease and cystic fibrosis. Birth Defects, 23: 115-149, 1987.

RENAL STONE DISEASE

Chapter 9

URINARY STONES WHICH REQUIRE ADJUNCTIVE MANAGEMENT FOR SUCCESSFUL EXTRACORPOREAL SHOCKWAVE LITHOTRIPSY

GERHARD J. FUCHS AND ANNA M. FUCHS

UCLA Stone Center, UCLA School of Medicine, Division of Urology, 10833 Leconte Ave, Los Angeles, Ca 90024, USA

DEVELOPMENT OF EXTRACORPOREAL SHOCKWAVE LITHOTRIPSY OF RENAL STONES

In February 1980, extracorporeal shock wave lithotripsy [ESWL] was introduced clinically at the Department of Urology, University of Munich, as the first noninvasive method to treat patients suffering from upper urinary tract stones (1-15). The high efficacy, safety, and reliability of the method, dramatically changed the management of upper urinary stones. In 1991, approximately 70% of patients with renal and ureteral stones can be treated with ESWL-monotherapy and additionally 20% of patients with more complex stones can receive ESWL treatment in conjunction with endoscopic procedures. The remaining 10% of patients either require percutaneous or ureteroscopic endoscopic surgery alone or open surgery.

Ten years of clinical experience with ESWL have led to the identification of the stone- and patient-related parameters governing the treatment outcome of the ESWL method. The ease with which the technique of ESWL can be performed by the urologist and the virtual absence of complications in the initial clinical series of highly selected patients have gradually led to an overutilization of this technology. Parallel to this trend, the technically more involved techniques of endoscopic stone surgery - ureteroscopy and percutaneous stone surgery - are being underutilized and the pool of urologists with skill in these techniques does not appear to be increasing. Therefore, an increasing number of patients with unnecessary complications from indiscriminate use of ESWL are being seen at academic institutions. It has to be stated clearly that ESWL, when performed according to the guidelines which have evolved over the 11 years of its clinical use, is safe, reliable, and the results are reproducible (8, 12-15).

211

SELECTION OF APPROPRIATE TREATMENT FOR RENAL STONES

The major determinants for the selection of the appropriate treatment for renal stones are [1] stone-burden, [2] intrarenal and upper urinary tract anatomy and [3] patient compliance.

A small number of exclusion criteria (Table 1) still have to be observed, such as uncorrected bleeding disorder, uncorrected hypertension, and aortic or renal artery aneurysms. Exclusion from ESWL treatment for technical reasons is rare and depends on the type of lithotripter used. However, patient habitus and renal anatomy may present problems because of the stone location relative to the energy source and the patient positioning system (e.g. patient size, patient obesity, skeletal anomalies and ectopic kidneys).

Table 1. Exclusion criteria for ESWL

Medical:	- uncorrected bleeding disorder
	- uncorrected hypertension
	- pregnancy (stone treatment rarely necessary, placement of internal stent or percutaneous nephrostomy)
	- aortic or renal artery aneurysm (calcifications of aorta and renal artery are relative contraindications)
	- pacemakers (standby - cardiologist recommended)
Technical:	- depending on type of lithotripter
	- general problems: stone location relative to energy source and patient positioning system (determinants: patient size, patient obesity, skeletal anomalies and ectopic kidneys, radioopacity of stone)
Urological:	- severe anatomical or functional alterations precluding proper elimination of debris
	- stenosis distal to the stone (calyceal neck, ureteropelvic junction, ureter, hypertrophy of prostate requiring surgical correction, urethral stricture)
	- stone bearing calyx grossly distended (especially dependent calyces)
	- functional impairment of ureteral mobility (neurogenic, immobile patient)

Urological contraindications to ESWL are severe anatomical or functional alterations precluding proper elimination of debris, stenosis distal to the stone, such as at the calyceal neck, the ureteropelvic junction, the ureter, hypertrophy of the prostate requiring surgical correction, urethral stricture, a grossly distended stone bearing calyx (especially dependent calyces), and severe functional impairment of ureteral mobility (neurogenic, immobile patient). In these situations percutaneous surgery or open surgery may be preferable (13, 16, 17).

The variables which govern treatment decisions are shown in Table 2 and are discussed below.

Table 2. Selection criteria for extracorporeal shockwave lithotripsy of renal stones.

Variables determining treatment approach:
- stone-burden (period of stone passage and rate of auxiliary procedures increase proportionally with stone size)
- intrarenal stone distribution (pelvis vs calyces)
- presence of intrarenal stenosis
- isolated dilatation of calyces
- stone composition (Calcium-oxalate monohydrate and Cystine stones respond poorly to ESWL)
- patient compliance (prolonged period of time before treatment is completed, depending on stone size)

Stone-burden

Solitary stones or multiple stones of an added diameter of up to 2.5 cm are considered ideal for ESWL treatment provided there is no hindrance to the spontaneous elimination of gravel. Stone clearance rates between 90%, for stones of 1 cm, and 70%, for stones of up to 2.5 cm, can be expected (9, 11, 16, 18-20). For such stones the clinical experience does not identify significant differences in terms of success and complication rates comparing first and later generation lithotripters. Fluoroscopy localizing lithotripters offer the advantage of a better assessment of stone fragmentation, whereas ultrasound localizing lithotripters allow treatment of radiolucent and semiopaque stones without auxiliary administration of contrast dye. Most newer, so-called second generation machines enable anesthesia-free ESWL; however, this is done at the expense of a higher retreatment rate than the first generation lithotripters (30% vs 10%).

Although it has been proven that even staghorn stones can be treated with ESWL monotherapy, increasing stone-burden resulting in lesser stone-free rates and higher complication rates (ureteral obstruction, obstructive pyelonephritis, prolonged period of stone passage, unpredictability of outcome) have significantly dampened the initial enthusiasm for ESWL treatment of staghorn stones (9, 11, 13, 16-23). Controversy still exists in the treatment of staghorn stones and different treatment strategies have evolved (monotherapy with extracorporeal shock wave lithotripsy vs the combined treatment of endourological procedures and subsequent extracorporeal shock wave lithotripsy) (16-23). In partial and complete staghorn stones, monotherapy with extracorporeal shock wave lithotripsy (in conjunction with the use of indwelling ureteral catheters) is only preferable to other treatment modalities in cases where the stone is filling a nondilated collecting system and in the absence of intrarenal stenosis or isolated gross distension of the dependent calyces (13, 16-22). When staghorn stones are filling a slightly dilated collecting system, i.e. have a slightly larger stone-burden, a planned staged extracorporeal shock wave lithotripsy procedure (2 treatment sessions spaced apart at least 2 days) is usually performed (20, 21). It has to be pointed out, however, that with increasing stone-burden the rates for second ESWL sessions and follow-up complications (ureteral obstruction, infection) are considerably higher than those encountered with smaller stones (22).

Also, the period of stone passage after ESWL monotherapy is significantly prolonged compared to percutaneous stone surgery or the combination therapy of percutaneous endoscopic stone debulking followed by ESWL. The liberal use of indwelling ureteral catheters has not had any proven effect on these parameters; however, it reduces perioperative morbidity and the need for auxiliary procedures to relieve ureteral obstruction. Auxiliary procedures, namely percutaneous nephrostomy tube placement and ureteroscopic ureteral manipulations are required in approximately 60% of patients after the ESWL treatment of large branched stones (20-22).

In staghorn stones with a large stone mass, filling a dilated renal collecting system, and with intrarenal anatomical alterations, a percutaneous procedure is performed first for de-bulking the stone. In a second session, extracorporeal shock wave lithotripsy is employed for the disintegration of the remaining calyceal stone parts and, under the same anesthesia, the patient undergoes a second percutaneous procedure for removal of the stone gravel (16-33). Although inherently more invasive than monotherapy with extracorporeal shock wave lithotripsy, this approach is of great benefit for the patient with regard to stone-free rates, hospitalizations, and time lost from work.

For these reasons, major stone referral centers with experience in endourology prefer percutaneous debulking for these patients, using ESWL as an auxiliary procedure for stone parts which cannot be reached from the percutaneous access. Average stone-free rates of approximately 50% for ESWL alone vs approximately 85% for percutaneous surgery combined with ESWL, as well as annualized recurrence rates of 25% and 10%, respectively, speak in favor of the combined or primary percutaneous approach.

Nephrolithiasis is a relatively rare incident in the pediatric age group. ESWL has become particularly advantageous in this patient population as clinical experience has shown no deleterious effects, even when multiple sessions are required. Concerns have been raised with regard to the effect of high energy shock waves on immature bony tissue, growing renal tissue, long-term renal function, or the induction of hypertension. The available clinical data indicate that extracorporeal shock wave lithotripsy does not lead to deterioration of renal function, or altered renal development, and no juvenile hypertension has been noted after extracorporeal shock wave lithotripsy. Recently conducted research on the effects of high energy shock waves on immature bony tissue and renal growth confirms the safety of this treatment modality. Cautious use of the energy with adherence to certain limits, however, is advocated and treatment should be performed at major referral centers where all treatment options are readily available (13, 17, 34).

Upper urinary tract anatomy

Anatomical alterations of the renal collecting system or ureter precluding spontaneous passage of fragmented stone material may require endourological or open surgical procedures only to be followed by ESWL as an auxiliary procedure. Such conditions are listed in Table 3. Depending on stone size, location, and severity of the anatomical alteration, either retrograde ureteroscopic intrarenal surgery (RIRS) or, in more complex cases, percutaneous endoscopic renal surgery is employed. Retrograde intrarenal surgery is performed with flexible ureteroscopes through the intact upper urinary tract. Percutaneous renal surgery is performed through a percutaneous access (usually performed by the radiologist or urologist under fluoroscopic and/or ultrasound control).

Table 3.   Indications for retrograde intrarenal surgery and percutaneous renal surgery.

A. RETROGRADE INTRARENAL SURGERY FOR RENAL STONE DISEASE:
    Failed ESWL (stones <1.5 cm or 5 particles up to 5 mm each)
    Radiolucent (stones <1.5 cm)
    Concomitant ureteral and renal stones (renal stone < 1.0 cm.)
    Stones in calyceal diverticuli
    Stones and nephrocalcinosis
    Stones and urinary diversion (supravesical)
    Staghorn stones (rare, when ESWL and PCNL may not be technically feasible, coagulopathy)
B. PERCUTANEOUS RENAL SURGERY FOR RENAL STONE DISEASE
    Staghorn Stones
    Intrarenal or ureteropelvic junction stenosis
    Struvite, matrix and cystine stones

Patient compliance

ESWL therapy consists of two parts, fragmentation of the stone and spontaneous elimination of the stone debris. Depending on the size of the original stone, a large amount of stone debris may have to clear the ureter, resulting in a prolonged period of stone passage. During this period of time, the patient is at theoretical risk of ureteral obstruction and obstructive pyelonephritis, which may result in loss of renal function or a life threatening septic complication, if not treated appropriately. Patients need to be made aware of this possibility and the need for compliance with a timely follow-up protocol has to be stressed. Patients who appear unfit to comply with the follow-up protocol should not receive ESWL treatment of complex stones, but should undergo percutaneous or open surgery instead.

INDICATIONS FOR RETROGRADE INTRARENAL SURGERY (RIRS)

For a number of stone patients who are not ideal candidates for ESWL, retrograde intrarenal surgery (RIRS) has become a highly successful alternative to the more invasive percutaneous approach. This minimally-invasive endoscopic approach has become possible due to the advent of new smaller caliber actively deflecting endoscopes and matching operating accessories. In our practice in a comprehensive stone center with referral of predominantly complex cases the following applications of RIRS have become routine procedures (Table 3):

a. Residual stones post ESWL

Residual stones following ESWL, such as occurs after insufficient fragmentation or delayed passage due to anatomical alterations (dilated lower calyceal group, intrarenal stenosis) are candidates for RIRS. The size limits at present are 1.5 cm for solitary stones and up to 5 particles of an individual size of 5 mm or less. Solid stones larger than 5 mm are fragmented using the 1.6 Fr EHL probe (alternative: Laser probe), and smaller fragments are retrieved using a three-pronged grasper or a flat wire stone basket [3.6 Fr]. Limiting factors for the use of the RIRS technique are stone-burden and anatomy of the lower calyceal group. Stone-burden directly correlates with treatment time and at times direct access to the lower calyceal group is technically not feasible due to the angle of bend of the scope. In the latter situation the stone or particle can be dislodged at times by careful hand irrigation and aspiration and thus repositioned in a location better suitable for direct removal.

b. Radiolucent and semiopaque stones

Radiolucent and semiopaque stones are difficult to localize with fluoroscopy-based lithotripters and need administration of contrast for stone localization. With ultrasound-based lithotripters such stones can be localized directly. Therefore, when no ultrasound localizing lithotripter is available (as in >90% of institutions), renal stones with the above size and number specifications are preferably approached with RIRS. This is usually done after a trial with conservative dissolution has failed (35-43).

216

c. Impacted proximal ureteral stones with ipsilateral renal stone

Impacted ureteral stones which fail retrograde manipulation with ureteral catheters are best treated with ureteroscopy and direct contact lithotripsy. In the past 4 years flexible ureteroscopy and electrohydraulic fragmentation have replaced rigid ureteroscopy (and ultrasound fragmentation) for stones in the upper half of the ureter. In cases with ipsilateral renal stones not larger than 1.0 cm or 3 fragments not larger than 5 mm each, RIRS stone removal can be performed under the same anesthesia. The limiting factors are: stone size in the kidney and time spent for fragmentation and removal of the ureteral stone (29-33, 43).

d. Renal stones associated with intrarenal stenosis

Absence of intrarenal stenosis distal to the stone is of basic importance for the success of stone elimination with ESWL. If repair of the condition is necessary the options have traditionally included percutaneous management or open surgery. RIRS affords a less invasive technique for the removal of such stones and repair of the condition by balloon dilation or incision with the 2 Fr Bugby electrode. This technique is ideal for intrarenal stenosis in the upper and mid calyceal group and also for selected cases of strictures of the ureteropelvic junction. When a calyceal diverticulum of the lower calyceal group is encountered, percutaneous renal surgery is the treatment of choice. This is due to the difficulty of deflecting the flexible ureteroscope sufficiently to reach the lower calyces once an operating accessory is passed through the work channel (36-38, 43).

e. Renal stones and nephrocalcinosis

Utilizing the basic technique of selective evaluation of the intrarenal collecting system under direct visual and fluoroscopic control, RIRS allows for easy differentiation of stones in the renal collecting system, submucosal calcifications and parenchymal calcifications. The result of the evaluation is based on the preoperative retrograde pyelogram, the treatment of smaller renal stones being with RIRS while larger stones are treated with ESWL and/or by percutaneous removal (43).

f. Renal stones and supravesical urinary diversion

Endoscopy of the upper urinary tract after supravesical urinary diversion is difficult and with rigid instrumentation often not feasible. Flexible endoscopy has been employed at our institution extensively for diagnostic purposes in such situations and, due to the good results especially with regard to gaining access to the upper urinary tract, RIRS has been utilized increasingly for these patients. When stone formation occurs in these patients the common problem is the fact that these patients tend to form infection-induced stones which are difficult to localize with fluoroscopy lithotripters. This is accentuated by the copious amount of intestinal air which is also found in many of those patients. Retrograde evaluation of the uretero-enteric anastomosis is possible in the majority of cases using a combination of flexible endoscopes (cystoscopes, ureteroscopes), contrast dye and fluoroscopy, and administration of methylene blue if renal function permits. With the exception of patients with antirefluxive pouches, identification of the anastomosis and instrumentation in the upper urinary tract are possible. Although the majority of cases is performed for the treatment of stones, an increasing number of patients with stenosis of the uretero-enteric anastomosis are now being treated. The indications are identical to the indications under *a-e* (17, 41, 43).

g. Patients with the need for complete stone removal

RIRS appears to be particularly beneficial for a subsegment of patients who need to be stone-free to keep up with specific requirements of their profession (pilots) or patients who may be at an increased risk of injury secondary to attacks of stone colic, such as circus artists, chimney sweeps. Also included in this group are young women planning pregnancy and patients who intend to go to countries with inferior medical infrastructure. In patients being prepared for organ transplantation or implantation of artificial materials RIRS is being increasingly used (43).

INDICATIONS FOR PERCUTANEOUS RENAL SURGERY

A. Large stones >2.5 cm and staghorn stones

Most of these stones are best approached by a primary percutaneous procedure as has been mentioned before. A one-stage procedure is preferred (access to the kidney, dilation of the percutaneous access tract, and percutaneous surgery in one sitting) which in the hands of the experienced endourologist results in stone-free rates greater than 85% and minimal morbidity (7, 9, 13, 17-25, 27).

B. Cystine, matrix, and infection-induced stones

Cystine stones tend to be rather difficult to fragment with ESWL and the results are not predictable (fragmentation rate approximately 60%). Therefore a primary percutaneous approach is preferred (stone-free rates greater than 90%). Matrix stone, i.e. poorly calcified proteinaceous material which is commonly found concomitantly with urinary tract infection, does not respond to ESWL and needs direct percutaneous removal. Struvite stone, i.e. magnesium-ammonium phosphate, is usually found as a result of urea splitting bacterial infection. This type of stone requires complete eradication since otherwise the persistent infection is difficult to control and regrowth of the residual debris necessitating further treatment is a common occurrence. The percutaneous technique with ultrasound aspiration of the fragmented stone material is the treatment of choice (17, 40).

C. Abnormal renal anatomy

Stones associated with intrarenal stenosis or stenosis of the ureteropelvic junction are not good candidates for ESWL monotherapy. Percutaneous surgery, however, in many instances can solve these problems. Also stones harbored in parts of the kidney which are grossly distended secondary to obstruction should be primarily removed by endoscopic surgery (Table 3).

INDICATIONS FOR OPEN RENAL SURGERY

Extensive intrarenal stenosis requiring correction may be too severe for endoscopic management and in these instances open surgery is the choice. Such cases (less than 3% of all stone patients) and nephrectomy of functionless kidneys (less than 1%) are the only open surgical procedures performed at our institution during the past 6 years (17, 26).

TREATMENT INDICATIONS FOR URETERAL STONES

Approximately 80% of all urinary stones pass spontaneously and only 20% need interventional therapy. The basic indications for surgical treatment of ureteral stones are [1] unresolving pain, [2] stone size too large for spontaneous passage, [3] persistent obstruction regardless of stone size, [4] anatomic alterations, such as stricture distal to the stone, and [5] emergent treatment to avoid severe complications. Indications for emergency treatment of ureteral stones are obstructive pyelonephritis (because of the impending risk of sepsis) and anuria (in the case of either bilateral ureteral obstruction or obstruction of a solitary kidney). Unremitting pain, unresponsive to oral analgesics and antispasmodics may become an indication for a more urgent treatment strategy, especially in the elderly and debilitated patient because of the risk of severe pain triggering a myocardial infarction or a stroke via hypertension secondary to the pain. The treatment strategy for patients with obstructive pyelonephritis is geared towards immediate renal

219

decompression via ureteral drainage or percutaneous nephrostomy tube placement and initiation of broad-spectrum intravenous antibiotic coverage. After resolution of the acute symptoms, further treatment follows the established guidelines for elective treatment of ureteral stones (Table 4).

Table 4.   Selection criteria for extracorporeal shock wave lithotripsy of ureteral stones

---

Variables determining treatment approach:
   - approach individualized according to expansion space and stone location
   - no standard treatment protocol for all ureteral stones available
   - depending on lithotripter used (X-ray or ultrasound stone localization)
   - depending on endourological experience

SELECTION CRITERIA FOR THE TREATMENT OF URETERAL STONES

Elective treatment of ureteral stones (Table 4) is determined by the stone location, stone size, degree of stone impaction, the anatomy of the upper urinary tract, and the availability of modern technology such as extracorporeal shock wave lithotripsy (ESWL) and ureteroscopy. Assuming that all the new technologies are available to the operator, the strategy for elective treatment of ureteral stones is mostly directed by the stone location and the technical features of the lithotripter available (anesthesia vs anesthesia-free, fluoroscopy vs ultrasound localization). Endourological skills, such as ureteroscopy and percutaneous antegrade access to the ureter, are important for the management of complicated stone disease and ESWL failures. Open surgical procedures are reserved for the concomitant repair of severe anatomical anomalies of the upper urinary tract and for the management of complications (28-33).

A. Stone location

Three different areas in the ureter, namely the proximal ureter above the iliac crest, the mid ureter between iliac crest and pelvic brim, and the lower ureter below the pelvic brim, are distinguished, and different protocols for the management of ureteral stones in each of these locations have to be implemented.

1. STONES IN PROXIMAL URETER

The factors determining the selection of the best treatment strategy for the management of proximal ureteral stones are the existence of a sufficient expansion space near the stone if ESWL is to be utilized, the availability of "anesthesia-free" lithotripters, and the availability of ureteroscopic lithotripsy.

For a patient with a proximal ureteral stone, i.e. above the iliac crest, the preferred treatment in the United States in 1991 is retrograde stone manipulation with the intent to reposition the stone into the renal collecting system followed by ESWL fragmentation under the same anesthesia. This treatment philosophy is based on the use of a first generation fluoroscopy localizing lithotripter which in a one-stage procedure yields the highest success rates, however, at the expense of the need for regional anesthesia and an auxiliary endoscopic procedure with limited invasiveness. Retrograde stone manipulation is successful in >80% of cases, and a greater than 90% stone-free rate is seen after ESWL of the repositioned stone. Whenever retrograde repositioning of the stone into the kidney is not feasible, creation of an artificial expansion chamber using ureteral stents yields stone-free rates of up to 92%. If the stone cannot be successfully manipulated using the above approach, the success with *in situ* ESWL is approximately 50% and these patients therefore are not good candidates for ESWL; instead they are best treated by direct contact lithotripsy with electrohydraulic, Laser, or ultrasonic fragmentation for a success rate of close to 100% in experienced hands (29, 31-33). Operators of the newer "anesthesia-free" lithotripters mostly favor direct *in situ* treatment of stones in the proximal ureter in order to capitalize on the anesthesia-free feature. This is especially true when fluoroscopy localizing lithotripters are used which allow successful localization of the stone in most of the cases. *In situ* treatment without attempted retrograde manipulation can result in a stone-free rate of up to 75%; however, a significant number of patients need multiple treatments and subsequent auxiliary endoscopic procedures which require regional or general anesthesia. Technical difficulties in ultrasonic identification of proximal ureteral stones below the lower margin of the kidney preclude *in situ* ESWL treatment of such patients with the newer lithotripters featuring ultrasound stone localization. To overcome this impasse a number of recently introduced lithotripters are equipped with dual imaging capabilities of ultrasound and fluoroscopy. No larger clinical series using these machines have been published, so that assessment of this approach is not possible at the present time.

2. STONES IN THE MID URETER

Originally called the "stone-cracker's no-mansland", stones located in the mid ureter, i.e. between the iliac crest and the pelvic brim, can now be treated with the newer, fluoroscopy localizing lithotripters. The patient can be positioned prone, so that no bone is interposed between the shock wave source and the targeted stone and shock wave energy is directly delivered top the stone. Stone-free rates of up to 60% can be achieved using this approach (31). Although the anesthesia-free feature makes this approach appealing, the treatment outcome is less than certain due to imaging problems (stone overlying bony pelvis). This approach requires the use of X-ray table version second generation lithotripters, which are not yet widely available. Most urologists still prefer the classic approach of retrograde stone manipulation followed by ESWL, which, for stones in this area, allows successful repositioning into the kidney in approximately 75% and ESWL stone-free rates of approximately 90%. Direct contact ureteroscopic lithotripsy is yet another approach which, in experienced hands, results in success rates of almost 100% at the expense of slightly increased invasiveness (33).

3. STONES IN THE DISTAL URETER

Stones in the distal and prevesical ureter were the first ureteral stones which were approached using the *in situ* ESWL treatment technique with the first generation lithotripters. Despite the difficulty of patient positioning for stone visualization with the fluoroscopy imaging systems, stone-free rates of up to 90% have been reported (29, 30). Alternatively, direct ureteroscopic stone retrieval or ureteroscopic lithotripsy can be employed which has yielded success rates close to 100% with minimal complications in almost all larger series published. Localization of the stone with ultrasound localizing lithotripters is feasible, but technically difficult and time-consuming. Using these lithotripters, the distal ureter can be imaged through a full bladder with the patient in the prone position. In these instances, the stone-free rates are similar to those with fluoroscopy localizing ESWL, i.e. up to 90%.

B. Stone size

Stone size of greater than 8 mm precludes spontaneous stone passage in greater than 90% of cases. Therefore in our experience conservative management using the strategy of watchful waiting is limited to smaller stones. Stones larger than 8 mm with preserved kidney function are scheduled for elective treatment. When the kidney is nonfunctioning on IVP studies, renal function studies are performed and the obstruction is relieved prior to the definite stone treatment.

C. Stone impaction

The degree of impaction of ureteral stones has been shown clinically and experimentally to be an important predictor of the outcome of ESWL when ESWL is employed to treat these stones *in situ* (28). The more a stone is wedged in the reactive edema surrounding it, the lesser are the chances for spontaneous stone passage after ESWL. Unfortunately, there are no accurate imaging studies to correctly assess the degree of stone impaction and therefore no prediction of the outcome of *in situ* ESWL is possible. Even a very recent intravenous pyelogram (IVP) demonstrating contrast passing by the stone does not ensure a successful treatment outcome. Overall, *in situ* ESWL of ureteral stones yields stone-free rates between 50% and 70% in one treatment session. In our health care environment in the United States this is poorly accepted. We therefore rely on retrograde ureteral stone manipulation as a minimally invasive and time-efficient adjunct to ESWL. Retrograde stone manipulation is successful in approximately 80% of all upper and mid ureteral stones. Stones resisting attempts at retrograde manipulation at best have a 50% clearance rate after *in situ* ESWL and therefore should be directly treated with ureteroscopic lithotripsy. The major advantages of ureteroscopy are consistently high success rates of greater than 90% with more than 95% of patients having only one treatment session. This is achieved at the expense of an anesthetic with an overall complication rate of less than 5%. For these reasons the above approach has become the treatment of choice for ureteral stones in the United States. The use of anesthesia-free ESWL appears to offer no advantages in our health system (relatively high costs because of secondary treatment required) as far as the treatment of ureteral stones is concerned.

D. Upper urinary tract anatomy

Anatomical alterations of the ureter precluding retrograde ureteral stone manipulation or spontaneous passage of fragmented stone material may require corrective endourological or open surgical procedures with ESWL being utilized as an auxiliary procedure at best.

SELECTION FOR URETEROSCOPY

Ureteroscopic removal of ureteral stones with or without direct contact fragmentation is the treatment of choice when [1] ESWL is not available, [2] ESWL is not the most appropriate choice, or [3] when ESWL has failed. Review of several larger series reveal average success rates with ureteroscopic ureteral stone removal of 70%, 85% and 95% in the upper, mid, and lower ureter, respectively. However, the higher invasiveness compared to ESWL and the rate of complications of 10%, 5% and 3% respectively have to be considered.

Ureteroscopy, especially for more complex stones which cannot be repositioned or have failed ESWL, requires special endoscopic skills and should be reserved for the more experienced endourologists. Antegrade ureteroscopy utilizing a percutaneous approach is indicated when retrograde access to the stone cannot be gained (stricture, urinary diversion) and when open surgery is not necessary for correction of an anatomical problem.

RESULTS OF EXTRACORPOREAL SHOCK WAVE LITHOTRIPSY

The initial results of the Munich group for the first three years (stone size limited to 2.5 cm) revealed a success rate of 99%. Ninety percent of patients became completely stone-free within a three month period. Only small, spontaneously passable fragments remained in 9.3% of patients. In 0.7% of cases an open surgical or endourological procedure was performed to relieve a persisting ureteral obstruction (6). Evaluation of pre- and post-lithotripsy renal function showed no evidence of any adverse effects of extracorporeal shock wave lithotripsy on renal function as evidenced by nuclear renogram. Over a four year period, it was found that the renal function of those patients treated with extracorporeal shock wave lithotripsy actually improved with time, which is attributable to those cases where obstructing stones had been successfully treated. Comparison of these results with the results from other institutions using the same lithotripter and those achieved with different machines are difficult since there is no commonly accepted nomenclature or stratification system. It would therefore seem reasonable to agree on a nomenclature appreciating stone size, location, anatomy of the urinary tract, and stone composition. At the present time, overall stone-free rates with ESWL of renal stones range from 90% for stones of 1 cm size to approximately 50% for staghorn stones (ESWL monotherapy). The reported annual stone recurrence rates of 4-8% is reassuringly low and compare favourably to those of other treatment modalities. Approximately 25% of residual stones increase in size over a 2 year follow-up period. Long-term observation of the clinical fate of these patients is necessary to decide whether or not the regrowth rate and the associated need for auxiliary procedures are acceptable.

Undoubtedly extracorporeal shockwave lithotripsy has become a most valuable asset to the urologist and greatly benefits urological stone patients. During the short period of time since its advent the management of urinary stone disease has completely changed. Extracorporeal shock wave lithotripsy has almost completely supplanted open surgical and to a lesser extent endourological approaches.

Experience has shown that approximately 70% of patients can benefit from extracorporeal shock wave lithotripsy as monotherapy. More complex stones require auxiliary procedures, namely endourological procedures or at times open surgery. Those 25% to 30% of cases, which require combined endourological or open surgical techniques, are technically demanding and should be reserved for the stone centers where extensive experience with all alternative techniques of urinary stone treatment exists.

REFERENCES

1. Chaussy C, Eisenberger F, Wanner K, Forssmann B, Hepp W: The use of shock waves for the destruction of renal calculi without direct contact. Urological Research, 4: 175, 1976.
2. Eisenberger F, Chaussy C, Wanner K, Forssmann B: Extracorporale Anwendung von hochenergetischen Stosswellen - ein neuer Aspekt in der Behandlung des Harnsteinleidens. Teil 1 Aktuel Urol, 8: 3-15, 1977.
3. Eisenberger F, Schmiedt E, Chaussy C, Wanner K, Forssmann B, Hepp W, Pielsticker K, Brendel W: Beruhrungsfreie Harnsteinzertummerung. Stand der Forschung. Deutsches Arzteblatt, 74: 1-5, 1977.
4. Chaussy C, Eisenberger F, Wanner K: Extracorporale Anwendung von hochenergetischen Stosswellenein neuer Aspekt in der Behandlung des Harnsteinleidens. Aktuel Urol, 9: 95-101, 1978.
5. Chaussy C, Brendel W, Schmiedt E.: Extracorporeally induced destruction of kidney stones by shock waves. Lancet, 12.3: 1265, 1980.
6. Chaussy C, Schmiedt E, Jocham D, Brendel W, Forssmann B, Walther W: First clinical experience with extracorporeally induced destruction of kidney stones by shock waves. J Urol, 417-420, 1981.
7. Fuchs G, Miller K, Rassweiler J, Eisenberger F: Alternatives to open surgery for renal calculi: percutaneous nephrolithotomy and extracorporeal shock wave lithotripsy. In: "Klinische und Experimentelle Urologie" (Ed W. Schilling), Zuckschwerdt, Munchen, 1984.
8. Fuchs G, Miller K, Rassweiler J, Eisenberger F: Extracorporeal shock wave lithotripsy: One-year experience with the Dornier Lithotripter. Eur Urol, 11: 145, 1985.
9. Eisenberger F, Fuchs G, Miller K, Rassweiler J: Extracorporeal shock wave lithotripsy and endourology - an ideal combination for the treatment of kidney stones. World J Urol, 3: 41-47, 1985.
10. Miller K, Fuchs G, Rassweiler J, Eisenberger F: Treatment of ureteral stone disease: the role of ESWL and endourology. World J Urol, 3: 445, 1985.
11. Fuchs G., Chaussy C.: Extracorporeal shockwave lithotripsy: an update. Endourology, 2: 1, 1987.
12. Drach G, Dretler S, Fair W, Finlayson B, Gillenwater J, Griffith D, Lingeman J, Newman D: Report of the United States cooperative study of extracorporeal shock wave lithotripsy. J Urol, 135: 1127, 1986.
13. Chaussy C, Schmiedt E, Jocham D, Fuchs G, Brendel W: Extracorporeal shock wave lithotripsy. (2nd Edition) (Ed C.G. Chausssy), Karger, Munich-Basel, 1986.
14. Lingeman J, Newman D, Mertz J, et al: Extracorporeal shock wave lithotripsy: The Methodist Hospital of Indiana experience. J Urol, 135: 1134, 1986.
15. Riehle R, Fair W, Vaughan D: Extracorporeal shock wave lithotripsy for upper urinary tract calculi - one year experience at a single center. JAMA, 255: 2043-2048, 1986.
16. Fuchs G, Chaussy C: Worldwide experience with, and future concepts of ESWL. In: "Principles of Extracorporeal Shock Wave Lithotripsy" (Eds R Riehle, D Newman) Livingstone, New York, 1987.
17. Chaussy C, Fuchs G: Extracorporeal shock wave lithotripsy (ESWL) for the treatment of urinary stones. In: "Textbook on Adult and Pediatric Urology". (Ed J Gillenwater), Year Book Publishers, 1986.
18. Rassweiler J, Gumpinger R, Miller K, Hoelzermann F, Eisenberger F: Multimodal treatment (extracorporeal shock wave lithotripsy and endourology) of complicated renal stone disease. Eur Urol, 12: 294, 1986.

19. Kahnoski R, Lingeman J, Coury T, Steele R, Mosbaugh P: Combined percutaneous and extracorporeal shock wave lithotripsy for staghorn calculi: an alternative to anatrophic nephrolithotomy. J Urol, 135: 679, 1986.

20. Fuchs G, Chaussy C, Lupu A, Royce P: Treatment of staghorn stones: emerging treatment strategies. Endourol Newsletter, 2, 1987.

21. Fuchs G., Chaussy C.: Extracorporeal shock wave lithotripsy of staghorn stones: reassessment of our treatment strategy, World J Urol, 5: 237-244, 1987.

22. Winfield H, Clayman R, Chaussy C, Weyman P, Fuchs G, Lupu A: Monotherapy of staghorn calculi: Comparative study between percutaneous nephrolithotomy and extracorporeal shock wave lithotripsy. J Urol, 139: 895, 1988.

23. Woodbury P, Lingeman J: Management of staghorn calculi: should there be any controversy? J Urol, 139: 186 A, 1988.

24. Rosciszewski A, Fuchs G, Chaussy C, et al: Staghorn stone treatment with extracorporeal shock wave lithotripsy (ESWL): the fate of residual stones. J Urol, 139: 264 A, 1988.

25. Egghart G, Miller K, Bachor R: Percutaneous nephrolithomy/ESWL versus ureteral stent/ESWL for the treatment of large renal calculi and staghorn stones - A prospective randomized study. J Urol, 139: 282 A, 1988.

26. Assimos D, Boyce W, McCullough D, et al: Role of open stone surgery since ESWL. J Urol, 139: 291 A, 1988.

27. Le Roy J, Segura J, Williams H, Patterson D: Percutaneous renal calculus removal in extracorporeal shockwave lithotripsy practice. J Urol, 138: 703, 1987.

28. Mueller S, Wilbert D, Thueroff J, Alken P: Extracorporeal shock wave lithotripsy of ureteral stones: clinical experience and experimental findings. J Urol, 135: 1083, 1986.

29. Fuchs G, Chaussy C, Riehle R: The Use of ESWL for ureteral stones. In: "Principles of Extracorporeal Shock Wave Lithotripsy" (Eds R Riehle, D Newman), Livingstone, New York, 1987.

30. Chaussy C, Fuchs G: Extracorporeal shockwave lithotripsy of distal ureteral calculi: is it worthwhile? J Endourol, 1: 1, 1987.

31. Jenkins A, Gillenwater J: Extracorporeal shock wave lithotripsy in prone position: treatment of stones in distal ureter or anomalous kidney. J Urol, 139: 911, 1988.

32. Lingeman J, Shirrell L, Newman D, Mosbaugh P, Steele R, Woods J: Management of upper ureteral calculi with extracorporeal shock wave lithotripsy. J Urol, 138: 720, 1987.

33. Fuchs G, Chaussy C, Lupu A: Treatment of ureteral stones: controversies and emerging concepts. J Urol, 139: 188 A, 1988.

34. Newman D, Coury T, Lingeman J, et al: Extracorporeal shockwave lithotripsy experience in children. J Urol, 136: 238, 1986.

35. Royce P, Fuchs G, Lupu A, Chaussy C: The treatment of uric acid stones with extracorporeal shock wave lithotripsy. Brit J Urol, 1987.

36. Psihramis K, Dretler S: Extracorporeal shock wave lithotripsy of calyceal diverticula calculi. J Urol, 138: 707, 1987.

37. Mee S, Thueroff J: Small calyceal calculi: is extracorporeal shock wave lithotripsy justified? J Urol, 139: 908, 1988.

38. Lingeman J, Mosbaugh G, Knapp P, et al: Percutaneous management of calyceal diverticula. J Urol, 139: 187 A, 1988.

39. Stenzl A, Randazzo R, Fuchs G: Extracorporeal shock wave lithotripsy for treatment of symptomatic nephrocalcinosis. J Urol, 139: 264 A, 1988.

40. Stenzl A, Zimmern P, Fuchs G: Technique and results of treatment of uric acid and cystine calculi with Extracorporeal Shock Wave Lithotripsy (ESWL). J Urol, 139: 264 A, 1988.

41. Boyd S, Everett R, Schiff W, Fugelso P: Treatment of unusual Kock pouch urinary calculi with extracorporeal shockwave lithotripsy. J Urol, 139: 805, 1988.

42. Rosciszewski A, Stenzl A, Fuchs G: The treatment of urinary calculi in transplant kidneys with extracorporeal shock wave lithotripsy. J Urol, 139: 261 A, 1988.

43. Fuchs A, Fuchs G: Retrograde intrarenal surgery for calculus disease: new minimally invasive treatment approach. J Endourol, 4: 337, 1990.

CHRONIC RENAL FAILURE

Chapter 10

METABOLIC AND CLINICAL EFFECTS OF LONG-TERM CONSERVATIVE TREATMENT IN PATIENTS WITH CHRONIC RENAL FAILURE

LAMBERTO OLDRIZZI, CARLO RUGIU AND GIUSEPPE MASCHIO

Division of Nephrology, University Hospital, Verona, Italy

INTRODUCTION

A great deal of interest has recently been focused on the effects of conservative treatment on the progression of chronic renal failure (CRF) (1, 2). Both dietary and non-dietary intervention have been suggested for preventing the evolution of chronic renal disease towards uremia. Dietary measures include restriction of protein, phosphate and supplementation with polyunsaturated fatty acids.

Several Countries have initiated multicentre clinical trials to assess whether long-term restriction of the two dietary components most widely believed to accelerate progression (protein and phosphate) may blunt the decline in renal function observed in the vast majority of patients with chronic renal diseases.

The deleterious effect of protein and phosphate on renal structure has been observed both in experimental and clinical studies. In 1928 Newburgh and Curtis (3) observed the occurrence of glomerular sclerosis in rats fed a high protein diet for 12 months. Similar lesions were found in rats with reduced renal mass after development of nephrotoxic serum nephritis (4). These results have eventually been confirmed in different models of experimental renal disease, in which both protein and phosphate appeared to be important factors in the progression of functional deterioration and for the mediation of structural damage, proteinuria and renal failure (5).

LIPID METABOLISM AND PROGRESSION OF CRF

Recently, it has been hypothesized that progressive kidney disease may also be mediated by abnormalities of lipid metabolism (6, 7): an initial glomerular injury may result in proteinuria, loss of lipoprotein lipase activators and lipoproteinuria. The first two abnormalities are eventually followed by increased synthesis and decreased catabolism of lipoproteins. Filtered lipoproteins may neutralize the negative charges of glomerular basement membrane, further increasing its permeability, and, in addition, may accumulate in mesangial cells and stimulate them to proliferate. Some of the filtered lipoproteins may be metabolized by proximal tubular cells, and apoproteins may precipitate in tubular lumens, thus initiating or aggravating tubulointerstitial damage. The combination of such lipid-mediated damage (glomerular and tubulointerstitial) eventually accelerates the progression of chronic renal failure.

Table 1. Clinical studies with low-protein diets (LPD).

Ref #	Statistic Design	pts/cnt	Follow-up (months)	SCr Increase (mg/dl/mo)		Effect on Progression
				LPD	Free Diet	
14	one-group	30/25	48	0.012	0.3	POSITIVE
15	with non	31/31	18	0.5	1.17	POSITIVE
16	equivalent	20/19	11	-0.015	0.064	POSITIVE
17	comparison	12/13	91	0.016	0.075	POSITIVE
18		78/22	44	0.016	0.25	POSITIVE
19		15/15	15	0.062	0.229	POSITIVE
20	self	8/8	12	-0.001	0.022	POSITIVE
21	controlled	39/39	12	0.016	0.067	VARIABLE
22		24/24	12	(*)	(*)	POSITIVE
23		7/7	30	-0.02	0.05	POSITIVE
24	random	118/110	18	0.015	0.062	POSITIVE
24		230/226	24	5.9% (°)	9.2% (°)	POSITIVE

pts = patients; cnt = controls; LPD = low-protein diet
(*) changes in renal function were assessed with GFR
(°) = per cent of patients reaching end-points during follow-up

Clinical support for the lipid hypothesis is available from data obtained in patients with the nephrotic syndrome, in whom the rate of decline in renal function is faster than in non nephrotic patients with glomerulonephritis (8), and is proportional to the amount of proteinuria and hence to the severity of lipid abnormalities (9).

PROTEIN AND PHOSPHATE RESTRICTION IN EXPERIMENTAL RENAL DISEASE

Dietary protein and phosphate restriction reduces renal injury in virtually all models of experimental renal disease (5). Protective effects with this dietary regimen have been observed in the severity of functional and structural damage after subtotal or partial nephrectomy, in the progression of nephrotoxic serum nephritis, in structural damage in adriamycin glomerulonephritis, in the development and extent of tubulointerstitial nephritis, in post-ischemic kidney function, and in glomerular injury in non-clipped kidney of Goldblatt hypertensive rats. These protective effects were obtained either by using protein restriction alone, phosphate restriction alone, or, more often, some combination thereof.

There are several mechanisms that may explain the efficacy of dietary protein and phosphate restriction. They include: [a] the blunting of adaptive increases in glomerular capillary pressures and flows after reduction in renal mass (5); [b] the modulation of glomerular response to several hemodynamic and humoral stimuli (10); [c] the modification of structural changes after reduction of renal mass (5); [d] the reduction of proteinuria by preservation of basement membrane permeability (5); [e] the prevention of secondary hyperparathyroidism, increased phosphaturia per nephron, and renal calcification (11); [f] the modification of humoral and cellular mechanisms of immune response (12); [g] the attenuation of lipid abnormalities (13).

LOW-PROTEIN DIET IN MAN WITH CRF

In man, after some early reports showing positive effects of low-protein diet - with or without aminoacid supplementation - on the course of CRF, in the last 8 years several clinical studies on the protective role of low-protein diets in patients with reduced renal function have been published (14-25) (Table 1). They include one-group design with non-equivalent comparison, self-controlled studies, and randomized clinical trials.

Virtually, all these reports have concluded that dietary protein restriction slowed the progressive course of renal disease, and almost all of them have been criticized for their inadequate statistic design (26). As far as this last point is concerned, it is beyond question that the randomized study is the gold standard, but, at least for studies performed in renal patients, too many variables have to be taken into account: age, sex, underlying renal disease, magnitude of proteinuria and presence of the nephrotic syndrome, duration and severity of hypertension, degree of functional deterioration, rate of progression of CRF and, finally, techniques to measure progression. All these parameters considerably increase the number of patients to be assigned between treated and untreated groups. Additional problems are logistic (clinical trials have to be performed as multicentre trials) and statistic in nature (high rate of drop-outs has to be handled), the most critical one being always the patients' compliance with the diet.

Final conclusions from randomized trials are partly available. The results of the Groningen Study (27) show significant differences between control and treatment in the subgroup of patients with more advanced renal failure. The authors stated that only glomerular disease benefit from low-protein diet; however, this conclusion seems difficult to accept, as in the subgroup the sample size is extremely small. The preliminary results of Northern Italian Trial (28) offer support to the hypothesis that protein restriction is efficacious in slowing down the progression of renal failure mainly in patients with serum creatinine below 5 mg/dl. Major problems with compliance have been observed. Ihle and coworkers (29) showed, in a smaller sample of patients, that low-protein diet blunts the progression of renal disease and they conclude that "...unlimited protein intake is no longer appropriate for most patients with chronic renal failure...". Finally, no data on progression are still available from neither of the three on-going trials (French, MDRD and European Study Group).

LIPID AND CARBOHYDRATE RESTRICTION IN CRF

Only a few studies on the efficacy of dietary lipid manipulation on progression of experimental renal disease have been published. They show protective effects of either reduction of fatty acids or supplementation by polyunsaturated fatty acids (PUFA), especially linoleic acid (30).

In patients with CRF, the simple dietary restriction in carbohydrate and cholesterol (CHOL) may result in a significant reduction in serum triglycerides (TG) and in TG production rate (31).

On the other hand, low-protein diets - supplemented by essential amino acids (EAA) or their ketoanalogues (KAA) - have been shown to reduce serum TG and CHOL even in patients with overt diabetic nephropathy (32), and supplementation by PUFA reduces serum TG and increases the HDL:total CHOL ratio in patients with CRF (33).

The potential mechanisms for these effects are linked (34): [1] to the low CHOL, high polyunsaturated (P) to saturated (S) fatty acid ratio of low-protein diet (higher than 1.4); [2] to a decrease in serum concentrations of both parathyroid hormone and growth hormone, with a consequent enhancement of insulin effect on lipoprotein lipase; [3] to an increase in serum thyroid hormone and testosterone levels which, in turn, potentiate the lipolytic activity and the hepatic production of HDL-CHOL; [4] to a reduction in the serum concentrations of many uremic toxins.

It should be reminded, however, that disappointing results have been reported by some German and Swedish authors (34, 35). Interesting results have been reported in a large population of patients with early CRF of different etiology, all kept on long-term low-protein diet (36). This diet provides 35 Kcal/kg b.w./day, 0.6 g/kg b.w./day of protein and 108 g of lipids, with a low CHOL content (less than 300 mg per day) and a high P:S fatty acid ratio. The long-term administration of the diet induced no change in serum levels of both CHOL and TG; however, when compared to patients on free diet and with similar degree of renal failure, those on low-protein diet had significantly lower serum TG levels and a higher percentage of HDL-CHOL. In addition, a protein restricted diet may be followed by favorable changes in lipid composition of erythrocyte membrane (Table 2).

Table 2.   Lipid composition of erythrocyte membrane in patients with CRF treated with low-protein diet.

Acid composition	LOW-PROTEIN DIET	FREE DIET	NORMAL VALUES
	%	%	%
SF	45.0	45.8 (*)	44.0
PUFA	37.2	35.4 (*)	35.8
Palmitic	27.6	26.9 (*)	26.5
Oleic	17.5	18.4 (*)	18.9
Linoleic	14.1	12.2 (*)	12.6
RATIOS			
SF/PUFA	0.82	0.77 (*)	0.80
Linoleic/Oleic	0.81	0.67 (*)	0.66

SF = saturated fatty acids; PUFA = polyunsaturated fatty acids
(*) $p < 0.01$ vs patients on low-protein diet

Admittedly, however, large prospective studies are needed to assess the effect of dietary manipulation on both the lipid abnormalities and the rate of progression of functional deterioration in patients with CRF.

In CRF, carbohydrate metabolism is affected by the interplay of many hormones. Of all these, the peripheral resistance to the action of insulin plays a preponderant role, secondary hyperparathyroidism, deficiency in 1,25 vitamin D and increased levels of cortisol, growth hormone and glucagon being additional pathogenic factors of the observed carbohydrate intolerance. It has been shown that low-protein diets may correct this metabolic derangement and increase both the metabolic rate and the insulin sensitivity in children with CRF.

The potential mechanisms by which low-protein diets may correct carbohydrate abnormalities in CRF include the prevention or the reversal of secondary hyperparathyroidism, the increase in serum thyroid hormones, and the reduction in serum levels of GH, beta-endorphin and several uremic toxins (37).

ABNORMALITIES OF PROTEIN METABOLISM IN CRF

Several abnormalities of protein metabolism may occur in patients with CRF. They include defective protein synthesis in the liver, increased gluconeogenesis, abnormalities of aminoacid metabolism, resistance to insulin-mediated aminoacid uptake in skeletal muscle, impaired polyamine formation, low-protein turnover rate in children, and low muscle RNA:DNA and Alkali-Soluble Proteins (ASP):DNA ratios (38, 39).

Besides the direct effects of reduced dietary protein intake and protein metabolism, a number of consequences on other metabolic and/or clinical parameters have been reported (40).

Low-protein diet has been shown to reduce proteinuria in patients with early to moderate CRF, and to decrease fractional clearances of albumin, IgG and neutral dextrans in those with moderate CRF. Similarly, more severe protein restriction resulted in a significant reduction in proteinuria and in fractional albumin clearance in patients with advanced CRF. The beneficial effect of low-protein diets may be linked to the influence of protein intake on plasma renin activity. It has been shown that low-protein diets may blunt the activity of the renin-angiotensin system. In addition, they decrease erythropoietin synthesis and haematocrit value and hence they may improve, to some extent, a previously abnormal blood rheology. Furthermore, it has been suggested that low-protein diets improve the size-selectivity defect in glomerular permselectivity.

Additional effects of these diets have been reported on serum oxalic acid and endogenous glucocorticoid production. Severe dietary protein restriction reduces serum oxalic acid levels, probably by lowering the intake of its metabolic precursor and by inhibiting its intestinal absorption due to high calcium carbonate content of the diet (41). The same diet may suppress endogenous glucocorticoid production, apparently an important factor in mediating progression of renal failure (42).

GUIDELINES FOR DIETARY TREATMENT OF CRF

Two preliminary considerations have to be kept in mind to optimize the dietary treatment and thus the patients' compliance: the characteristics of the diet and the patient's attitude toward the diet, depending, in turn, on his psychosocial profile.

The general guidelines for the dietary treatment of CRF must satisfy the following policies: [a] to reduce the nitrogen intake; [b] to cover essential aminoacids requirements; [c] to give a sufficient energy intake and [d] to be palatable.

In line with these statements, nephrologists face three possibilities: the unsupplemented low nitrogen diet with proteins of high biologic value, the EAA-supplemented diets and KAA supplemented diets.

The unsupplemented low-protein diet implies some characteristics (palatability, simplicity, cheapness, long-term safety) which make it easy to follow, and therefore improves compliance. In this sense, its use appears suitable for early CRF patients.

The supplemented (EAA or KAA) low-protein diets have been shown to be quite useful in more advanced stages of CRF. Many positive effects are due to their use: [1] a blunted progression rate of CRF; [2] a significant improvement in metabolic state as well as in uremic neuropathy; [3] a nitrogen sparing effect; [4] a decrease in proteinuria and in serum parathyroid hormone levels; [5] a well being of patients.

A number of negative aspects, however, must be considered: high cost, monotony, risk of malnutrition, need of careful dietary education, decreasing family support with time. A careful balance between the pros and cons suggests that their use would be limited in patients with far advanced stages of CRF (serum creatinine higher than 5 mg/dl) (43).

Therefore, the potential use of unsupplemented low-protein diet, when compared with EAA-KAA supplemented diets, is suitable for a higher percentage of renal patients. Thus, it is useful to review some metabolic and nutritional characteristics of this diet.

It provides 35 Kcal/kg b.w./day, 0.6 g/kg b.w./day of protein, 615 mg/day of phosphate, 110 g/day of lipids and 320 g/day of carbohydrates. As to the trace elements and vitamins, the respective requirements are satisfied; thus, even if some authors suggest that supplementation of water-soluble vitamins is necessary when low-protein diets are used (44), no sign of vitamin abnormalities are observed in patients treated with this diet.

With respect to proteins, 75% are of high biologic value. A quite peculiar aspect of this diet is represented by the partition of proteins: 64% are from vegetable and 46% from animal origin. The plant/animal proteins ratio is 1.77, a value much higher than that recorded in the current eating habits of European Countries (usually less than 1.0) (45). Such a typical protein profile allows a low CHOL and saturated fatty acids intake. In addition, vegetable proteins might play a more effective protective role on the surviving nephrons, as already clinically and experimentally described (46), even if in nutritional field they have a score lower than animal proteins.

The energy intake of a low-protein diet must aim at well established nutritional guidelines (47). Patients with CRF ingesting 0.55 to 0.60 g/kg b.w./day of protein may have a neutral nitrogen balance and a reduced net urea generation only when the energy intake is higher than 30 Kcal/kg b.w./day. The caloric support is given mainly by lipids (40%) and by carbohydrates (53%).

This partition of energy supplies might arise some nutritional controversy due to the fact that the lipid and carbohydrates fractions are higher than that pointed out in nutritional standards. As to lipids, however, in the unsupplemented low-protein diet they are mostly from non-animal origin, the P:S fatty acids ratio is higher than 1.0 and the CHOL intake is small (less than 300 mg per day). Moreover, there is so far no clinical evidence that abnormalities of lipid metabolism (mainly of lipoproteins catabolism) in patients with CRF limit the usefulness of fat as energy source. In fact, apolipoprotein pattern and lipolytic activities are not influenced by low-protein diets in patients with CRF. On the contrary, low-protein diet improves the erythrocyte membrane lipid composition (36).

Carbohydrates must be provided as complex carbohydrates. The most likely metabolic effect of a high percentage of such dietary components might be a detrimental effect on TG levels. But, in our (47) as well as in other authors'(13) experience, the mean TG level was not increasing over time in patients on low-protein diet. It has been hypothesized that a low-nitrogen intake, by an improvement in the uremic metabolic state, makes the patient able to deal successfully with the increased intake of lipids and carbohydrates with no further aggravation of lipoproteins disturbances (13).

At variance with some more restricted low-protein diets, the essential aminoacid requirements are satisfied by the unsupplemented diet that provides nearly 32 g/day of high biologic value proteins. A negative aspect, on the other hand, might be the rather high amount of sulfur-containing aminoacids, especially because of their acidotic effect (47) (Table 3).

The total daily amount of protein (0.6 g/kg b.w./day) is adequate to nutritional requirements (47). Many studies clearly demonstrated that the daily protein requirement in patients with CRF is close to 0.6 g/kg b.w. per day. Since 1958 Herndorn showed that to maintain a patient in nitrogen balance, near to 0.5 g/kg b.w./day of protein were required, with a high:low quality protein ratio as high as 70%. These results were repeatedly confirmed in the following years. More recently, in a self-controlled study, it has been shown that patients with early CRF switched from a 0.6 g/kg b.w./day to a 0.8-0.9 g/kg

236

b.w./day of protein intake and under a strict metabolic and dietary control, experienced over a 9-month period a decrease in glomerular filtration rate and an increase in daily proteinuria.

Table 3. Aminoacid contents of unsupplemented low-protein diet.

AMINOACID	LOW-PROTEIN DIET (mg/day)	RECOMMENDED DAILY ALLOWANCES (mg/day)
VALINE	1800	1200
LEUCINE	2300	1500
ISOLEUCINE	1450	1100
METHIONINE and CYSTINE	850	650
PHENYLALANINE and TYROSINE	2500	1250
TRYPTOPHAN	250	200
THREONINE	1100	750
LYSINE	2000	1500
HISTIDINE	850	800

A diet providing less than 0.6 g/kg b.w./day of protein and the same energy supply as the unsupplemented low-protein diet, probably implies problems concerning the possibility of a negative nitrogen balance, and requires, to be nutritionally adequate, some supplement with non-natural foods, the latter point being probably linked with a progressively worsening compliance (47). Such a possibility seems, to some extent, supported by various authors (27, 48): patients advised to have a 0.4-0.5 g/kg b.w./day protein intake, showed a daily protein intake (estimated on the basis of the daily urinary urea excretion) averaging 0.6 g/kg b.w.

PATIENT'S COMPLIANCE

It seems clear, with this premise, that the most critical point in dietary treatment is the patient's compliance with the diet.

This is for the nephrologist an intriguing as well as a puzzling aspect, mostly because the estimation of patients' dietary intakes is not reliable and because factors improving compliance vary in different Countries (43). Thus, the satisfactory results we observe in the daily practice are probably improved by the similarity between Italian dietary habits (the so-called Mediterranean diet) and the low-protein diet scheme. With respect to the assessment of dietary compliance, the recent recommendations, based mostly on a feasibility criterion, indicate that the best estimate of the true protein consumption is given by the mean of two consecutive measurements of daily urinary urea excretion (49).

Table 4. Methods to assess nutritional status in CRF patients

1. PHYSICAL EXAMINATION
2. ASSESSMENT OF DIETARY INTAKES
     . dietetic interviews
     . dietetic diaries
3. BIOCHEMISTRY
     . serum/urine urea and creatinine
     . urinary 3-methylhistidine
     . serum visceral proteins (albumin, transferrin, retinol binding protein ...)
     . plasma aminoacids
     . nitrogen balance
4. ANTHROPOMETRY
     . body weight and height
     . skinfold thickness
     . mid-arm circumferences
5. BODY COMPOSITION
     . body fat and cell mass
     . total body water
     . extracellular water
     . intracellular water
     . muscle biopsy
     . bone biopsy
6. IMMUNOLOGY
     . lymphocyte count
     . antibody production
     . skin tests

MALNUTRITION

One of the most important characteristic of dietary treatment of chronic renal failure is represented by its safety (50), in other words by the proof that low-protein diet does not provoke malnutrition in renal patients. Actually, the nutritional adequacy of the long-term dietary therapies has so far scarcely assessed. Historically, malnutrition has been shown to be very common as in uremic patients as in those receiving hemodialysis or peritoneal dialysis.

Table 5. Nutritional status of patients on long-term dietary protein restriction. Anthropometric and biochemical evaluation after 5 and 10 years of low-protein diet. The study was performed in 12 patients.

ANTHROPOMETRY	5 year	10 year	
Body mass index	24.0	23.0	
Skinfold thickness triceps (mm)	11.6	9.0	
Arm muscle circumference (mm)	244	249	
Arm muscle area (mm²)	4.75	4.93	

VISCERAL PROTEINS	5 year	10 year	lower normal values
Albumin (mg/dl)	4.59	3.34	3.50
Transferrin (mg/dl)	243	145	205
C3 (mg/dl)	75	46	55
C3 activator (mg/dl)	14	11	10

The causes of such a malnutrition are mainly metabolic, due to the interactions of nitrogen wastes and toxins with hormonal and/or metabolic pathways.

A number of methods have been proposed to evaluate the nutritional status of chronic patients (50) (Table 4). Some of them have been evaluated in a group of patients with CRF on long-term dietary protein restriction (unsupplemented diet), after a 5- and 10-year follow-up (39).

The results obtained by anthropometric measurements and biochemical determinations (Table 5) and direct skeletal muscle analysis (Table 6), show that the nutritional state of the patients is normal at 5-year evaluation and tended to be only slightly worse than normal controls after a long-lasting treatment (10 years). Anthropometric indices were not significantly decreased in treated patients and notably they did not have any change in the very long-term evaluation. On the contrary, serum levels of proteins of hepatic origin were decreased after a 10-year follow-up, thus indicating that a 0.6/kg b.w./day of protein intake implies some influence on the liver production of protein.

Muscle protein synthesis (RNA:DNA ratio) and content (ASP:DNA ratio) were normal in the two assessments. Muscle protein degradation (evaluated as cathepsin D activity) was decreased in patients on dietary treatment at the 10-year check. The global figure of muscle data suggest that the decreased protein catabolism, in the presence of a normal synthesis and content, may represent an adaptive mechanism of protein sparing. The above cited abnormalities in visceral protein metabolism probably derives from an energy intake lower than that prescribed, thus indicating that a careful monitoring of nutritional and metabolic state of renal patients on long-term dietary therapy must be scheduled. At the same time, it is necessary, in order to have the best compliance, to repeatedly instruct the patients on the diet. All these clinical necessities make it imperative to integrate the work of the nephrologist, nutritionist, dietitian and psychologist.

Table 6. Nutritional status of patients on long-term dietary protein restriction. Muscle composition after 5 and 10 years of low-protein diet. The study was performed in 12 patients.

	5 year	10 year	normal values
DNA mg/100 g wet wt	39.0	37.0	34.0
RNA mg/100 g wet wt	83.0	71.0	77.0
ASP g/100 g wet wt	19.0	17.0	18.0
RNA:DNA mg/mg	2.0	2.0	2.3
ASP:DNA mg/mg	472	499	554
Cathepsin D activity mU/100 g wet wt	80	68	94

wt: = weight

REFERENCES

1.   Oldrizzi L, Maschio G, Rugiu C, Campese VM: The progressive nature of renal disease: myths and facts. Contrib Nephrol, Karger, Basel, 1989, 75.
2.   Proceedings of 3rd Verona Seminar on Nephrology: Emerging risk factors for the progression of renal disease. Am J Kidney Dis, 17, suppl 1, 1991.
3.   Newburgh LH, Curtis AC: Production of renal injury in the white rat by the protein of the diet. Dependance of the injury on the duration of feeding, and on the amount and kind of protein. Arch Int Med, 42: 801-821, 1928.
4.   Farr LE, Smadel JE: The effect of dietary protein on the course of nephrotoxic nephritis in the rat. J Exp Med, 70: 615-627, 1939.
5.   Diamond JR: Effects of dietary interventions on glomerular pathophysiology. Am J Physiol, 258: F1-F8, 1990.
6.   Keane WF, Kasiske BL, O'Donnel MP: Lipids and progressive glomerulosclerosis: a model analogous to atherosclerosis. Am J Nephrol, 8: 261-271, 1988.
7.   Moorhead JF, Wheeler DC, Varghese Z: Glomerular structures and lipids in progressive renal disease. Am J Med, 87: 12N-20N, 1989.
8.   Maschio G, Oldrizzi L, Rugiu C: Factors affecting progression of renal failure in patients on long-term dietary protein restriction. Kidney Int, 32, suppl 22: S49-S52, 1987.
9.   Williams PS, Fass G, Bone JM: Renal pathology and proteinuria in untreated mild/moderate chronic renal failure. Q J Med 252: 343-354, 1988.
10.   Murray BM, Brown GP: Effect of protein intake on the autoregulation of renal blood flow. Am J Physiol, 258: F168-F174, 1990.

11. Hostetter TH: Dietary protein restriction in control of progressive renal failure. In: "Nephrology, Proceedings of the Xth International Congress of Nephrology", Bailliere Tindall Publish, London, 1988, pp 1195-1205.

12. Agus D, Mann R, Cohn D, Michaud L, Kelly C, Clayman M, Neilson G: Inhibitory role of dietary protein restriction on the development and expression of immune-mediated antitubular basement membrane-induced tubulointerstitial nephritis in rats. J Clin Invest, 76: 930-936, 1985.

13. Attman PO, Alaupovic P: The role of lipid metabolism in dietary treatment of chronic renal failure. Contrib Nephrol, Karger, Basel, 81: 35-41, 1990.

14. Maschio G, Oldrizzi L, Tessitore N: Effects of dietary protein and phosphorus restriction on the progression of early renal failure. Kidney Int, 22: 371-376, 1982.

15. Bennet SE, Russel GI, Walls J: Low-protein diets in uraemia. Br Med J, 287: 1344-1345, 1983.

16. Barsotti G, Morelli E, Giannoni A: Restricted phosphorus and nitrogen intake to slow the progression of chronic renal failure. A controlled trial. Kidney Int, 24 (Suppl 16): S278-S284, 1983.

17. Giordano C: Early dietary protein restriction protects the failing kidney. Kidney Int, 17 (Suppl 17): S56-S57, 1985.

18. Oldrizzi L, Rugiu C, Valvo E: Progression of renal failure in patients with renal disease of diverse etiology on protein restricted diet. Kidney Int, 27: 553-557, 1985.

19. Acchiardo SR, Moore LW, Cockrell S: Does low-protein diet halt the progression of renal insufficiency?. Clin Nephrol, 25: 289-294, 1986.

20. Evanoff GV, Thompson CS, Braun J: The effect of dietary protein restriction on the progression of diabetic nephropathy. Arch Int Med, 147: 492-495, 1987.

21. El Nahas AM, Master-Thomas A, Brady SA: Selective effect of low-protein diets in chronic renal diseases. Br Med J, 289: 1337-1341, 1984.

22. Schaap GH, Bilo HJG, Alferink THR: The effect of a high protein intake on renal function in patients with chronic renal insufficiency. Nephron, 47: 1-6, 1987.

23. Oldrizzi L, Rugiu C, Maschio G: Different protein diets in renal failure: a self-controlled study. Am J Nephrol, 9: 184-189, 1989.

24. Rosman JB, Mejir S, Slujiter WJ: Prospective randomised trial of early dietary protein restriction in chronic renal failure. Lancet, II: 1291-1296, 1984.

25. Locatelli F, Alberti D, Gentile MG: Effects of two different protein prescriptions on progression of chronic renal failure. Cooperative Study. Proc Xth Internat Congress of Nephrology, London, 1987, A20.

26. Walser M: Progression of chronic renal failure in man. Kidney Int, 37: 1195-1210, 1990.

27. Rosman JB, Longer K, Brandl M, Piers-Becht TPM, van Derhem GK, ter Wee P, Donker AJM: Protein restricted diets in chronic renal failure: a four years follow up shows limited indications. Kidney Int, 3 (Suppl 27): S96-S102, 1989.

28. Locatelli F: Controlled study of protein restricted diet in chronic renal failure. Contrib Nephrol, Karger, Basel, 75: 141-146, 1989.

29. Ihle BU, Becker GJ, Whitworth JA, Charlwood RA, Kincaid-Smith PS: The effect of protein restriction on the progression of renal insufficiency. N Engl J Med, 321: 1773-1777, 1989.

30. Golper TA: Therapy for uremic hyperlipidemia. Nephron, 35: 217-225, 1984.

31. Sanfelippo ML, Swenson RS, Reaven GM: Reduction of plasma triglycerides by diet in subjects with chronic renal failure. Kidney Int, 11: 54-61, 1977.

32. Barsotti G, Navalesi R, Giampietro O, Ciardella F, Morelli E, Cupisti A, Mantovanelli S: Effects of a vegetarian, supplemented diet on renal function, proteinuria, glucose metabolism in patients with overt diabetic nephropathy and renal insufficiency. Contrib Nephrol, Karger, Basel, 65: 87-94, 1988.

33. Tsukamoto Y, Wakabayashi Y Okubo M, Marumo F: Abnormal lipid profiles at various stages of uremia. Nephrol Dial Transplant, 4: S142-S145, 1988.

34. Ciardella F: Effects of nutritional treatment on hormonal and metabolic derangements on the uremic syndrome. In: "Nutritional treatment of chronic renal failure" (Ed S Giovannetti), Kluwer Academic Publish, Boston, 1989, pp 241-254.

35. Schafer B, Kluthe R: Fettstoffwechselstonungen bei chronischen niereninsuffizienz unter konservative behandlung. Med Klin, 69: 577-581, 1974.

36. Maschio G, Oldrizzi L, Rugiu C, Loschiavo C: Serum lipids in patients with chronic renal failure on long-term, protein restricted diets. Am J Med , 87: 51N-54N, 1989.

37. Ferrarini E, DeFronzo RA: Abnormalities of carbohydrate metabolism. In: "Nutritional treatment of chronic renal failure" (Ed S Giovannetti), Kluwer Academic Publish, Boston, 1989, pp 61-72.

38. Tizianello A, Deferrari G, Garibotto G, Robaudo C, Saffiotti S, Pontremoli R : Aminoacid imbalance in patients with chronic renal failure. Contrib Nephrol, Karger, Basel, 75: 185-193, 1989.
39. Toigo G, Oldrizzi L, Situlin R, Tamaro G, Faccini L, Russo M, Campanacci L, Rugiu C, Maschio G, Guarnieri GF: Nutritional and metabolic effects of ten years of protein restricted diet in patients with early renal failure. Contrib Nephrol, Karger, Basel, 75: 194-202, 1989.
40. Maschio G, Oldrizzi L, Rugiu C: Is there a "point of no return" in progressive renal disease?. J Amer Soc Nephrol, 1991 (in press).
41. Barsotti G, Cristofano C, Morelli E, Meola M, Lupetti S, Giovannetti S: Serum oxalic acid in uremia. Effect of a low-protein diet supplemented with essential aminoacids and ketoanalogues. Nephron, 38: 54-56, 1984.
42. Walser M: Weighted least square regression analysis of factors contributing to progression of chronic renal failure. Contrib Nephrol, Karger, Basel, 75: 127-133, 1989.
43. Oldrizzi L, Rugiu C, De Biase V, Maschio G: Factors influencing dietary compliance in patients with chronic renal failure on unsupplemented low-protein diet. Contrib Nephrol, Karger, Basel, 81: 9-15, 1990.
44. Gentile MG, Manna GM, D'Amico G, Testolin G, Porrini M, Simonetti P: Vitamin nutrition in patients with chronic renal failure and dietary manipulation. Contrib Nephrol, Karger, Basel, 65: 43-50, 1988.
45. Strauch M, Lasserre JJ, Jerabek A, Gretz N: The normal food intake. Contrib Nephrol, Karger, Basel, 72: 1-10, 1989.
46. Wiseman MJ, Hunt R, Goodwin A, Gross JL, Keen H, Viberti GC: Dietary composition and renal function in healthy subjects. Nephron, 46: 37-42, 1988.
47. Oldrizzi L, Rugiu C, De Biase V, Maschio G: Which diet and when to start it, in patients with chronic renal disease. In: "Nephrology- Proceedings XIth International Congress of Nephrology", Springer Verlag, Tokyo, 1991 (in press).
48. Bergström J, Alvestrand A, Bucht H, Gutierrez A: Stockholm clinical study on progression of chronic renal failure. An interim report. Kidney Int, 36 (Suppl 27): S110-S114, 1989.
49. Coles GA, Meadows JH, Bright C, Tomlinson K: The estimation of dietary protein intake in chronic renal failure. Nephrol Dial Transplant, 4: 877-882, 1989.
50. Guarnieri GF, Toigo G, Situlin R, Tamaro G, Giuliani V: The assessment of nutritional state. In: "Nutritional treatment of chronic renal failure" (Ed S Giovannetti), Kluwer Academic Publish, Boston, 1989, pp 133-142.

DIALYSIS

Chapter 11

TREATMENT OF SECONDARY HYPERPARATHYROIDISM BY INTRAVENOUS CALCITRIOL

FRANCISCO LLACH

Veterans Affairs Medical Center, West Los Angeles, UCLA School of Medicine, Wilshire & Sawtelle Blvds,.Los Angeles, CA 90073, USA

INTRODUCTION

Secondary hyperparathyroidism resulting in osteitis fibrosa is the most common bone abnormality observed in dialysis patients. Most recent data strongly suggest that a deficit of calcitriol is an important factor in the high parathyroid hormone (PTH) levels of these patients (1, 2). Thus, it is not surprising that the administration of calcitriol orally (3, 4) has resulted in the amelioration or even dramatic improvement of secondary hyperparathyroidism. What makes the use of intravenous calcitriol an attractive modality of therapy is the recent observation that calcitriol *per se*, in the absence of hypercalcemia inhibit both synthesis and secretion of PTH (5, 6). In the present chapter we will briefly review the physiological action of calcitriol in dialysis patients in regard to divalent ion metabolism, then we will discuss new data on calcitriol and PTH interaction and finally, the available clinical data on the intravenous use of calcitriol will be reviewed.

EFFECTS OF CALCITRIOL IN END STAGE RENAL FAILURE

There are several important effects of calcitriol in the uremic patient. It is these important biological effects what makes the use of calcitriol essential in the control of secondary hyperparathyroidism. First, it is well known that intestinal absorption of calcium is primarily dependent on calcitriol (7). Thus, in several studies the administration of calcitriol to patients with renal insufficiency always result in a marked increase of the low gut absorption of calcium (8). Likewise, intestinal absorption of phosphate also augments after calcitriol therapy (9). However, the magnitude of this increment is lower than that observed with calcium. A third major effect of calcitriol is to increase serum calcium from the hypocalcemic range to normo- or hypercalcemic range. Although this increment may be due to a multifactorial action of calcitriol, by far the increase in intestinal absorption of calcium is the major factor. Of interest is the fact that the rise in serum calcium may not occur for weeks, even months after commencement of calcitriol therapy (10), even though intestinal calcium absorption may be increased and calcium balances are positive. This may reflect active bone mineralization and marked movement of calcium from the extracellular to the intracellular space.

For years it has been known that calcitriol administration is followed by a decrease in PTH levels. However, until recently, this inhibitory effect of calcitriol on PTH was thought to be secondary to the ensuing hypercalcemia. As we will discuss shortly, a direct inhibitory effect of this sterol on PTH secretion may be its most important biological effect in the uremic patient.

Finally, various studies using both oral and intravenous calcitriol have shown marked improvement in the osteitis fibrosa observed in the bone histology of dialysis patients. However, it should be remembered that in a substantial number of patients, bone histology does not always return to normal, clearly indicating the presence of factors other that calcitriol in the pathogenesis of secondary hyperparathyroidism.

VITAMIN D AND PTH INTERACTIONS

Historically, an increase of plasma calcium following calcitriol was thought to be the only mechanism influencing PTH secretion and improving the secondary hyperparathyroidism observed in dialysis patients. However, recent studies have shown calcitriol to decrease PTH gene transcription in the rat (11) and in primary cultures of parathyroid gland cells (11, 12). In the past, it had been assumed that the decrease in PTH secretion observed in dialysis patients treated with Vitamin D was the result of the ensuing hypercalcemia. New studies in dialysis patients demonstrate a direct inhibitory effect of calcitriol on PTH secretion.

Very recent studies have evaluated the regulation of parathyroid cell gene expression in experimental uremia (13). The effect of calcitriol on PTHmRNA in uremic rats in doses as low as 25 mmol/100 g body weight decreases significantly with no greater effect at 100 pmol/100 g, unlike in normal rats. Neither hypo- or hypercalcemia seemed to change PTHmRNA. The explanation for this lack of response is unclear, but it is likely that the prevailing levels of calcitriol may determine the response of the parathyroid gland to changes in Ca concentration.

Silver et al (5) recently demonstrated a suppressive effect of calcitriol on cytoplasmic mRNA coding for preproparathyroid hormone in isolated parathyroid cells; they have recently shown *in vivo* in the rat that calcitriol decreases PTH gene transcription by more than 90% after a single injection of 100 pmol (11). Similar results have been observed *in vitro* in primary cultures of parathyroid cells (6).

Slatopolsky et al (14) compared the effects of oral and intravenous administration calcitriol on the circulating plasma levels of calcitriol as well as on PTH secretion. They observed that oral administration of calcitriol in doses adequate to maintain serum calcium in the upper limits of normal did not alter PTH levels, whereas a marked suppression (70.1±3.2%) of PTH levels was observed in all 20 patients receiving intravenous calcitriol. The studies by these authors suggest that a 20.1±5.2% decrease in PTH resulted with administration of i.v. calcitriol without significant changes in serum calcium. However, by the second month of therapy, hypercalcemia developed as PTH secretion decreased. Thus, the possibility that hypercalcemia *per se* may also have been a factor in the PTH suppression could not be ruled out.

Delmez et al (15) evaluated the inhibitory effect of intravenous calcitriol on PTH synthesis in uremic patients undergoing maneuvers designed to avoid changes in serum calcium concentration. In addition, the response of the parathyroid gland in patients undergoing hypercalcemic suppression and hypocalcemic stimulation of PTH before and after two weeks of intravenous calcitriol was evaluated. In patients undergoing hypercalcemic suppression, PTH values fell from 376±66 to 290±50 pg/ml after calcitriol administration. During hypercalcemic suppression, the set point of Ca for PTH secretion fell from 5.25±0.14 to 5.06±0.15 mg/dl after calcitriol. A similar decline in PTH levels using intravenous, administration of calcitriol was noted in those patients undergoing hypocalcemic stimulation of PTH. The authors concluded that intravenous calcitriol directly suppresses PTH secretion in the uremic patient, and this suppression in part was due to increased sensitivity of the gland to ambient plasma calcium levels.

Recently, we have evaluated the direct inhibitory effect of calcitriol on parathyroid function in dialysis patients with secondary hyperparathyroidism (16). Following a baseline evaluation of parathyroid function, we administered 2 mcg of calcitriol intravenously after dialysis three times weekly for 10 weeks. Parathyroid function was assessed by inducing hypo- and hypercalcemia using a low and a high Ca dialysate during two separate dialysis performed a week apart. In order to avoid hypercalcemia during calcitriol administration, the dialysate calcium concentration was reduced to 2.5 mEq/l.

Parathyroid hormone values after dialysis induced by hypo- and hypercalcemia were plotted against serum ionized calcium for each patient, and the sigmoidal relationship

247

between PTH and calcium was evaluated. A sigmoidal relationship was established for each patient and the true set point of calcium (i.e. the level of serum calcium which induces a 50% inhibition of maximal PTH stimulation) was determined. The basal PTH levels fell from 902±126 pg/ml to 466±152 pg/ml (P<0.01) after 10 weeks of calcitriol therapy. This occurred in the absence of any significant changes in serum calcium concentration. The serum ionized calcium/PTH sigmoidal curve shifted to the left and downward after calcitriol therapy. Thus, the maximum PTH response during hypocalcemia decreased after calcitriol therapy from 1661±485 pg/ml to 1031±280 pg/ml (P<0.05).

The slope of the sigmoidal curve changed from -2125±487 to -1563±385 (P<0.05). The set point of ionized calcium (4.6±0.11 at baseline vs 4.4±0.07 mg/dl at ten weeks) did not change significantly with calcitriol therapy. However, if one patient with severe hyperphosphatemia was excluded from the study, there was a statistically significant change in the set point of calcium after calcitriol therapy (Figure 1). In summary, 10 weeks of intravenous calcitriol therapy decreased PTH secretion across a wide range of serum ionized calcium concentrations, shifting the ionized calcium/PTH sigmoidal curve toward normal (left and downward). Most likely, the set point of calcium also changed. There were no significant changes in basal serum calcium concentration throughout the study. These results clearly demonstrate a direct, inhibitive effect of intravenous calcitriol on parathyroid function in dialysis patients with secondary hyperparathyroidism.

CLINICAL EFFECTS OF INTRAVENOUS CALCITRIOL

Preliminary data from Norris et al (17) demonstrated the beneficial effect of intravenous calcitriol in 10 patients with overt secondary hyperparathyroidism. These investigators administered 1-5 mcg calcitriol intravenously to the patients three times per week following each dialysis for 13 months. They observed a decrease in PTH levels of 42±4%, an increase in serum calcium from 10.1 to 11.2±.1 mg/dl and a 62±4% decrease in serum alkaline phosphatase.

Andress et al (18) showed the beneficial effect of intravenous calcitriol on the bone lesion of secondary hyperparathyroidism. These authors evaluated 12 hemodialysis patients with significant osteitis fibrosa who were refractory to conventional oral calcitriol therapy. They received 1-2.5 mcg of calcitriol intravenously thee times a week. After one year of therapy, an increase in serum ionized calcium was observed from 2.5 to 2.6 mmol/l and a decrease in PTH from 172±34 to 69±16 pg/ml. Most importantly, there was a significant improvement in bone histology after one year of calcitriol therapy.

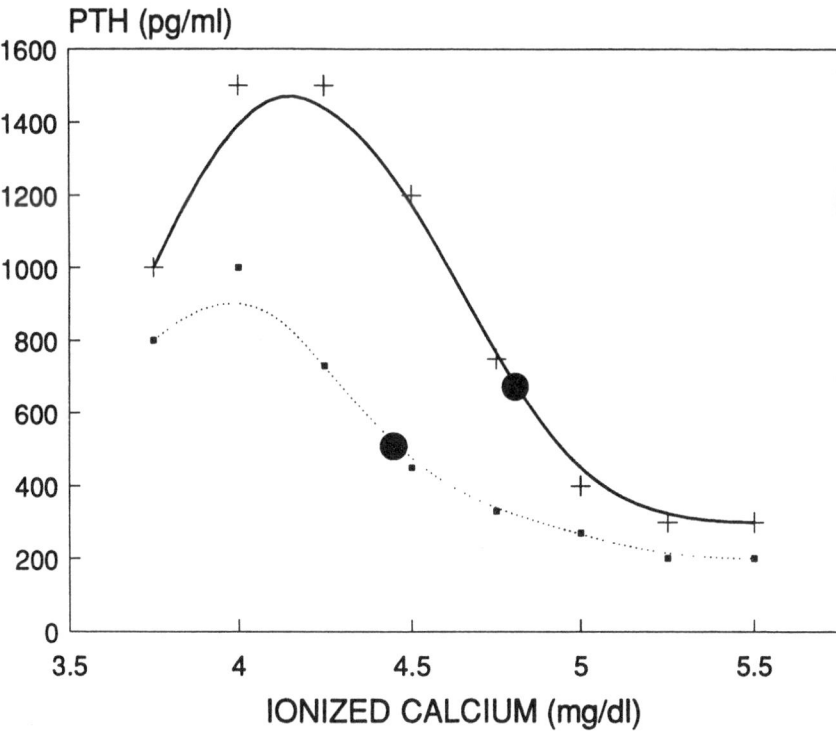

Figure 1. The sigmoidal serum ionized calcium-PTH curve before (solid line) and after (dotted line) ten weeks of intravenous calcitriol therapy is shown. The set point is represented by a solid circle before and after calcitriol.

Hamdy et al (19) evaluated the effect of intravenous calcitriol in four uremic patients with persistent hypercalcemia and marked secondary hyperparathyroidism. These patients had been shown to be intolerant to oral administration of calcitriol. After each dialysis, calcitriol was administered intravenously in doses of 0.5-2.5 mcg for 2 months. Calcitriol therapy continued for 7 and 8 months respectively, in 2 of the 4 patients. After 2 weeks of therapy, a significant decrease in serum calcium was observed which was maintained throughout treatment as i.v. calcitriol dosage was increased. This was associated with a decrease in serum of PTH. During the long-term administration of calcitriol, serum calcium values increased but lower concentrations of PTH were maintained. The authors concluded that the increment in serum calcium was not a prerequisite for the suppression of PTH secretion by calcitriol and that the presence of hypercalcemia does not preclude the use of intravenous calcitriol.

Similar observations have been made of the effect of intravenous 1-alphahydroxy-D_3 [$1\alpha(OH)D_3$] on secondary hyperparathyroidism in chronic uremic patients undergoing maintenance dialysis. Brandi et al (20) evaluated the effect of this sterol on PTH levels in 21 patients on chronic hemodialysis. The patients were treated for 3 months with increasing dose of $1\alpha(OH)D_3$ while serum calcium was carefully controlled. The sterol was given intravenously at doses of up to 4 mcg three times a week, and blood samples were obtained weekly. After 3 months, intact PTH levels were reduced by an average of $67\pm6\%$, serum calcium was kept within normal levels but there was a net increase from 1.17 to 1.30 mmol/l. The authors concluded that although high normal levels of Ca may have influenced PTH secretion, an effect of the alpha sterol, independent of serum calcium concentration, was also observed. This effect, in their opinion, may be mediated by calcitriol as it is assumed that $1\alpha(OH)D_3$ is converted in the liver into calcitriol by the enzyme 25-hydroxylase. Another possibility is that the parathyroid gland may possess receptors for $1\alpha(OH)D_3$ with an effect similar to that of $1,25(OH)_2D_3$ receptors.

In summary, although the beneficial effect of intravenous calcitriol is apparent, it is difficult at present to reach any conclusion with regard to its therapeutic role in dialysis patients. Before final recommendations are possible, certain issues have to be elucidated, such as the net effect of higher plasma calcitriol levels observed with oral calcitriol therapy as compared to intravenous therapy, and the effect of a given plasma level of calcitriol on target organs which can be achieved by oral versus intravenous administration.

In our opinion, patients who may benefit from intravenous calcitriol are:

[1] The noncompliant patients who are not taking oral calcitriol.

[2] The patient with overt hyperparathyroidism who cannot be treated with oral calcitriol therapy because of induced hypercalcemia. In the past, this type of patient has surgical parathyroidectomy. Theoretically, it is conceivable that sufficient intravenous calcitriol may induce a medical rather than a surgical parathyroidectomy.

[3] The patient who develops hyperphosphatemia immediately after oral administration of calcitriol may respond to intravenous calcitriol with a lesser degree of hyperphosphatemia.

[4] Those patients with severe osteitis fibrosa who must undergo parathyroidectomy to ameliorate bone abnormalities may benefit from intravenous calcitriol prior to parathyroidectomy (21). In the post-parathyroidectomy period, hypocalcemia may be accompanied by high morbidity and mortality because of tetany and bone fractures. In these patients, administration of intravenous calcitriol one or two weeks prior to

parathyroidectomy may render them less prone to severe hypocalcemia and decrease morbidity and mortality.

REFERENCES

1. Wilson L, Felsenfeld A, Drezner MK, Llach F: Altered divalent ion metabolism in early renal failure: role of 1,25(OH)$_2$D. Kidney Int, 27: 565-573, 1985.
2. Llach F, Massry SG: On the mechanism of secondary hyperparathyroidism in moderate renal insufficiency. J Clin Endocrinol Metab, 61: 601-606, 1985.
3. Brickman AS, Coburn JW, Norman AW: Action of 1,25-dihydroxycholecalciferol, a potent, kidney-produced metabolite of vitamin D$_3$ in uremic man. N Engl J Med, 287: 891-895, 1972.
4. Chan JCM, Oldham SB, Holick MF et al: Alpha hydroxyvitamin D$_3$ in chronic renal failure: A potent analogue of the kidney hormone 1,25 dihydroxycholecalciferol. JAMA, 234: 47-52, 1975.
5. Silver J, Naveh-Many T, Mayer H, Schmelzer HJ, Popovtzer MM: Regulation by vitamin D metabolites of parathyroid hormone gene transcription *in vivo* in the rat. J. Clin Invest, 78: 1296-1301, 1986.
6. Russell J, Lettieri D, Sherwood LM: Suppression by 1,25 (OH)$_2$D$_3$ of transcription of the pre-proparathyroid hormone gene. Endocrinology, 119: 2864-2866, 1986.
7. Kanis JA, Cundy J, Smith R et al: Possible function of different renal metabolites of vitamin D in man. Contrib Nephrol, 18: 192-211, 1980.
8. Henderson RG, Ledingham JGG, Oliver DO et al: Effects of 1,25 dihydroxycholecalciferol on calcium absorption, muscle weakness, and bone disease in chronic renal failure. Lancet, I: 379-384, 1974.
9. Coburn JW et al: Intestinal phosphate absorption in normal and uremic man: Effects of 1,25(OH)$_2$ vitamin D$_3$ and 1(OH) vitamin D$_3$. In: "Phosphate Metabolism" (Eds SG Massry, E Ritz), Plenum Press, New York, 1977, p 549.
10. Coburn JW et al: Clinical efficacy of 1,25 di-hydroxyvitamin D$_3$ in renal osteodystrophy. In: "Vitamin D: Biochemical, Chemical and Clinical Aspects Related to Calcium Metabolism" (Eds AW Norman et al), Walter de Gruyter, Berlin, 1977, p 657.
11. Silver J, Naveh-Many T, Mayer H, Schmelzer HJ, Popovtzer MM: Regulation by vitamin D Metabolites of parathyroid hormone gene transcription *in vivo* in the rat. J Clin Invest, 78: 1296-1301, 1986.
12. Silver J, Russell J, Sherwood LM: Regulation by vitamin D metabolites of messenger ribonucleic acid for preproparathyroid hormone in isolated bovine parathyroid cells. Proc Natl Sci, 82: 4270-4273, 1985.
13. Shuil Y, Naveh-Many T, Barach P, Silver J: Regulation of parathyroid cell gene expression in experimental uremia. J Am Soc Nephrol, 1: 99-104, 1990.
14. Slatopolsky E, Weerts C, Thielan J, Horst R, Harter H, Martin KJ: Marked suppression of secondary hyperparathyroidism by intravenous administration of 1,25-dihydroxycholecalciferol in uremic patients. J Clin Invest, 74: 2136-2140, 1984.
15. Delmez JA, Tindira C, Grooms P, Dusso A, Windus DW, Slatopolsky E: Parathyroid hormone suppression by 1,25-dihydroxyvitamin D. A role for increased sensitivity to calcium. J Clin Invest, 83: 1349-1355, 1989.
16. Dunlay R, Rodriguez M, Felsenfeld AJ, Llach F: Direct inhibitory effect of calcitriol on parathyroid function (sigmoidal curve) in dialysis. Kidney Int, 36: 1093-1098, 1989.
17. Norris KC, Kraut JA, Andress DL, Agre KL, Sherrard DJ, Coburn JW: Intravenous calcitriol: Effect in severe secondary hyperparathyroidism. J Bone Mineral Research, 1 (Suppl 1): 374, 1986.
18. Andress DL, Norris KC, Coburn JW, Slatopolsky E, Sherrard DJ: Intravenous calcitriol in the treatment of refractory osteitis fibrosa of chronic renal failure. N Engl J Med, 321: 274-279, 1989.
19. Hamdy NAT, Brown CB, Kanis JA: Intravenous calcitriol lowers serum calcium concentrations in uremic patients with severe hyperparathyroidism and hypercalcemia. Nephrol Dial Transplant, 4: 545-548, 1989.

20. Brandi L, Daugaad H, Tvedegaard E, Storm T, Olgaard K: Effect of intravenous 1-alpha-hydroxyvitamin D_3 on secondary hyperparathyroidism in chronic uremic patients on maintenance hemodialysis. Nephron, 53: 194-200, 1989.
21. Llach F: Parathyroidectomy in chronic renal failure: Indications, surgical approach and the use of calcitriol. Kidney Int, 38 (Suppl 29): 62-68, 1990.

Chapter 12

NON-A, NON-B HEPATITIS IN DIALYSIS PATIENTS: DIAGNOSIS, PREVENTION AND TREATMENT

MICHEL JADOUL, CHANTAL CORNU* AND CHARLES VAN YPERSELE DE STRIHOU

Divisions of Nephrology and Virology*, University of Louvain Medical School, Cliniques Universitaires St-Luc, 1200 Bruxelles, Belgium

INTRODUCTION

The concept of non-A, non-B hepatitis (NANBH) developed as accurate serologic tools became available to recognize various etiologic agents of hepatitis such as the hepatitis A and B viruses, the Epstein Barr virus and the cytomegalovirus (1). NANBH was recognized in the 80's as the most common type of post-transfusion hepatitis (2). In hemodialysis patients, it emerged as the main cause of liver dysfunction once the spread of hepatitis B in dialysis units was controlled (3, 4).

During the past three years, a new virus responsible for the development of NANBH has been identified, the hepatitis C virus (HCV) (4). Now that serological tests allow its recognition (5) HCV appears responsible for most, if not all, cases of parenteral or sporadic NANBH (5). Interestingly, almost simultaneously, the discovery of the hepatitis E virus has elucidated outbreaks of waterborne NANBH, a disease observed in developing countries (6, 7).

In this review, we summarize the characteristics of the HCV, describe the various tests available for its detection with an emphasis on their sensitivity and specificity. We review the epidemiological and clinical characteristics of hepatitis C, first in the general population and then in patients on renal replacement therapy. Practical guidelines for the prevention of HCV transmission in dialysis patients are eventually discussed.

THE "HCV STORY"

The identification of the HCV has set a landmark in biomedical research: the viral genome has been sequenced prior to the isolation of the virus itself (4). In the process, parts of the viral RNA have been retrieved and expressed providing the clinician with various serological tools to diagnose infection.

The Chiron Corporation initiated in 1982 the search for the etiologic agent of parenteral NANBH. Pooled chimpanzee plasma known to be highly infectious was ultracentrifuged so as to include in the pellet even the smallest infectious particles (4). Total nucleic acid was extracted from the pellet and denatured. Complementary DNA (cDNA) was then prepared by use of random primers of reverse transcriptase. The various cDNA strands were cloned into a bacteriophage vector providing thus a large cDNA library. Subsequent transfer to E. Coli, allowed the expression of the coded peptides. The search for the viral peptides then began. Screening was performed with serum obtained from a patient with a firm clinical diagnosis of NANBH and thus expected to have antibodies against viral proteins. A million different clones had to be screened to find a protein that reacted with the patient's serum (4). The 155 base pair insert (identified as C5-1-1) in this clone was then cut out and used as a hybridization probe to extract from the original library a larger, 353 base pair, overlapping clone (identified as C100) (5). This cDNA did not hybridise to human or chimpanzee DNA but was shown to be derived from a single stranded RNA molecule of approximately 10,000 nucleotides. Comparative sequence analysis of this single strand RNA suggests that HCV is a distant relative of the flaviviridae (4, 8).

The C100 clone was then fused to the human gene encoding for superoxide dismutase (SOD), an enzyme promoting the expression of foreign proteins in plasmids. The resulting polypeptide C-100-3 was expressed first in recombinant E. Coli and subsequently yeast (5) and used to capture HCV antibodies. The diagnostic characteristics of the C-100-3 derived radioimmunoassay (5) proved very encouraging. The first tests were conducted blind, with a well characterized panel of non-A, non-B sera. Of seven non-A, non-B serum samples shown to be infectious in chimpanzees, six contained antibodies that reacted with C-100-3 while seven non-infectious control sera were negative (5). In serial samples from ten well-characterized cases of post-transfusion NANBH, the antibody appeared approximately 6 months after the transfusion in all but one case. The assay proved positive in 71% of a further 24 patients with post-transfusion NANBH, and 58% of 59 patients with sporadic NANBH (5).

Recombinant antigens C100 and its subsegment C5-1-1 are fragments of the nonstructural part (NS3-NS4) of the HCV polyprotein. Further work led to the identification of other peptides coded for by other segments of the viral RNA: C33-c located in another non structural region (NS3) and C-22 located in a structural part, putatively the core of HCV (9). These new recombinant antigens are currently utilized in

254

HCV immunodiagnostic tests whose characteristics, sensitivity and specificity are discussed in the next section.

TESTS FOR THE DIAGNOSIS OF HCV INFECTION

ELISA

The first commercially available test subsequently referred to as ELISA relies on the recognition of antibodies to the C-100-3 polypeptide expressed in yeast, coating wells of microtitre trays (Table 1). The presence in the tested serum of specific IgG antibodies is detected by an enzyme linked immunosorbent assay (Ortho Diagnostic Systems, Raritan, New Jersey). Results were similar to those obtained with the original RIA (5): the test was positive in about 80% of patients with a firm clinical diagnosis of chronic post-transfusion NANBH (10, 11). A high prevalence of ELISA(+) subjects was identified in various subgroups of patients known to be at high risk for NANBH such as intravenous drug abusers, hemodialysis patients and hemophiliacs (12, 13).

Table 1. Tests for the diagnosis of HCV infection.

Test	Antigens				
ELISA	C-100-3				
2-RIBA	C-100-3	C5-1-1	SOD		
4 RIBA	C-100-3	C5-1-1	SOD	C-33c	C-22
second generation ELISA	C-100-3			C-33c	C-22

The limits of the test became quickly apparent. Sensitivity is suboptimal as the test remains negative in one fifth of the cases with clear-cut evidence of chronic post-transfusion NANBH (10, 11). In some of these ELISA negative patients, the presence of HCV in liver cells or serum was verified by polymerase chain reaction (13, 14). Furthermore, the detected antibody appears late after the onset of infection, the delay extending up to one year, leaving a diagnostic "window" of uncertainty (15, 16). Finally, the antibody is obviously not neutralizing as ELISA(+) blood products proved infective in 15 to 30% of the cases in several studies (17, 18) and even up to 88% in another study (19). This characteristic probably derives from the fact that C-100-3 polypeptide is not part of the virus envelope.

255

The specificity of the test is also wanting. Unexpectedly high prevalences of positive ELISA tests have been reported in some patient groups who were not at high risk of infectious hepatitis, but who were characterized by severe hypergammaglobulinemia such as type 1 and type 2 autoimmune active hepatitis with liver kidney microsomal type I antibodies (20-22), rheumatoid arthritis associated with rheumatoid factor (23), primary biliary cirrhosis (24), malaria, schistosomiasis, hydatidosis (25, 26), and in 15% of patients with paraproteinemia (27). In these series, false positivity of the ELISA test appeared related to the elevated IgG levels.

Indeed, in different groups, optical density values of the ELISA correlated significantly with the patients' IgG level (22, 26, 28). Although a positive ELISA test might reflect in some of these patients past or present HCV infection, this hypothesis has been ruled out by the lack of HCV-RNA in the serum of 7 ELISA positive patients with primary biliary cirrhosis (28). In Boudart et al's (27) study of 28 ELISA(+) cases with paraproteinemia, the confirmatory 2-RIBA test described below, proved negative in 86% of the cases.

Further evidence for false positive ELISA tests accrues from the observation that the results fluctuate with the activity of some autoimmune disorders: 65% of patients with chronic autoimmune hepatitis type I had a positive ELISA test when the disease was active versus only 5% if the disease was in remission. Furthermore the test became negative in six patients after initiation of immunosuppressive therapy (22).

Several explanations have been proposed to account for false (+) tests: low-avidity cross-reacting antibodies (29), antibodies against bacterial proteins contaminating the recombinant C-100-3 fusion polypeptide (18), antibodies against superoxide dismutase (30) or against an unrelated protein sharing an epitope with C-100-3 (18) such as those produced by other flaviviruses or pestiviruses (8).

First generation RIBA (2-RIBA)

A first generation Recombinant ImmunoBlot Assay (RIBA), referred to as 2-RIBA (Ortho Diagnostic Systems), was developed as a confirmatory test (Table 1). Three recombinant antigens are coated in distinct bands on nitrocellulose strips: the same C-100-3 peptide than in the ELISA, the C5-1-1, fused to SOD and expressed in E. Coli, and SOD itself as control. Two additional bands of gammaglobulins (high and low concentration) act as controls. The presence in the patient's serum of IgG antibodies is detected by a goat anti-human IgG labelled with peroxidase (31). The presence of antibodies reacting with both C5-1-1 and C-100-3 defines a positive result whereas reactivity against a single viral antigen or against both SOD and HCV antigens is called an indeterminate result. This new test proved positive in about 80% of the ELISA(+) patients belonging to a high risk group (hemophiliacs, HD patients) (32, 33) but in only 16-45% of ELISA(+) subjects belonging to low risk groups such as blood donors (31, 34, 35). The 2-RIBA test is not more sensitive than the ELISA test as it relies on the same antigen, the C-100-3 and its subsegment C5-1-1. By contrast, it is more specific as it verifies that the reactivity seen is not due to a contaminant.

Second generation RIBA (4-RIBA)

A second generation RIBA, also called 4-RIBA (Ortho Diagnostic Systems), has been recently developed (Table 1): it relies on the presence of 4 recombinant HCV antigens all fused to SOD: besides the recombinant antigens used in the 2-RIBA, the C-33c and C-22 antigens expressed in E. Coli or yeast are added. A positive test is defined by the presence of antibodies against at least 2 HCV antigens. Preliminary results suggest that the sensitivity, specificity and prediction of infectivity of this test are much higher than those of the first generation tests. Marcellin et al (36) evaluated 100 patients with well documented chronic NANBH: 96 were positive with the 4-RIBA test versus only 76 with the ELISA test. In another study van der Poel et al (37) re-examined stored samples of 37 ELISA(+) blood products obtained in a previous post-transfusional NANBH study. Eight samples proved 4-RIBA reactive, 7 of whom had been implicated in post-transfusion NANBH and/or HCV infection (confirmed by polymerase chain reaction) of their recipients. By contrast, none of the 29 ELISA(+) but 4-RIBA(-) products had apparently caused a post-transfusional NANBH. Ebeling et al (38) confirmed the infectious potential of 4-RIBA(+) blood: they further showed that it was associated with the presence of antibodies against C-33c and C-22.

The increased sensitivity and specificity of the 4-RIBA is due to the presence of C-33c or C-22 (37). In clinical practice, ELISA tests are less cumbersome and expensive than the RIBA technology.

Second generation ELISA test

At the present time, a second generation ELISA test, including C-100-3, C-33c and C-22 is available (Table 1). Very preliminary data suggest that this newer technique retains most qualities of the 4-RIBA test (39).

Polymerase chain reaction (PCR)

Viral RNA may be detected directly after amplification through the polymerase chain reaction (PCR), a technique now widely used in clinical medicine. PCR relies on the ability of an enzyme, Taq polymerase, to copy minute amounts of genetic material (40). Repetition of the reproduction cycle yields large quantities of material to be subsequently analysed. This highly sensitive technique requires, in order to remain specific, strict methodological rules to avoid contamination of the reaction mixture (40). At present, it is too cumbersome to be applied in routine. However it provides a golden standard for the critical assessment of serological tests.

With the help of PCR, Weiner and Zanetti (13, 41) have detected HCV-RNA in the liver and/or serum of ELISA(-) patients with NANBH, and thus demonstrated the limited sensitivity of the ELISA test. Garson et al (42) have studied the temporal relationship between the development of NANBH, the appearance of ELISA HCV antibodies and the detection of serum HCV-RNA in previously untreated hemophiliacs. In 3 patients, HCV-RNA preceded the onset of liver function abnormalities and/or the detection of ELISA antibodies. The presence of serum HCV-RNA also predicts infectivity of blood products: the one out of 6 ELISA(+) blood donors who transmitted post-transfusional non-A, non-B hepatitis was also the only one in whom serum HCV-RNA was detected (18). Simmonds et al (14) have demonstrated that many high-risk patients with a positive ELISA still harbour the HCV.

PCR has also yielded important information on the variability of the viral genome. This information is particularly relevant to the field of vaccine development.

Kato et al (43) sequenced 37 nucleotides of the viral RNA in 15 patients with chronic NANBH. They found only 68-78% homology with the prototype HCV nucleotide sequence. However, the translated aminoacid sequence had a 83-100% homology with the prototype translated sequence.

From 4 HCV isolates, Ulrich et al (44) observed a much smaller nucleotide diversity, less than 9%, with a resulting homology of translated amino acids exceeding 96%.

HEPATITIS C: INCUBATION AND MODES OF TRANSMISSION, PREVALENCE AND HIGH-RISK GROUPS, PROGNOSIS AND TREATMENT

As might be anticipated, many conclusions drawn from studies of NANBH (1) apply to hepatitis C.

Incubation

Incubation time ranges from 2 to 13 weeks as demonstrated in 2 longitudinal studies of 15 and 59 cases of post-transfusion hepatitis C respectively (15, 16).

Transmission

HCV is transmitted mainly through blood transfusion (including plasma, and factor VIII concentrates) or through blood contaminated needles [surgeons (45), intravenous drug abusers, etc]. HCV is also probably transmitted by sexual contacts but certainly less readily than the hepatitis B virus (HBV) or human immunodeficiency virus (HIV). Indeed, the prevalence of ELISA antibodies in long-term sexual partners (>3 years) of HCV(+) patients remains low, ranging from 0 to 7% (46). The seroconversion rate of a cohort of 250 homosexual men followed for 3 to 8 years was ≤ 2.5% for HCV versus 12-15% for HBV or 8-16% for HIV (47). The prevalence of HCV ELISA antibodies was higher (4.7%) among 191 patients with heterosexually transmitted diseases than among control blood donors (0.5%), but markedly lower than that of antibodies against HBV (31%) (48). In that respect it is noteworthy that HCV has been isolated from the saliva of ELISA(+) patients (49) and of infected chimpanzees (50). The possibility of HCV transmission through household contact with HCV(+) patients has been suggested by some investigators reporting a higher prevalence of HCV antibodies (3 to 15%) in household contact of HCV(+) patients than in the general population (46, 51, 52) but this has been denied by others (53). Transmission in such cases might occur through sharing of personal objects like razors, toothbrushes, nail scissors, etc. Finally, mother to infant HCV transmission remains equally controversial (54, 55).

Prevalence

The prevalence of ELISA HCV antibodies differs among groups. Among blood donors, the prevalence varies among countries. In Europe, a North to South gradient is apparent, the prevalence increasing from 0.4% in Germany (56) and 0.7% in France (57) and Northern Italy (58), to 1.2% in Spain (12) and 1.4% in Southern Italy (58). Prevalences of 1.2 to 1.4% have been reported in the US and Japan (56).

Prevalence of ELISA antibodies rises in specific at risk groups: 64 to 85% in hemophiliacs given unheated blood products (12, 59), 48 to 81% (10, 12, 60) in i.v. drug abusers, 1-33% in dialyzed patients (discussed in subsequent section), 4-24% in multitransfused patients with acute leukemia (61) or thalassemia major (62).

259

Interestingly, a similar high prevalence of HCV antibodies has been reported in patients with hepatocellular carcinoma: 29 to 65% (63, 64). If confirmed by PCR, this finding suggests that just as HBV, HCV might play a role in the pathogenesis of this tumor.

Clinical presentation and prognosis

The clinical picture of acute hepatitis C is frequently mild, without jaundice in about 2/3 of cases (16). Serum ALT levels peak in the hundreds rather than thousands range (15). By contrast, the long-term prognosis of hepatitis C is a cause of major concern (65, 66). Longitudinal studies on post-transfusion NANBH have indeed reported that the actuarial probability of normalizing serum ALT levels is only 50% even after 10 years of follow-up (67). Thus up to 50% of patients show biochemical evidence of chronicity (66). Liver cirrhosis has been documented (67, 68) in 9 to 24% of patients with biochemical signs of chronicity. In patients with chronic hepatitis C, liver biopsies have been performed in 166, 41 and 56 patients, prior to the enrollment in three therapeutic trials with interferon-α (65, 66, 69). Histological evidence of cirrhosis was obtained in 55, 17 and 14% of the cases respectively, thus confirming the tendency of chronic hepatitis C to progress to cirrhosis.

Treatment

This gloomy prognosis has recently changed as a result of new treatment strategies relying on the use of cytokines. In three randomized placebo controlled trials, interferon-α was injected subcutaneously thrice weekly (respectively 10^6 or 3×10^6 units in the first two trials and 2×10^6 units in the third one) for 24 to 26 weeks and treatment normalized ALT serum level in 46% and 39% of patients treated with 3×10^6 U respectively, versus in 28% and 45% of patients treated with 10^6 U and 8% and 0% of placebo treated patients (65, 69). In the third trial, treatment normalized ALT serum level in 48% of 2×10^6 U treated patients versus 10% of placebo treated patients (66). The high doses (2 or 3×10^6 U) also significantly improved liver histology (64, 65, 69). Unfortunately, 6 months after the completion of treatment, ALT had returned to pre-treatment level in at least 50% of responding patients (65, 66, 69). The long-term benefits of short term interferon-α remain thus to be established.

The mechanism of the interferon-α action remains unclear. The drug has been shown to reduce HCV-RNA serum levels (70) and to normalize the hepatic levels of transforming growth factor ß1 mRNA, an effect likely to decrease hepatic fibrogenesis (71). It should be stressed that interferon-α is currently not recommended for all patients with chronic hepatitis C. Indeed, the drug is not devoid of side effects, sometimes severe (flulike syndrome, psychological side effects, bone marrow suppression, induction of autoimmunity) (72), is expensive and lacks proven long-term effects in many patients. Di Bisceglie et al (72) thus currently recommend to treat only patients with severe disease (aminotransferase levels ≥ 5 times above normal or symptoms interfering with daily life or severe histological changes). Patients with milder disease might indeed benefit from the current evaluation of alternative regimens in this rapidly evolving field (72).

Very recently, ribavirin, a nucleotide analogue with broad antiviral activity, was administered orally for 12 weeks to 10 patients with chronic hepatitis C in an open study (73). It decreased significantly ALT levels which returned to pretreatment level within 6 weeks after the end of treatment. If confirmed in placebo-controlled studies of larger groups of patients, it would offer a potentially effective oral treatment for chronic hepatitis C (73). Interestingly, both interferon-α and ribavirin decrease ALT levels in chronic hepatitis C without first inducing a short-lived ALT increase analogous to that observed upon initiation of antiviral treatment in chronic hepatitis B (74). This suggests that the deleterious effect of HCV results from a direct cytopathic effect on hepatocytes and is not related to the viral induced immune response.

Such therapies should be undertaken only in patients in whom chronic autoimmune active hepatitis has been excluded as autoimmune hepatitis may be exacerbated by interferon-α (75). Likewise non-A, non-B hepatitis and thus probably hepatitis C might be adversely influenced by immunosuppressive drugs, the choice treatment for autoimmune hepatitis. An accurate etiologic diagnosis of hepatitis is thus mandatory before initiating any form of therapy.

EPIDEMIOLOGY AND CLINICAL CHARACTERISTICS OF HEPATITIS C IN HEMODIALYSIS PATIENTS

Prevalence of HCV antibodies

Studies of the prevalence of ELISA HCV antibodies in hemodialysis (HD) patients report figures ranging from 1 to 33% (60, 76-89). The prevalence is in the range of 10 to 30% in Japan, the US and Southern Europe but markedly lower in Northern Europe (UK and FRG) (1-9%), a pattern analogous to that observed in the general population (60, 77, 89).

The actual prevalence of HCV antibodies will probably increase as more sensitive tests become available: in our dialysis population, the prevalence of HCV(+) rose from 14% with the ELISA test to 22% with a second generation ELISA (personal contribution). By contrast, the specificity of the ELISA test appears satisfactory in HD patients. Three studies (33, 85, 90) report positive or indeterminate results with either the 2-RIBA or the 4-RIBA test in 87.5 to 100% of the ELISA(+) subjects. Interestingly, as the 4-RIBA test has been considered as a marker associated to infectivity (37), this suggests that most HD patients with a positive ELISA are infective.

Factors influencing HCV antibodies' prevalence

Several factors influence the prevalence of HCV antibodies. Duration of dialysis has been indicted in several studies (33, 76, 78, 82, 83, 86, 89, 91). In our own series (76) the prevalence rose from 0% in 20 patients dialyzed for less than 12 months to 35% in 20 patients dialyzed for more than 6 years (Table 2).

Table 2 Effect of dialysis duration on the prevalence of ELISA HCV(+) patients (76)

	Months on dialysis			
	< 12	12-36	37-72	> 72
number of patients at risk	20	18	18	20
% of ELISA HCV(+) patients	0	6	22	35

This trend is undoubtedly related, at least in part, to the transfusional transmission of HCV. Indeed in several studies the number of transfusions was significantly higher in the HCV(+) than in the HCV(-) patients (78, 80, 87, 91), the fraction of patients who have never received a transfusion was markedly lower in the HCV(+) than HCV(-) patients (33). Still these observations should not obscure the fact that HCV positivity has been reported in up to 5 to 22% of never transfused dialyzed patients (78, 80-83) a figure much higher than that observed in the general population. Nosocomial transmission, unrelated to transfusion, is thus very likely. The respective contributions of transfusion and nosocomial transmission remain to be defined. Finally, in some urban areas in the US, intravenous drug abuse is a significant risk factor (87, 88).

Nosocomial transmission may affect staff members. HCV transmission has been documented in 2 nurses after needlestick injury (92, 93). These events must be rare as the prevalence of HCV positivity is low in hemodialysis staff members; we compiled a prevalence of less than 2% (3/171) from four studies (76, 85, 87, 94).

Clinical characteristics and prognosis

The clinical picture of hepatitis C is as indolent in HD as in non uremic patients. It is often accompanied by a mild elevation of serum ALT levels as illustrated by significantly higher mean ALT levels in HCV(+) than in HCV(-) patients (91).

The prevalence of patients with elevated ALT levels among HCV(+) subjects depends both on the criteria defining raised ALT levels and on the sensitivity and specificity of the HCV test.

Among 16 patients who had HCV antibodies detectable by a first and/or second generation ELISA test, we found 12 cases with at least two abnormal ALT values over a period of 24 months, i.e. a prevalence of 75% (personal observations).

Elevation of serum ALT levels in HD patients is multifactorial. HBV may coincide with HCV infection (84). In the absence of HBV infection, chronically elevated ALT levels are mainly if not exclusively due to HCV infection. In our series, all 7 patients with at least three values of ALT exceeding 150% of normal over 6-24 months proved HCV(+) by first and/or second generation ELISA tests (personal observations).

The long-term prognosis of hepatitis C in dialyzed patients has not yet been delineated. No liver histological data are available and no trial with interferon-α or ribavirin has yet been reported. Preliminary data concerning the chronicity of ALT and other liver function markers alterations suggest that the disease course is not different in HD than in non uremic patients (78).

EPIDEMIOLOGY AND CLINICAL CHARACTERISTICS OF HEPATITIS C IN RENAL TRANSPLANT RECIPIENTS

Prevalence of HCV antibodies

The prevalence of HCV antibodies (ELISA) in renal transplant recipients ranges from 6.5 to 42% (95-99). In this limited number of studies, no geographical trend is apparent.

Factors influencing HCV antibodies prevalence

Just as for the HBV, infection by HCV seems to occur mainly prior to transplantation. HCV(+) patients have dialyzed for a longer period than HCV(-) subjects (95, 97). Not unexpectedly, in some (95) but not all (96, 97) reports the presence of HCV antibodies is also related to the number of transfusions.

The determinants of HCV antibodies first detected after transplantation also remain moot both as a result of the inadequate sensitivity of the ELISA assay, the frequent peroperative transfusions and the unknown HCV status of the renal graft. Gomez et al (95) have reported that one out of 3 patients who seroconverted after transplantation (ELISA test) had received a graft from an HCV(+) donor, raising the possibility of graft transmitted HCV infection. Roth et al (98) have observed the development of ELISA HCV antibodies in only one out of 23 HCV(-) patients given an HCV(+) renal graft, a finding compatible with the relatively low infectivity of ELISA(+) blood products (17). None of these studies ruled out the role of potentially infectious perioperative blood transfusion. Recently, however, Otero et al (100) analyzed 3 HCV(-) recipients, transfused pre- and post-operatively with HCV(-) packed red blood cells and given HCV(+) grafts. One of them became HCV(+) 7 months post transplant.

The possibility of HCV transmission by the graft has led many transplantation centers to refuse to transplant HCV(+) kidneys, a policy recently criticized as it might further limit the availability of organs. Transplantation of HCV(+) kidneys has been proposed in recipients with antibodies to HCV as determined by RIBA or in relatively untransplantable patients (e.g. hyperimmunized) (101).

Prognosis

The fate of HCV(+) transplanted patients remains ill defined. It is not yet clear whether transplantation and its attendant immunosuppressive therapy modifies the natural history of hepatitis C. Preliminary results are too fragmentary to provide yet a coherent picture. Stempel et al (101) reported that the majority of 35 HCV(+) patients have normal aspartate aminotransferase levels 3 years after transplantation. Graft survival, overall and liver related mortality after a mean 39 months follow-up is similar in HCV(+) and HCV(-) patients. Roth et al (98) find no difference in patients and graft survival over a ten year period between HCV(+) and HCV(-) patients. Morales et al (102) analyzed 60 grafted patients and observed biochemical evidence of chronic hepatitis (abnormal liver tests for more than 6 months) in 50% of them, several of whom had severe histologic liver abnormalities, a pattern similar to that observed in HCV(+) non uremic patients.

The role of HCV in the genesis of HBV unrelated elevation of serum ALT levels after transplantation appears limited. Goffin et al (97) observed HCV antibodies in only 3 of 23 HBV(-) renal graft recipients with a chronic rise of serum ALT levels.

Final answers to these various questions will have to await the generalized use of more sensitive and specific serological tests of HCV infection.

PRACTICAL GUIDELINES FOR THE PREVENTION OF HCV TRANSMISSION TO HD PATIENTS AND STAFF MEMBERS.

Routine screening of blood donors for HCV is already applied in several European countries (56). It should decrease post-transfusional HCV infection to the extent that the test is able to detect early immune response. The widespread availability of erythropoietin reduces transfusional requirements and thus should reduce the incidence of hepatitis C.

The usefulness of providing separate facilities for HCV(+) patients is a more controversial issue. This procedure has been advocated to avoid nosocomial transmission of the disease (94). In a retrospective study, Arici et al (94) found a fall in the incidence of NANBH (most cases of which were later found to correspond to hepatitis C) once patients with suspected NANBH had been separated from the other patients. However, the possibility that other measures were introduced simultaneously and explain the reduction of NANBH incidence cannot be ruled out.

Segregation of HD patients into different facilities (B+C+, B+C-, B-C-, B-C+ !) is difficult to implement in practice. Its effectiveness depends on several prerequisites. First, it should be demonstrated that past infection with one HCV strain protects from subsequent infection with another strain. Second, only tests allowing an early identification of infected patients should be utilized. The available ELISA test does not satisfy this requirement. Until these requirements are met, it seems reasonable to rely mainly on the "universal precautions for prevention of transmission of bloodborne pathogens in health-care settings" (103) and on the "recommended precautions for patients undergoing hemodialysis who have AIDS or NANBH" (104). They include the prevention of injuries by needles and other sharp instruments (no recaping of used needles by hand, puncture-resistent containers for disposal as close to the use area as is practical), the use of protective barriers (gloves for phlebotomy and, more importantly, during HD even in emergency cases) and immediate and thorough skin and hand washing after blood contamination (103). A recent study from the USA has clearly shown that these guidelines are frequently not followed but that staff compliance can be improved by appropriate training (105).

265

In addition, particular attention should be paid to the cleaning and disinfection of instruments, machines and environmental surfaces that are routinely touched. No articles should be shared between patients (104).

CONCLUSIONS

The hepatitis C virus has recently been identified and recognized as the etiologic agent of most, if not all, cases of NANBH, a significant complication of HD. Increasingly sensitive and specific tests are introduced into clinical medicine to detect HCV infection and to recognize infectivity.

The prevalence of HCV antibodies among HD and renal transplant patients is much higher (10 to 20%) than in the general population; risk factors include dialysis duration and/or blood transfusions. The presence of HCV antibodies in HD patients who have never been transfused suggests the existence of nosocomial HCV transmission in addition to the transfusion route. In patients on renal replacement therapy, hepatitis C appears to follow the same indolent course as in non uremic subjects. Although it seems likely that it will eventually lead to a high incidence of chronic hepatitis and possibly of cirrhosis, its long-term prognosis remains to be documented.

New treatment strategies are developed for hepatitis C. Their benefit in dialyzed or transplanted patients has not yet been tested. The apparently gloomy long-term prognosis of hepatitis C justifies scrupulous preventive measures, such as the widespread use of erythropoietin, in order to reduce blood transfusions, screening of blood donors for HCV, and strict observation of guidelines for the prevention of transmission of bloodborne pathogens and precautions for patients undergoing hemodialysis who have AIDS or NANBH as edicted by the CDC (Atlanta, Ga, USA).

REFERENCES

1. Dienstag JL: Non-A, non-B hepatitis. I. Recognition, epidemiology and clinical features. Gastroenterology, 85: 439-462, 1983.
2. Koretz RL, Stone O, Mousa M, Gitnick G: The pursuit of hepatitis in dialysis units. Am J Nephrol, 4: 222-226, 1984.
3. Seaworth BJ, Garrett LE, Stead WW, Hamilton JD: Non-A, non-B hepatitis and chronic dialysis - another dilemma. Am J Nephrol, 4: 235-239, 1984.
4. Choo QL, Kuo G, Weiner AJ, Overby LR, Bradley DW, Houghton M: Isolation of a cDNA clone derived from a bloodborne non-A, non-B viral hepatitis genome. Science, 244: 359-364, 1989.
5. Kuo G, Choo QL, Alter HJ, Gitnick GL, Redeker AG, Purcell RH, Miyamura T, Dienstag JL, Alter MJ, Stevens CE, Tergtmeier GE, Bonino F, Colombo M, Lee WS, Kuo C, Berger K, Shuster JR, Overby LR, Bradley DW, Houghton M: An assay for circulating antibodies to a major etiologic virus of human non-A, non-B hepatitis. Science, 244: 362-364, 1989.
6. De Cock KM, Bradley DW, Sandford NL, Govindarajan S, Maynard JE, Redeker AG: Epidemic non-A, non-B hepatitis in patients from Pakistan. Ann Int Med, 106: 227-230, 1987.

7. Reyes GR, Purdy MA, Kim JP, Luk KC, Young LM, Fry KE, Bradley DW: Isolation of a cDNA from the virus responsible for enterically transmitted non-A, non-B hepatitis. Science 247: 1335-1339, 1990.

8. Miller RH, Purcell RH: Hepatitis C virus shares amino acid sequence similarity with pestiviruses and flaviviruses as well as members of two plant virus supergroups. Proc Natl Acad Sci, 87: 2057-2061, 1990.

9. Mimms L, Vallari D, Ducharme L, Holland P, Kuramoto IK, Zeldis J: Specificity of anti-HCV ELISA assessed by reactivity to three immunodominant HCV regions. Lancet, 336: 1590-1591, 1990.

10. Roggendorf M, Deinhardt F, Rasshofer R, Eberle J, Hopf U, Möller B, Zachoval R, Pape G, Schramm W, Rommel F: Antibodies to hepatitis C virus. Lancet, II: 324-325, 1989.

11. van der Poel CL, Reesink HW, Lelie PN, Leentvaar-Kuypers A, Choo QL, Kuo G, Houghton M: Anti-hepatitis C antibodies and non-A, non-B post-transfusion hepatitis in The Netherlands. Lancet, II: 297-298, 1989.

12. Esteban JI, Viladomiu L, Gonzalez A, Roget M, Genesca J, Esteban R, Lopez-Talavera JC, Hernandez JM, Vargas V, Buti M: Hepatitis C virus antibodies among risk groups in Spain. Lancet, II: 294-297, 1989.

13. Weiner AJ, Kuo G, Bradley DW, Bonino F, Saracco G, Lee C, Rosenblatt J, Choo QL, Houghton M: Detection of hepatitis C viral sequences in non-A, non-B hepatitis. Lancet, 335: 1-3, 1990.

14. Simmonds P, Zhang LQ, Watson HG, Rebus, Ferguson ED, Balfe P, Leadbetter GH, Yap PL, Peutherer JF, Ludlam CA: Hepatitis C quantification and sequencing in blood products, haemophiliacs and drug users. Lancet, 336: 1469-1472, 1990.

15. Alter HJ, Purcell RH, Shih JW, Melpolder JC, Houghton M, Choo QL, Kuo G: Detection of antibody to hepatitis C virus in prospectively followed transfusion recipients with acute and chronic non-A, non-B hepatitis. N Engl J Med, 321: 1494-1500, 1989.

16. Tremolada F, Casarin C, Tagger A, Ribero ML, Realdi G, Alberti A, Ruol A: Antibody to hepatitis C virus in post-transfusion hepatitis. Ann Intern Med, 114: 277-281, 1991.

17. van der Poel CL, Reesink HW, Schaasberg W, Leentvaar-Kuypers A, Bakker E, Exel-Oehlers PJ, Lelie PN: Infectivity of blood seropositive for hepatitis C virus antibodies. Lancet, 335: 558-560, 1990.

18. Garson JA, Tedder RS, Briggs M, Tuke P, Glazebrook JA, Trute A, Parker D, Barbara JAJ, Contreras M, Aloysius S: Detection of hepatitis C viral sequences in blood donations by "nested" polymerase chain reaction and prediction of infectivity. Lancet, 335: 1419-1422, 1990.

19. Esteban JI, Gonzalez A, Hernandez JM, Viladomiu L, Sanchez C, Lopez-Talavera JC, Lueca D, Martin-Vega C, Vidal X, Esteban R, Guardia J: Evaluation of antibodies to hepatitis C virus in a study of transfusion-associated hepatitis. N Engl J Med, 323: 1107-1112, 1990.

20. Lenzi M, Ballardini G, Fusconi M, Cassani F, Selleri L, Volta U, Zauli D, Bianchi FB: Type 2 autoimmune hepatitis and hepatitis C virus infection. Lancet, 335: 258-259, 1990.

21. Dussaix E, Maggiore G, De Giacomo C, Mondelli M, Martres P, Alvarez F: Autoimmune hepatitis in children and hepatitis C virus testing. Lancet, 335: 1160-1161, 1990.

22. McFarlane IG, Smith HM, Johnson PJ, Bray GP, Vergani D, Williams R: Hepatitis C virus antibodies in chronic active hepatitis: pathogenetic factor or false-positive result? Lancet, 335: 754-757, 1990.

23. Theilmann L, Blazek M, Goeser T, Gmelin K, Kommerell B, Fiehn W: False-positive anti-HCV tests in rheumatoid arthritis. Lancet, 335: 1346, 1990.

24. Fusconi M, Lenzi M, Ballardini G, Miniero R, Cassani F, Zauli D, Bianchi FB: Anti-HCV testing in autoimmune hepatitis and primary biliary cirrhosis. Lancet, 336: 823, 1990.

25. Aceti A, Taliani G, De Bac C, Sebastiani A: Anti-HCV false positivity in malaria. Lancet, 336: 1442, 1990.

26. Aceti A, Taliani G: Hepatitis C virus antibodies in parasitic infections. Ann Int Med, 113: 560, 1990.

27. Boudart D, Lucas JC, Muller JY, Le Carrer D, Planchon B, Harousseau JL: False-positive hepatitis C virus antibody tests in paraproteinaemia. Lancet, 336: 63, 1990.

28 Bertolini E, Zermiani P, Battezzati PM, Bruno S, Villa E, Manenti F, Marelli F, Moroni GA, Zuin M, Podda M: Lack of association between circulating HCV-RNA and anti-HCV positivity in primary biliary cirrhosis. Lancet, 337: 675-676, 1991.

29. Gray JJ, Wreghitt TG, Friend PJ, Wight DGD, Sundaresan V, Calne RY: Differentiation between specific and non-specific hepatitis C antibodies in chronic liver disease. Lancet, 335: 609-610, 1990.

30. Ikeda Y, Toda G, Hashimoto N, Kurokawa K: Antibody to superoxide dismutase, autoimmune hepatitis, and antibody tests for hepatitis C virus. Lancet, 335: 1345-1346, 1990.

31. Skidmore S: Recombinant immunoblot assay for hepatitis C antibody. Lancet 335: 1346, 1990.

32. Colombo M, Rumi MG, Mannucci PM: Specificity of hepatitis C antibody ELISA in patients with haemophilia. Lancet, 335: 1345, 1990.

33. Mondelli MU, Cristina G, Filice G, Rondanelli EG, Piazza V, Barbieri C: Anti-HCV positive patients in dialysis units? Lancet, 336: 244, 1990.

34. van der Poel CL, Reesink HW, Lelie PN, Exel-Oehlers P, Winkel I, Schaasberg W, Polito A, Houghton H: Anti-HCV and transaminase testing of blood donors. Lancet, 336: 187-188, 1990.

35. Weiner AJ, Truett MA, Rosenblatt J, Han J, Quan S, Polito AJ, Kuo G, Choo QL, Houghton M, Aguis C, Page E, Nelles MJ: HCV testing in low-risk population. Lancet, 336: 695, 1990.

36. Marcellin P, Martinot-Peignoux M, Boyer N, Pouteau M, Aumont P, Erlinger S, Benhamou JP: Second generation (RIBA) test in diagnosis of chronic hepatitis C. Lancet, 337: 551-552, 1991.

37. van der Poel CL, Cuypers HTM, Reesink HW, Weiner AJ, Quan S, Di Nello R, van Boven JJP, Winkel I, Mulder-Folkerts D, Exel-Oehlers PJ, Schaasberg W, Leentvaar-Kuypers A, Polito A, Houghton M, Lelie PN: Confirmation of hepatitis C virus infection by new four-antigen recombinant immunoblot assay. Lancet, 337: 317-319, 1991.

38. Ebeling F, Naukkarinen R, Myllylä G, Leikola J: Second-generation RIBA to confirm diagnosis of HCV infection. Lancet, 337: 912-913, 1991.

39. Bassetti D, Cutrupi V, Dallago B, Alfonsi P: Second-generation RIBA to confirm diagnosis of HCV infection. Lancet, 337: 912, 1991.

40. Carman WF: The polymerase chain reaction. Quart J Med, 78: 195-203, 1991.

41. Zanetti AR, Tanzi E, Zehender G, Magni E, Incarbone C, Zonaro A, Primi D, Cariani E: Hepatitis C virus RNA in symptomless donors implicated in post-transfusion non-A, non-B hepatitis. Lancet, 336: 448, 1990.

42. Garson JA, Tuke PW, Makris M, Briggs M, Machin SJ, Preston FE, Tedder RS: Demonstration of viraemia patterns in haemophiliacs treated with hepatitis-C-virus contaminated factor VIII concentrates. Lancet, 336: 1022-1025, 1990.

43. Kato N, Yokosuka O, Omata M, Hosoda K, Ohto M: Detection of hepatitis C virus ribonucleic acid in the serum by amplification with polymerase chain reaction. J Clin Invest, 86: 1764-1767, 1990.

44. Ulrich PP, Romeo JM, Lane PK, Kelly I, Daniel LJ, Vyas GN: Detection, semiquantitation, and genetic variation in hepatitis C virus sequences amplified from the plasma of blood donors with elevated alanine aminotransferase. J Clin Invest, 86: 1609-1614, 1990.

45. Vaglia A, Nicolin R, Puro V, Ippolito G, Bettini C, de Lalla F: Needlestick hepatitis C virus seroconversion in a surgeon. Lancet, 336: 1315-1316, 1990.

46. Opolon P: Transmission sexuelle du virus de l'hépatite C. Gastroenterol Clin Biol, 14: 903-905, 1990.

47. Melbye M. Biggar RJ, Wantzin P, Krogsgaard K, Ebbesen P, Becker NG: Sexual transmission of hepatitis C virus: cohort study (1981-9) among European homosexual men. Br Med J, 301: 210-212, 1990.

48. Hess G, Massing A, Rossol S, Schütt H, Clemens R, Meyer zum Büschenfelde KH: Hepatitis C virus and sexual transmission. Lancet, II: 987, 1989.

49. Takamatsu K, Koyanagi Y, Okita K, Yamamoto N: Hepatitis C virus RNA in saliva. Lancet, 336: 1515, 1990.

50. Abe K, Inchauspe G: Transmission of hepatitis C by saliva. Lancet, 337: 248, 1991.

51. Idéo G, Bellati G, Pedraglio E, Bottelli, Donzelli T, Putignano G: Intrafamilial transmission of hepatitis C virus. Lancet, 335: 353, 1990.

52. Pérez-Romero M, Sanchez-Quijano A, Lissen E: Transmission of hepatitis C virus. Ann Int Med, 113: 411, 1990.

53. Everhart JE, Di Bisceglie AM, Murray LM, Alter HJ, Melpolder JJ, Kuo G, Hoofnagle JH: Risk for non-A, non-B (type C) hepatitis through sexual or household contact with chronic carriers. Ann Int Med, 112: 544-545, 1990.

54. Reesink HW, Wong VCW, Ip HMH, van der Poel CL, van Exel-Oehlers PJ, Lelie PN: Mother-to-infant transmission and hepatitis C virus. Lancet, 335: 1216-1217, 1990.

55. Giovannini M, Tagger A, Ribero ML, Zuccotti G, Pogliani L, Grossi A, Ferroni P, Fiocchi A: Maternal-infant transmission of hepatitis C virus and HIV infections: a possible interaction. Lancet, 335: 1166, 1990.

56. Editorial: Hepatitis C virus upstanding. Lancet, 335: 1431, 1990.

57. Janot C, Couroucé AM, Maniez M: Antibodies to hepatitis C virus in French blood donors. Lancet, II: 796-797, 1989.
58. Sirchia G, Bellobuono A, Giovanetti A, Marconi M: Antibodies to hepatitis C virus in Italian blood donors. Lancet, II: 797, 1989.
59. Ludlam CA, Chapman D, Cohen B, Litton PA: Antibodies to hepatitis C virus in haemophilia. Lancet, II: 294-297, 1989.
60. Mortimer PP, Cohen BJ, Litton PA, Vandervelde EM, Bassendine MF, Brind AM, Hambling MH: Hepatitis C virus antibody. Lancet, II: 798, 1989.
61. Murphy MF, Waters AH, Grint PCA, Hardiman AE, Lister TA: Hepatitis C infection in multitransfused patients with acute leukaemia. Lancet, 335: 58-59, 1990.
62. Wonke B, Hoffbrand AV, Brown D, Dusheiko G: Antibody to hepatitis C virus in multiply transfused patients with thalassaemia major. J Clin Pathol, 43: 638-640, 1990.
63. Colombo M, Kuo G, Choo QL, Donato MF, Del Ninno E, Tommasini MA, Dioguardi N, Houghton M: Prevalence of antibodies to hepatitis C-virus in Italian patients with hepatocellular carcinoma. Lancet, II: 1006-1008, 1989.
64. Kew MC, Houghton M, Choo QL, Kuo G: Hepatitis C virus antibodies in southern African blacks with hepatocellular carcinoma. Lancet, 335: 873-874, 1990.
65. Davis GL, Balart LA, Schiff ER, Lindsay K, Bodenheimer HC, Perrillo RP, Carey W, Jacobson IM, Payne J, Dienstag JL, VanThiel DH, Tamburro C, Lefkowitch J, Albrecht J, Meschievitz C, Ortego TJ, Gibas A: Hepatitis Interventional Therapy Group: Treatment of chronic hepatitis C with recombinant interferon alfa. N Engl J Med, 321: 1501-1506, 1989.
66. Di Bisceglie AM, Martin P, Kassianides C, Lisker-Melman M, Murray L, Waggoner J, Goodman Z, Banks SM, Hoofnagle JH: Recombinant interferon alfa therapy for chronic hepatitis C. N Engl J Med, 321: 1506-1510, 1989.
67. Koretz RL, Stone O, Mousa M, Gitnick GL: Non-A, non-B posttransfusion hepatitis - a decade later. Gastroenterology, 88: 1251-1254, 1985.
68. Realdi G, Alberti A, Rugge M, Rigoli AM, Tremolada F, Schivazappa L, Ruol A: Long-term follow-up of acute and chronic non-A, non-B post-transfusion hepatitis: evidence of progression to liver cirrhosis. Gut, 23: 270-275, 1982.
69. Marcellin P, Boyer N, Giostra E, Degott C, Couroucé, Degos F, Coppere H, Cales P, Couzigou P, Benhamou JP: Recombinant human α-interferon in patients with chronic non-A, non-B hepatitis: a multicenter randomized controlled trial from France. Hepatology, 13: 393-397, 1991.
70. Kanai K, Iwata K, Nakao K, Kako M, Okamoto H: Suppression of hepatitis C virus RNA by interferon-α. Lancet, 336: 245, 1990.
71. Castilla A, Prieto J, Fausto N: Transforming growth factors ß1 and α in chronic liver disease. Effects of interferon alfa therapy. N Engl J Med, 324: 933-940, 1991.
72. Di Bisceglie AM, Hoofnagle JH: Therapy of chronic hepatitis C with α-interferon. The answer? Or more questions? Hepatology, 13: 601-603, 1991.
73. Reichard O, Andersson J, Schvarz R, Weiland O: Ribavirin treatment for chronic hepatitis C. Lancet, 337: 1058-1961, 1991.
74. Dusheiko G, Dibisceglie A, Bowyer S, Sachs E, Richie M, Schoub B, Kew M: Recombinant leukocyte interferon treatment of chronic hepatitis B. Hepatology, 5: 556-560, 1985.
75. Vento S, Di Perri G, Luzzati R, Garofano T, Concia E, Bassetti D: Type 2 autoimmune hepatitis and hepatitis C virus infection. Lancet, 335: 921-922, 1990.
76. Jadoul M, Cornu Ch, Lamy ME, van Ypersele de Strihou C: Prevalence and clinical significance of hepatitis C virus antibodies in haemodialysis patients. Nephrol Dial Transpl, 5: 705, 1990.
77. Kallinowksi B, Theilmann L, Gmelin H, Rambausek M, Andrassy H, Mehls O, Moehring H, Ritz E: Prevalence of HCV antibodies in haemodialysis and kidney transplant patients. Nephrol Dial Transpl, 5: 706, 1990.
78. Vandelli L, Medici G, Savazzi AM, Lusvarghi E: Emergency of hepatitis C virus (HCV) infection in haemodialysis units: must the patients be dialysed in segregated sections? J Am Soc Nephrol, 1: 380, 1990.
79. Nishi T, Kurai K, Iino S, Kuwata S, Nosaka K, Kurokawa K: Hepatitis C virus antibodies among haemodialysis patients in Japan. Nephrol Dial Transpl, 5: 707, 1990.
80. Tamura I, Kobayashi Y, Koda T, Ichimura H, Kurimura O, Takasugi T, Kurimura T: Hepatitis C virus antibodies in haemodialysis patients. Lancet, 335: 1409, 1990.
81. Teruel JL, Maren R, Gamez C, Rivera M, Munoz RF, Celma ML, Ortuno J: Antibody to hepatitis C virus in patients on haemodialysis and after kidney transplantation. Nephrol Dial Transpl, 5: 714, 1990.

82. Yamaguchi K, Nishimura Y, Fukuoka N, Machida J, Ueda S, Kusumoto Y, Futami G, Ishii T, Takatsuki: Hepatitis C virus antibodies in haemodialysis patients. Lancet, 335: 1409-1410, 1990.
83. Susanna F, Tagariello G, Gaio G, Dugo M, Cascone C: Hepatitis C-virus prevalence and transmission in patients on regular dialytic treatment. Nephrol Dial Transpl, 5: 714, 1990.
84. Elisaf M, Tsianos E, Mavridis A, Pappas M, Masalas K, Siamopoulos KC: Antibodies against hepatitis C virus (anti-HCV) in haemodialysis patients: correlation with hepatitis B serologic markers. Nephrol Dial Transpl, 5: 701-702, 1990.
85. Couroucé AM, Chauveau Ph, Le Marrec N, Naret C, Delons S: Infection par le virus de l'hépatite C dans une unité d'hémodialyse parisienne. Presse Méd, 20: 609, 1991.
86. Gilli P, Moretti M, Soffritti D, Menini C: Anti-HCV positive patients in dialysis units? Lancet, 336: 243-244, 1990.
87. Jeffers LJ, Perez GO, De Medina MD, Ortiz-Interian CJ, Schiff ER, Reddy KR, Jimenez M, Bourgoignie JJ, Vaamonde CA, Duncan R, Houghton M, Choo GL, Kuo G: Hepatitis C infection in two urban hemodialysis units. Kidney Int, 38: 320-322, 1990.
88. Zeldis JB, Depner TA, Kuramoto IK, Gish RG, Holland PV: The prevalence of hepatitis C virus antibodies among hemodialysis patients. Ann Int Med, 112: 958-960, 1990.
89. Schlipköter U, Roggendorf M, Ernst G, Rasshofer R, Deinhardt F, Weise A, Gladziwa U, Luz N: Hepatitis C virus antibodies in haemodialysis patients. Lancet, 335: 1409, 1990.
90. Léon A, Canton R, Elia M, Mateos M: Second-generation RIBA to confirm diagnosis of HCV infection. Lancet, 337: 912, 1991.
91. Alonso MC, Novoa D, Romero R, Arcocha V, Sanchez-Guisande D: Antibodies to hepatitis C virus in patients on haemodialysis. Nephron, 57: 247, 1991.
92. Cariani E, Zonaro A, Primi D, Magni E, Incarbone C, Scalia P, Tanzi E, Zehender G, Zanetti AR: Detection of HCV-RNA and antibodies to HCV after needlestick injury. Lancet, 337: 850, 1991.
93. Schlipköter U, Roggendorf M, Cholmakow K, Weise A, Deinhardt F: Transmission of hepatitis C virus (HCV) from a haemodialysis patient to a medical staff member. Scand J Infect Dis, 22: 757-758, 1990.
94. Arici C, Gregis GP, Marchesi D, Mingardi G, Mecca G, Bellavita P: Effectiveness of a preventive programme for non-A, non-B hepatitis in a large dialysis unit. Nephrol Dial Transpl, 5: 902-903, 1990.
95. Gomez E, Aquado S, de Oña M, Martinez A, Cimadeville R, Sanchez L, Cago E, Alvarez-Grande. Hepatitis C virus antibodies in renal transplant patient. Nephrol Dial Transpl, 5: 748-749, 1990.
96. Ponz E, Andreu J, Bruguera M: Incidence and role of hepatitis C virus in liver disease of renal transplant recipients. Nephrol Dial Transpl, 5: 751, 1990.
97. Goffin E, Pirson Y, Cornu C, Lamy ME, van Ypersele de Strihou C: Prevalence and significance of anti-HCV antibodies in kidney graft recipients. Nephrol Dial Transpl 5: 1057-1058, 1990.
98. Roth D, Fernandez JA, Burke GW, Esquenazi V, Miller J: Detection of antibody to hepatitis C virus in renal transplant recipients. Transplantation, 51: 396-400, 1991.
99. Stempel CA, Lake JR, Vincenti FG. Hepatitis C: Prevalence in endstage renal failure patients and course after kidney transplant. J Am Soc Nephrol, 1: 772, 1990.
100. Otero J, Rodriguez M, Escudero D, Gomez E, Aguada S, de Oña M: Kidney transplants with positive anti-hepatitis virus C donors. Transplantation, 50: 1087-1088, 1990.
101. Mizrahi S, Hussey JL, Hayes DH, Boudreaux JP: Organ transplantation and hepatitis C virus infection. Lancet, 337: 1100, 1991.
102. Morales JM, Campo C, Castellanos G, Colina F, Fuertes A, Andres A, Moreno F, Prieto C, Rodicio JL: Clinical implications of the presence of antibody to hepatitis C positive after renal transplantation. Nephrol Dial Transpl, 5: 749, 1990.
103. Leads from the MMWR: Update: Universal precautions for prevention of transmission of human immunodeficiency virus, hepatitis B virus, and other bloodborne pathogens in health-care settings. JAMA, 260: 462-465, 1988.
104. Favero MS: Recommended precautions for patients undergoing hemodialysis who have AIDS or non-A, non-B hepatitis. Infection Control, 6: 301-305, 1985.
105. Fahey BJ, Koziol DE, Banks SM, Henderson DK: Frequency of nonparenteral occupational exposures to blood and body fluids before and after universal precautions training. Am J Med, 90: 145-153, 1991.

Chapter 13

NEW DEVELOPMENTS IN CONTINUOUS ARTERIOVENOUS HEMOFILTRATION/DIALYSIS

RAVINDRA L. MEHTA

Division of Nephrology, Department of Medicine, University of California San Diego, San Diego, California 92103, USA

INTRODUCTION

There is a growing consensus that continuous renal replacement therapy (1-4) is preferable to intermittent renal replacement in treating patients with acute renal failure (ARF). Continuous therapies are not associated with the rapid "unphysiologic" shifts in fluid and solutes which characterize intermittent hemodialysis (IHD). Conventional IHD utilizes diffusion based transport of solutes and fluid across cellulose acetate and cuprophane membranes. New membranes which use polysulphone, polyacrylonitrile or polyamide as the basic material are more permeable than IHD membranes and have a higher molecular weight cut off for enhanced clearance of middle molecules (5). Alternate renal replacement therapies have evolved with the availability of these membranes (6). Continuous ArterioVenous Hemofiltration/HemoDialysis (CAVH/CAVHD) is a new therapy rapidly gaining acceptance worldwide as the treatment of choice for ARF in critically ill, hemodynamically unstable, patients (7-10). This review describes the current status and discusses new developments of these techniques.

EVOLUTION AND NOMENCLATURE

Although the concept of continuous dialysis was advocated as early as 1960 by Scribner and his colleagues (11), *Intermittent HemoDialysis* (IHD) became the standard therapy and remains the commonest form of treatment for ARF. *Peritoneal dialysis* was the first form of continuous renal replacement (CAPD, CCPD) and became available largely because of its highly permeable natural membrane. While useful for chronic renal replacement, its utility in ARF is limited (12). All continuous renal replacement methods

271

use membranes highly permeable to water and low molecular weight solutes. In its most basic form, termed *Slow Continuous Ultra-Filtration* (SCUF), fluid is removed by ultrafiltration. The ultrafiltrate has the composition of normal plasma and is not replaced. Solute clearance is minimal. SCUF is used predominantly for fluid management in patients undergoing cardiac surgery (13). In *Continuous ArterioVenous Hemofiltration* (CAVH), the ultrafiltrate removed is replaced by a solution with an electrolyte composition similar to that of plasma (14). Net fluid removal is determined by the amount of replacement fluid administered. One modification to improve clearance of small molecules, *Continuous Arterio-Venous Hemo-Dialysis* (CAVHD), incorporates diffusive transport by circulating dialysis fluid through the filter using gravity, thereby enhancing solute clearances (15). In standard CAVHD as described by Geronemus et al (15), fluid removal is tailored to individual requirements and a replacement fluid is not generally used. Solute clearances are thus more dependent on diffusive transport and less on convective transfer. *Continuous Arterio-Venous Hemo-DiaFiltration* (CAVHDF) further enhances ultrafiltration rates and maintains fluid balance by adjusting the amount of replacement fluid, thereby maximizing convective and diffusive mechanisms for solute clearance (16).

Table 1. Continuous renal replacement therapy: comparison of techniques.

	SCUF	CAVH	CVVH	CAVHD	CAVHDF	CVVHD
Access	A-V	A-V	V-V	A-V	A-V	V-V
Pump	No	No	Yes	No	No	Yes
Dialysate	No	No	No	Yes	Yes	Yes
Filtrate (ml/hr)	100	600	1000	300	600	800
Filtrate (l/day)	2.4	14.4	24	7.2	14.4	19.2
Replace. fluid (l/day)	0	12	21.6	4.8	12	16.8
Urea clearance (ml/min))	1.7	10	16.7	21.7	26.7	30
Simplicity (*)	4	3	2	3	3	2
Cost (°)	1	2	4	3	3	4

(*) 1 = least simple; 4 = most simple
(°) 1 = Least expensive; 4 = most expensive

If adequate arterial access is not available, the external blood pumps used in standard hemodialysis machines can provide the driving force and permit veno-venous access for blood delivery to the hemofilter. Counterparts of the above techniques are *Continuous Veno-Venous Hemofiltration* (CVVH) (17) (similar to CAVH), *Continuous Veno-Venous Hemo-Dialysis* (CVVHD) (18) (which simulates CAVHD), and *Continuous Veno-Venous*

Hemo-DiaFiltration (CVVHDF) (19) (which is similar to CAVHDF). Blood pumps permit continuous therapy in patients with poor arterial access but add complexity and cost to an otherwise simple procedure. Table 1 summarizes the key features of the above techniques.

Simpson et al (20) used a continuous, volumetrically controlled, machine-driven ultrafiltration device with continuous bicarbonate hemodialysis across a polysulphone membrane and termed the process *Continuous Ultrafiltration Plus Intermittent hemo-Dialysis* (CUPID). Hombrouckx et al (21) described *Go Slow-Dialysis*, which uses a single-needle blood pump with a blood flow of 80 ml/min and a closed recirculating low volume bicarbonate dialysate system to dialyze patients for 8-12 hours per day. Neither method has yet gained wide acceptance.

OPERATIONAL CHARACTERISTICS

All continuous renal replacement therapies seek to use highly permeable membranes to filter large volumes of fluid at relatively low pressures (5). The hemofilter offers a low resistance to blood flow and the driving force for ultrafiltration is the mean arterial pressure (MAP) of the patient, which is opposed by the oncotic pressure. Net filtration is dependent on the transmembrane pressure (TMP) difference generated. The generation of a TMP gradient within the filter is influenced by several factors including a patient's mean arterial pressure, serum protein concentrations, hematocrit and the length of the filtrate column (5). In general the goal is to minimize the hydrostatic pressure drop across the filter by using a large bore access and short lines. Ultrafiltration is also optimized by adjusting the filtrate bag height and reducing oncotic pressure and viscosity within the filter. Some recent investigations in this area are described below.

Component modifications

ACCESS

Blood flow is determined by hemodynamic status of the patient, site and type of vascular access (catheter, Scribner shunt, A-V fistula), and diameter of the device being used (22, 23). Olbricht et al (22) found blood flows were higher and overall pressure drop across the filter was smaller (70 ± 13 mm Hg) for femoral artery catheters as compared to a Scribner shunt (90 ± 12 mm Hg), confirming that femoral arterial access appears to be preferable. Ahmad (24) developed longer term access by externally connecting two catheters tunneled subcutaneously into the femoral artery and vein respectively. Venous access can be via single or double lumen catheters in the femoral or subclavian vein. A double lumen catheter offers flexibility for use in hemodialysis if CAVHD is discontinued (16).

MEMBRANE CHARACTERISTICS AND FILTER DESIGN

A variety of membranes are currently available in different configurations (5). Several investigators studied the role of filter design on filter performance. Yohay et al (25) compared the effect of filter geometry in CAVHD and found that parallel plate AN-69 dialyzer provided similar ultrafiltration rates but better diffusive clearance than the larger polyamide FH66 hollow fibers. When the resistance of the AN-69 0.6 m^2 PAN membrane was compared to a 0.23 m^2 polysulphone capillary dialyzer, the capillary geometry resulted in higher resistances (26). Ronco et al (27) found that an increase in the inner diameter of a polysulphone hollow fiber from 200 μ to 250 μ resulted in a 39% increase in blood flow with similar filtration rates, fewer clotting problems and lower heparin requirements. These data suggest that flat plate configuration offers less resistance to blood flow and may require less anticoagulation.

Ultrafiltration rates tend to decrease with time even when other factors are constant (28). First attributed to a decline in filter permeability, possibly related to protein coating the membrane, it now appears that permeability decay is not related to membrane protein exposure but depends on membrane characteristics (29). A large exponential decay in permeability within the first 6 hours is followed by a more gradual decay. Polysulphone membrane permeability appears to decrease most markedly, both initially and in later periods, while PAN and polyamide membranes have minimal decays after the initial decline. Other investigators (22) also demonstrated that hydraulic membrane permeability (Lp) significantly affects ultrafiltration rates; polyamide membranes had a higher Qf than polysulphone membranes. So, if the primary indication is fluid removal, a polyamide or polysulphone membrane would suffice, but if solute control is desired, a membrane with better diffusive characteristics [such as AN-69 (PAN)] is preferable.

Operational enhancements

FLUID BALANCE

Continuous therapy removes large volumes of fluid with relative ease even in hemodynamically unstable patients. Two approaches can be used to adjust the ultrafiltration rate. We maintain ultrafiltration rates of 8-12 ml/min by varying the length of the filtrate column (16); others regulate filtrate volume by a peristaltic pump placed on the dialysate outflow line (28). The former method is simple but requires more monitoring; the latter adds another pump to the system but maintains more consistent ultrafiltration rates. In CAVH and CAVHDF net fluid balance is achieved by varying the amount of replacement fluid administered. Replacement fluid always lags behind reconstitution of plasma volume, so there is a potential for volume depletion. Flow sheets can minimize this problem but this is labor intensive. Several new systems automate fluid balancing and allow for real time replacement of filtrate removed. Amicon's Equaline system (Amicon publication # 261) uses two load cells (one for the infusate and one for the filtrate) to continually provide weight data to a microprocessor programmed to control infusion rate. This system provides accurate real time fluid replacement, but was designed for CAVH and not CAVHD or CAVHDF, both of which require dialysate infusions. Additionally, the load cells are sensitive and lose their accuracy if bumped. Other balancing devices are used (30, 31) and other investigators (32, 33) have developed a computer operated system which gives graphical information of fluid balance.

SOLUTE CLEARANCES

Siegler at al (28) significantly enhanced our current understanding of the processes involved in solute removal in continuous renal replacement systems. In CAVH, solutes are removed purely by convective transport (5); additional diffusive transfer is added in CAVHD and CAVHDF (15). The total solute clearance in CAVHD and CAVHDF is the sum of the convective and diffusive clearances (28). Since the molecular weight cut off for the membranes is >20,000 daltons, most low and middle molecular weight substances have sieving coefficients (SC) of 1. Clearance is = Qf x SC for most middle molecules and is directly proportional to the amount of filtrate produced. Small molecules are less dependent on convective clearance and are more effectively transferred by diffusion (7). CAVHD and CAVHDF dialysate flow rates are between 16.7-33.2 ml/min (1-2 l/hr), which is much lower than blood flow rate (50-120 ml/min). This allows for complete saturation of the dialysate fluid with solutes. Thus the limiting factor for solute removal by diffusion is the dialysate flow rate and not the blood flow rate as is with conventional hemodialysis. Blood flow rates are not limiting until they are below 50 ml/min (34). Dialysate flow rates of up to 3 l/hr do not appear to affect the ultrafiltration rate in spite of higher pressure within the dialysate compartment. Such low dialysate flow rates usually prevent backfiltration of fluid to the blood compartment (35).

Several methods enhance solute clearance in CAVH. Kaplan (36) demonstrated that suction applied to the ultrafiltrate port enhanced filtrate volumes, increased effective filter life and was even more efficacious in conjunction with predilution. Replacement fluid administered prefilter dilutes blood prior to entry in the filter. This reduces the viscosity of blood within the filter, promotes superior filtration rates and increases urea clearances by facilitating transfer of BUN from the intraerythrocytic compartment. If an external pump is applied to the circuit (as in CVVH), the limitation of low ultrafiltration rates is overcome as 20-40 liters of filtrate can be easily produced in 24 hours (17). This method requires adequate monitoring to prevent volume depletion and air embolism. Dialysate used across the membrane markedly improves clearances and retains the simplicity of the procedure. Solute clearances can be further enhanced in CAVHD by increasing the dialysate flow rate to 2 l/hr (37); predilution with traditional CAVHD enhances convective and diffusive solute transport, resulting in CAVHDF. Using this method we have had mean BUN clearances in the range of 23-30 ml/min even in hypotensive patients (38). Other investigators reported similarly good results with CAVHDF. The advantage of this approach over CAVHD is that convective transfer contributes to middle molecule clearance, an important factor in removing mediators seen in ARF [such as tumor necrosis factor (TNF) and Interleukin 1 (IL1)] (38, 39).

DRUG CLEARANCES

The disposition of drugs in patients on CAVH largely depends on the sieving coefficient of the drug, the degree of protein binding, and the ultrafiltration rate since convective transfer is the main mechanism of solute removal. Several investigators described the pharmacokinetics of different drugs in CAVH and developed guidelines for dosing (40-42). Davies et al (37) measured the effect of dialysate flow rates on the removal of some of the commoner drugs in patients on CAVHD. They found that increasing dialysate flow rate from 1 to 2 liters per hour did not make a significant impact on clearance of most antibiotics. Other investigators found that clearances of theophylline, phenytoin, digoxin and vancomycin were progressively enhanced when dialysate flow rates were increased from 5 ml/min to 16.7 ml/min (43). Slugg et al (44) and others (45, 46) found that higher doses of vancomycin are required for both CAVH and CAVHD but no major kinetic differences appeared between CAVH and CAVHD. Tobramycin removal is well documented in CAVH (47) and in CAVHD appears to depend more on the Qf than on dialysate flow rate (48). The effect of these therapies on newer antibiotics was also studied (49, 50). Table 2 lists current recommendations on drug dosing in CAVHD.

276

Table 2. Effect of dialysate flow (Qd) on drug clearance (Cl) in CAVHD (*).

Drug	Qd 1 l/hr Cl (ml/min)	Qd 2 l/hr Cl (ml/min)	Recommended dose (mg/hr)
Cefuroxime	13.97	16.22	500-700/12
Ceftazidime	13.11	15.24	1000/24
Ciprofloxacin	16.31	19.93	200/8
Vancomycin	11.70	15.60	1000/48
Tobramycin	11.10	14.85	60-80/24
Gentamicin	20.50	25.90	80-100/24
Doxycycline	6.99	12.11	200/24

(*) Modified from Davies et al (37).

Anticoagulation

Insufficient anticoagulation leads to deterioration of filter performance and eventual clotting (51, 52), contributing to blood loss, while excessive anticoagulation may cause bleeding complications. The oldest and most frequently used anticoagulant in continuous dialysis procedures is heparin. Various other alternatives are now available and their relative advantages will be discussed.

HEPARIN

Heparin remains the most common anticoagulant used for continuous therapies (53). Its effects in CAVH are relatively localized to the circuit in contrast to its use in conventional machine dialysis, where anticoagulation occurs in the systemic circulation and the extracorporeal circuit (52). These differences may be due to the lower blood flow rate in CAVH; also, heparin is more likely to be removed across the filter's more permeable membrane as compared to conventional dialysis. Heparin doses depend on the presence or absence of coagulation abnormalities secondary to the underlying illness (52). We modified the basic protocol for heparin dosing (53) and use the circuit shown in Figure 1a. The filter is primed with 2 liters of saline containing 2400 U heparin. After a bolus of 5-10 U/kg b.w., heparin is infused pre-filter at 3-12 U/kg b.w./hr to maintain activated clotting times (ACT) between 200-250 seconds post-filter (for minimal changes in systemic PTT without any major impact on filter longevity) (16). In neonates Ronco et al (54) used a loading dose of 100 U/kg b.w. and maintained continuous infusion at 5-7 U/kg b.w./hr. Post-filter ACT's simplify monitoring and allow immediate comparison to PTT determinations. We found more filter clotting if post-filter ACT's were much below 200 seconds because of reduced blood flow rates. Major side effects of heparin are excessive bleeding [up to 30% (2)], thrombocytopenia and allergic reactions. If complications occur, heparin can sometimes be continued in markedly reduced doses, although usually non-heparin anticoagulation must be considered especially when thrombocytopenia develops (55).

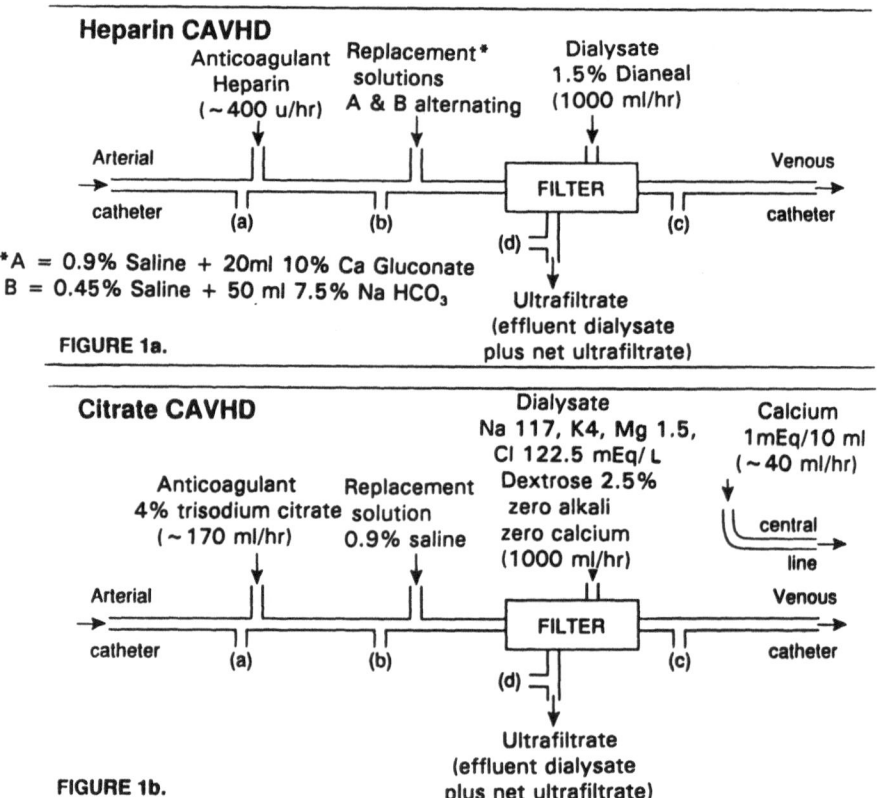

Figure 1. Comparison of circuit diagrams for heparin CAVHD (Figure 1a) and citrate CAVHD (Figure 1b). Sampling ports are marked (a) peripheral, (b) pre-filter, (c) post-filter, and (d) ultrafiltrate. See text for details [Reproduced from Mehta RL, McDonald BR, Aguilar MM, Ward DM: Regional citrate anticoagulation for continuous arteriovenous hemodialysis in critically ill patients. Kidney Int, 38: 976-981, 1990, with permission].

LOW MOLECULAR WEIGHT (LMW) HEPARIN

Regular heparin used clinically has several fractions with different molecular weights ranging from 4,000-50,000. Heparin's inhibiting effect on thrombin (measured by PTT) decreases with decreasing molecular weight, while Factor Xa (FXa) inhibition increases.

278

Heparin's antithrombotic activity depends on FXa inhibition and an increased PTT is associated with enhanced bleeding risk; low molecular weight heparin should improve the ratio between desirable antithrombotic effects and undesirable bleeding risk. This supposition led to separation by fractionation of low molecular weight (LMW) heparin (4000 to 7000 daltons). When LMW heparin was tested in conventional dialysis patients, it decreased complication rates (56-58) but experiences with LMW heparin as an anticoagulant in continuous therapy are few to date. Hory et al (59) treated two ARF patients with CAVH and LMW heparin (Fraxiparin R). The resulting anti-FXa activity indicated a successful antithrombotic effect. Wynckel et al (60) used enoxaparin in seven ARF patients treated with slow continuous hemodialysis (pump driven). Hemodialysis lasted from 26-120 hours. A 40 mg initial dose was followed by intermittent infusions of 10-40 mg every 4-6 hours. There were no bleeding episodes or thrombocytopenia; one episode of thrombosis occurred due to technical reasons. The half-life of LMW heparin is approximately twice that of unfractionated heparin. Effectiveness is monitored by a chromogenic test to measure anti-FXa activity. The anti-Fxa level should lie between 0.2 and 0.3 (or 0.4) IU/ml for patients with bleeding risk, and between 0.5 and 1.0 IU/ml for patients without bleeding risk (58). Neutralization of LMW heparin by protamine is reduced. Since PTT and thrombin times are not elevated, the PTT test is not useful. LMW heparin may have a role in continuous renal replacement therapy, but disadvantages include inadequate experience in continuous dialysis, reduced neutralization by protamine and few facilities able to monitor anti-Xa levels. Also dose recommendations of LMW heparin vary, depending on the manufacturer, and are not interchangeable (56, 57).

REGIONAL HEPARINIZATION AND NEUTRALIZATION WITH PROTAMINE

Heparin's anticoagulative effect can be neutralized by protamine (protamine hydrochloride), a basic protein and 1000 IU heparin is inactivated by 1 ml protamine 1000 (Roche). Protamine is an antithromboplastin with an anticoagulative effect in high doses (61). Kaplan and Petrillo (62) treated ten ARF patients with CAVH and regional heparin neutralization with protamine. Seven patients had preexisting coagulopathies (PTT >43 or platelets <50,000). After heparinization, the blood in the filter displayed an elevated PTT of >150 seconds, but systemic values did not differ significantly from pre-treatment values. Nevertheless, hemorrhaging was reported in two patients. Kaplan (62) used regional heparinization almost exclusively and found it a simple and easily monitored method. Other investigators have not attempted it extensively because protamine doses require meticulous

279

adjustment and it has potential side effects. Regional heparinization is an alternative but requires careful monitoring.

HEPARIN-FREE ANTICOAGULATION

Heparin-free anticoagulation in intermittent hemodialysis using saline flushes has been used previously and filter patency maintained (63, 64). Experience with heparin-free anticoagulation in non-pumped continuous therapy has not been very encouraging. Kaplan et al (3) dispensed with heparinization completely in CAVH patients with preexisting platelet counts of <100,000 platelets/mm^3 and elevated PTT. With pre-dilution, filter function could be maintained for up to 58 hours without anticoagulation. Geronemus et al (15) found that filters clot within 24 hours, and we had similar results in our series [median filter life of 16 hours for filters maintained with saline flushes (16)]. Saline flushes are best used with CAVHD at a dialysate flow rate of 2 liters/hour to maximize solute clearance during filter patency.

REGIONAL CITRATE ANTICOAGULATION

Citrate is an anticoagulant by virtue of its ability to chelate calcium. The anticoagulant effect is overwhelmed and neutralized when citrated blood from the extracorporeal circuit returns and mixes with central venous blood. Citrate has been used for conventional hemodialysis (65, 66), but not previously for CAVHD. Our method for using citrate anticoagulation in CAVHD (16) is depicted in Figure 1b. Four percent trisodium citrate solution is infused pre-filter at approximately 3-7% of blood flow rate, initially 170 ml/hr (range 100-200 ml/hr). Citrate flow rate is adjusted to maintain post-filter ACT at 200-250 seconds. Dialysis solution consists of zero calcium, zero alkali dialysate at a flow rate of 1 l/hr. Ten percent CaCl$_2$ is infused in a separate line to replace chelated calcium. The calcium and alkali free dialysate permits removal of calcium-citrate chelate. The majority of the citrate is free within the filter and both free and complexed citrate are effectively removed across the filter (67). A hyponatremic dialysate allows removal of the sodium load imposed by the trisodium citrate. Hourly ultrafiltration rates are maintained between 400-800 ml/hr. Desired fluid balance is attained by infusing 0.9% saline as replacement fluid pre-filter.

In our comparison of citrate (CIT-CAVHD) versus heparin (HEP-CAVHD) anticoagulation for more than 4000 hours of continuous therapy (68), we found the citrate group had significantly higher ultrafiltration rates and urea clearances than the heparin group [CIT-CAVHD mean urea clearance = 23.5 ml/min vs HEP-CAVHD mean urea clearance = 19.9 ml/min (p = 0.003)]. Both groups had adequate anticoagulation as evidenced by ACT and PTT determinations. The mean filter life for CIT-CAVHD (62.4 hrs) was superior to HEP-CAVHD (45.4 hrs) but was not statistically significant (p = 0.07). When all filters were considered, 72 hr patency was 40% for CIT-CAVHD vs 25% for HEP-CAVHD filters. Three (30%) HEP-CAVHD patients had serious bleeding and one developed heparin-induced thrombocytopenia. No bleeding or thrombocytopenia occurred with CIT-CAVHD. The major problems with citrate were transient metabolic alkalosis which developed in six patients (26%). This was easily corrected by infusion of 0.2 M HCl through a central vein. Peripheral ionized calcium levels ranged between 0.84 to 1.24 mmol/l in most patients and no patient developed symptomatic hypocalcemia. There was no evidence of EKG changes or myocardial depression. CIT-CAVHD allows adequate anticoagulation and the procedure is well tolerated by most patients, including those with hepatic insufficiency who metabolize citrate despite significant deterioration in liver function. The trade-offs of citrate vs heparin are increased complexity of the citrate procedure and higher risk of metabolic alkalosis in patients. This citrate anticoagulation protocol should also be applicable to pumped systems, such as CVVHD.

PROSTACYCLIN ANALOGUES

A metabolite of arachidonic acid, PGI_2, inhibits aggregation and adhesion of platelets by increasing adenylate cyclase activity and thereby increasing platelet cyclic-AMP levels. (69). Thus, contact with non-endothelial surfaces (e.g. dialysis membrane) does not result in degranulation and subsequent platelet aggregation. PGI_2 has a relaxing effect on the vascular muscles and a half-life of 2 minutes (51). PGI_2 has been used as an anticoagulant in chronic hemodialysis patients (51, 70, 71), but information on prostacyclin and its analogues in continuous therapy is limited. Zobel et al (72) treated 6 children with high bleeding risk with CAVH, and combined heparin (2.5-5 IU/kg b.w./min) and prostacyclin (4-8 ng/kg b.w./min) for anticoagulation. Urea clearance after 24 hrs was higher and filter life was longer than in patients treated with heparin alone. Bleeding, thrombosis or hypotension did not occur. Stevens et al (73) similarly used a combination of heparin and prostacyclin for anticoagulation in CAVHD. No studies have been reported on administering solely prostacyclin as an anticoagulant in CAVH/CAVHD. Journois et al (74) combined PGI_2 and LMW heparin. In comparison to standard heparin in 42 CVVH treatments, they found that the combination enhanced filter longevity by 55%. Similarly, Ponikvar et al (75) used prostacyclin at 5 ng/kg b.w./min in 7 patients for 630 hours of

CVVH and observed no alteration in hemodynamic stability. Prostacyclin appears to be a viable alternative to heparin in pumped systems, but is likely to be more expensive. For CAVH and CAVHD, most centers have used prostacyclin in combination with heparin. Prostacyclin administration can be monitored by measuring the ADP-stimulated platelet aggregation. The procedure must be calibrated individually for each patient, complicating the monitoring for intensive care patients. Limitations for this method are the high incidence of hypotension and lack of a specific antagonist. If preliminary results from Ota et al (76) regarding a prostacyclin derivative without hypotensive side effects are confirmed, the major argument against routine application of PGI_2 in CAVH procedures would be eliminated.

NAFOMOSTAT MESILATE

Serine proteinase inhibitors such as Gabexate mesilate have been used to reduce the risk of bleeding in hemodialysis patients (77). It was found to result in lesser transfusion requirements as compared to heparin in high risk patients. Nafomostat mesilate is a similar proteinase inhibitor with a molecular weight of 540 which has anticoagulative properties by virtue of its inhibition of thrombin and factor Xa and factor XIIa. Ohtake et al (78) described its use in CAVH and CAVHD. They administered it in a dose of 0.1 mg/kg b.w./hr and found a good correlation between this dose and the ACT levels. Bleeding incidence was as high as 67% in heparin anticoagulation, 29% for low molecular weight heparin and 5% for nafomostat mesilate. Although it appears that there is a reduction in bleeding, filter patency duration and filter efficacy parameters were not described. At the present time this method has limited utility.

Factors affecting anticoagulation in continuous renal replacement

Factors influencing the choice of an anticoagulant include its antithrombotic and hemorrhagic effects. The antithrombotic effect should be high, and the risk of hemorrhaging low. Drug action should be brief and ideally limited to the blood in the filter. Drug monitoring should be easy and suited for bedside use in the intensive care unit. Long-term treatment must be without severe systemic side effects. An antagonistic drug should be available in case of overdose. Table 3 summarizes the advantages and drawbacks of current anticoagulation methods in continuous therapies. The choice of anticoagulant depends on [a] the access site and whether an external pump is being used; [b] the nature and geometry of the membrane; [c] whether enhancements for ultrafiltration such as predilution are used; and [d] the clinical status of the patient and preexisting coagulation abnormalities. Since anticoagulation in continuous therapy is for a longer duration than in intermittent hemodialysis, careful selection and monitoring are essential to prevent complications.

Table 3. Anticoagulation modalities for continuous renal replacement.

Method	Filter Prime	Initial Dose	Maintenance Dose	Monitoring	Advantages	Disadvantages
Saline solution	2l saline	150-250 ml pre-filter	100-250 ml/hr pre-filter	Visual check	No anticoagulant used	Poor filter patency
Heparin	2,500-10,000	5-10 U/kg	3-12/kg/hr	ACT 200-250; PTT	Standard method	Bleeding risk
LMW heparin	2l saline	40 mg	10-40 mg/6hr	Factor Xa levels; maintained between 0.1-0.41 U/ml	Decreased risk of bleeding	Special monitoring; not available everywhere
Regional heparin	2500 U/2l saline	5-10 U/kg	3-12 U/kg/hr + protamine post-filter	PTT; post-filter ACT 200-250	reduced bleeding risk	complex; risk of thrombo-cytopenia; protamine effects; hypotension
Regional citrate	2l saline	4% trisodium citrate 150-180 ml/hr	100-180 ml/hr 3-7% of BFR Ca replaced by central line	ACT: 200-250 maintain ionized calcium 0.96-1.2 mmol/l	no bleeding; no thrombocyto-penia; improved filter efficacy, longevity	complex; needs Ca monitoring; alkalosis
Prosta-cyclin	2l saline + heparin	Heparin 2-4 U/kg	4-8 ng/kg/min	ACT,PTT, Platelet aggregation	reduced heparinization	needs heparin addition; hypotension
Nafomo-stat mesilate	2l saline	----------	0.1 mg/kg/hr	ACT	no heparin	new procedure; filter efficacy?

ACT = Activated Clotting Time; BFR = Blood Flow Rate

Monitoring of anticoagulation adequacy

Adequacy of anticoagulation should be monitored by continuous evaluation of the circuit and filter patency. Some signs of clotting include [a] a sustained (>3 hrs) reduction

283

in the volume of ultrafiltrate to less than 150-200 ml/hr not attributable to changes in hemodynamic status; [b] an alteration in the ratio of fluid urea nitrogen (FUN) to blood urea nitrogen (BUN) of <0.6, as under optimal operating conditions this should equal 1 (34); [c] coolness and darkening of the arterial and venous lines; [d] separation of serum from cells in the blood lines. Periodic monitoring of the post-filter ACT or PTT is necessary to assess anticoagulation efficacy. We routinely use the post-filter ACT's to adjust anticoagulation dosing and also check the FUN/BUN ratio every 12 hours. If this ratio is below 0.6 we change the filter as it suggests impending filter clotting. In this setting it is possible to use the filter for a few more hours but efficacy is markedly reduced. Early recognition of filter dysfunction is thus an important consideration.

INDICATIONS AND CONTRAINDICATIONS

Continuous therapies provide all of the common features of intermittent hemodialysis but are best utilized in the intensive care unit setting. Since fluid and solute removal can be controlled easily and are done continuously, these methods have a significant advantage in the hemodynamically unstable patient. In addition to providing renal replacement, these techniques permit unlimited fluid administration thereby allowing nutritional repletion in critically ill patients. Patients with ARF in the presence of multiple organ failure, sepsis, burns, cardiogenic shock are all likely to be better managed with these methods. Cosentino et al (79) recently described their results in a randomized trial of CAVH in adult respiratory distress syndrome and reported a trend of enhanced survival in CAVH recipients. CAVH has a particular advantage in reducing intracranial pressure in patients with oliguric ARF with fulminant hepatic failure as CAVH is more gradual and less likely to produce hypotension and reduced cerebral perfusion pressure (80). There has been some interest in combining continuous therapies with other methods of solute removal [such as hemoperfusion (81) and plasmapheresis (82)] to treat sepsis and multiple organ failure without the traditional indication of ARF. Initial results appear promising but using these methods for treating the sepsis syndrome remains experimental.

Although absence of adequate arterial access is a significant contraindication, pumped systems should be usable in this setting once they are developed further. Since large volumes of fluid can be removed quickly, meticulous monitoring is essential and requires a nurse-to-patient ratio of at least 1:1. These procedures are difficult to perform in the non-intensive care unit setting and are not recommended for the patient with uncomplicated ARF. Complications associated with continuous therapies are mostly due to the potential for volume depletion, particularly if monitoring is inadequate and calculations inaccurate.

Access related problems include peripheral embolism and dissection, resulting in limb ischemia with arterial catheters. Fortunately, this is rare but arterial catheters should be of an appropriate size and be placed by experienced personnel (22). Connections should be taped to prevent accidental disconnection.

RESULTS WITH CONTINUOUS THERAPIES

Continuous renal replacement modalities have been available for at least a decade but are not yet widely used. This is because these techniques are new, there is a learning curve and there is a lack of controlled comparisons with intermittent hemodialysis. As the techniques evolve results must be considered in the following categories: [a] the efficiency of these modalities to achieve solute and fluid balance; [b] effect on the nutritional status and [c] the impact on overall patient outcome.

[a] Efficacy

Several investigators have utilized CAVH to treat ARF in the intensive care unit setting. Over the last 10 years the procedure has been done in over 600 ARF patients for periods ranging from a few hours to several days (83). The majority of these investigators reported minimal difficulty in achieving fluid balance; however, solute balances were controlled only when high ultrafiltrate volumes could be maintained. In some patients CAVH is inadequate for small solute removal (10, 14) and in maintaining BUN concentrations below 120-150 mg/dl in severely catabolic patients. This is because the clearance achieved by CAVH is largely dependent on convective transport of solutes. Better solute clearances and metabolic control have been reported for CAVHD in comparison to CAVH (7, 84, 85). Seigler et al (28) studied solute transport characteristics in 15 critically ill patients treated with CAVHD and found whole blood clearances of urea, creatinine and phosphate averaged 25.3, 24.1 and 21.3 ml/min, respectively. These clearances are a marked improvement over those achieved with CAVH alone (BUN 8.1 ml/min) or CAVH with predilution replacement solution and suction (18 ml/min) (36). Pattison et al (86) were able to maintain BUN levels at 40-60 mg/dl and serum creatinine 1.4-4.0 mg/dl in hypercatabolic ARF patients. Similarly other investigators (8, 9, 73) used CAVHD to achieve solute and volume control and provide adequate nutrition in patients with multiple organ failure. In our experience CAVHDF provides better fluid and solute control than CAVHD. We have routinely achieved solute control with urea clearances ranging from 23-30 ml/min in hypercatabolic patients (16).

285

Table 4. Summary of results with CAVH (CVVH) for acute renal failure.

Author	Year	Ref. #	Patients	% Survival
Kramer	1981	1	20	40
Olbricht	1982	109	34	26
Kaplan	1984	3	15	27
Klehr	1985	110	182	22
Domoto	1985	111	36	25
Frisch	1986	112	27	41
Bartlett	1986	94	32	28
Mault	1987	113	61	18
Lieberman	1987	114	23	35
Paganini	1988	13	20	19
Weiss	1989	4	100	45
Wendon	1989	17	(28)	(52)
Alarabi	1990	115	112	52
Scherier	1990	117	49	35
Sluiter	1990	118	89	44
Zobel	1990	119	32 (15)	63 (27)
Bishof	1990	89	4	50
Canaud	1990	120	(32)	(16)
Korner	1990	121	(15)	(40)

Both CAVH and CAVHD have been used successfully in children (87) and have been associated with an improvement in pulmonary gas exchange in combined renal and respiratory failure (88). CAVHD was found to be more efficacious than CAVH in managing ARF in critically ill children (89). Zobel and co-investigators (90) reported their experience with 5 different A-V replacement modalities in 23 pediatric patients. Urea clearances were 5.6 ± 2.1 ml/min/m^2 for CAVH and 15.3 ± 3.7 ml/min/m^2 for CAVHD. Other investigators used this technique successfully in select patient populations, including those with congenital heart disease (91), hyperammonemia (92) and severe hyperkalemia (93).

[b] Effect on nutrition

Continuous therapies have a major advantage over intermittent hemodialysis in permitting unlimited nutrition as fluid removal is not a limiting factor. Bartlett et al (94) found that nutritional status was better in patients on CAVH and this factor may result in an improvement in survival. Similarly Chima et al (95) found that nutritional status improved in all 16 patients on CAVH, although 14 were in negative nitrogen balance. In our experience CAVHDF allowed better nutritional support and we were able to match or exceed the nutritional goals for patients treated with this modality; this was not possible in patients on intermittent hemodialysis (96). Other investigators have had similar results (88, 97). In the overall nutritional balance of the patient two other factors need to be recognized. The dialysate fluid used in CAVHD has 1.5-2.5% glucose which can be absorbed during the procedure (154-270 grams/day) and which contributes to the caloric load (28, 98). This must be considered in the nutritional prescription. A second factor is the loss of amino acids across the filter which ranges from 2.7 to 8.9 g/day at low infusion rates (i.e. when <102 grams of amino acids are infused per 24 hrs) and reaches 30 grams at higher infusion rates (i.e. when >102 grams of amino acids are infused per 24 hours) (99). Losses appear to depend more on the serum levels than the underlying clinical status of the patient (100).

Table 5. Summary of results with CAVHD (CVVHD) for acute renal failure.

Author	Year	Ref. #	Patients	% Survival
Schneider	1988	7	41	24
Pattison	1988	86	5	40
Barzilay	1988	122	6	50
Gibney	1988	8	15	33
Stevens	1988	73	36	31
Tam	1988	108	(16)	(56)
Voerman	1990	98	17	29
Geronemus	1990	123	111	24
Keller	1990	124	18	11
Hirasawa	1990	116	36	44
Schafer	1990	125	(38)	(33)
McDonald	1990	96	22	18
Bastien	1990	126	(34)	(50)
Di Carlo	1990	88	8	38
Bellomo	1990	9	12	42

[c] Outcome

Despite significant advances in the management of ARF over the last four decades, the associated mortality has not changed significantly (101). Mortality rates range from 30% in nephrotoxic drug induced ARF and 90% in severe multiple organ failure (102, 103). Intermittent hemodialysis has reduced the 100% mortality of ARF to its current level, but has not been without its own problems.

The effect of continuous renal replacement therapy (CAVH, CAVHD) on overall patient outcome is still unclear. Tables 4 and 5 summarize the major studies using CAVH and CAVHD and the actual mortality figures. Differences in mortality statistics arise because some investigators record hospital discharge as an outcome while others use a definition of intensive care unit survival. The absence of an effect on mortality may represent an initial bias in selection of patients since continuous therapies have generally only been used in hemodynamically unstable patients "too sick" for intermittent hemodialysis. A second consideration is that very few studies (8, 9, 13) have used severity of illness scoring systems (104) to assess the impact of renal replacement therapy for ARF. Paganini et al (13) calculated the APACHE II scores retrospectively in 162 patients treated with continuous, combined or intermittent therapy in the intensive care unit and found that patients with continuous therapy had a greater incidence of multisystem involvement and the highest scores. Dobkin et al (105) retrospectively calculated the APACHE II scores in 100 patients receiving hemodialysis in the intensive care unit between 1982-1986. The scoring system was found to accurately predict a risk of death greater than 70% with 100% specificity. A third factor is the role of nutrition on outcome. Bartlett et al (94) found that nutritional status was improved in 56 ARF patients treated with CAVH and resulted in an improved trend for survival in the CAVH group (CAVH 28% survivors, hemodialysis 12%). This area needs further investigation.

Critical evaluation of CAVH and CAVHD in comparison with intermittent hemodialysis is scanty (106). Recently Paganini et al (13) summarized their experience with 133 ARF patients. Nineteen percent were treated with continuous therapy (SCUF, CAVH or CAVHD) alone, 48% had combined continuous and intermittent hemodialysis therapy and 33% received intermittent hemodialysis only. The continuous group had better hemodynamic stability and lower BUN's, but overall mortality was similar in all three groups and ranged from 76% for the combined group to 81% of the intermittent group. Sieberth (107) found continuous therapies reduced mortality in high risk patients but were not superior to intermittent therapy. These data and other studies (7-9, 82) suggest an overall poor prognosis for patients with multisystem failure and ARF in the intensive care unit setting. However, there is little information regarding the impact of these therapies in a controlled trial.

Simpson et al (20) have an on-going study randomizing patients with ARF and multiorgan failure to receive either continuous ultrafiltration and paired intermittent dialysis (CUPID) or conventional hemodialysis. Sixty one patients have been entered and 13 out of 30 (57%) in the CUPID group have survived as compared to 7 out of 24 (77%) in the conventional dialysis group. These figures are encouraging but not statistically significant. We retrospectively analyzed the effect of CAVHD and intermittent hemodialysis (IHD) on the mortality of intensive care unit patients with ARF during two consecutive 8 month periods following initiation of a CAVHD program (96). In the initial 8 months, when CAVHD was used predominantly in hemodynamically unstable patients who would not tolerate IHD, mortality rates were 67% for IHD, 86% for IHD + CAVHD, and 91% for CAVHD alone. Overall mortality declined 13% during the second 8 month period. Those receiving only IHD had a 12% increase in mortality (67% to 75%); mortality decreased in patients crossing over from IHD to CAVHD (86% to 67%) and those receiving CAVHD initially (91% to 73%). Although our numbers are small and do not permit statistical comparison, we are encouraged by the trend in better outcomes. We believe that CAVHD is preferable to IHD in treating ARF in the intensive care unit setting and we are currently conducting a prospective randomized trial to further assess the relative efficacy of these two therapies.

FUTURE DIRECTIONS

Continuous renal replacement therapy is still evolving, and in the next few years new modifications should make the techniques applicable to a broader group of patients. One major concerns with these therapies is the requirement of arterial access. Currently available pumped systems have generally been conventional dialysis machines with minor modifications, so they are often bulky and relatively limited in capabilities. New pumped systems are being designed specifically for continuous therapies to control fluid removal and replacement and allow stable blood flows from a venous access. These systems will be smaller and more user friendly to allow for acceptance into the cramped intensive care unit arena. Another area of intense interest is the ability of these techniques to remove mediators of inflammation such as TNFα, Interleukin 1, and Interleukin 6. Since the membranes used for continuous therapies have much higher molecular weight cut-offs, these mediators are likely to be cleared from the circulation. If this area of investigation is successful it will open new applications for this therapy. Randomized trials comparing this technique with standard intermittent hemodialysis are already underway, but will need to be done at several centers. The impact of these therapies on outcome and nutritional status will be awaited with great interest.

SUMMARY

Continuous renal replacement therapies have emerged as treatment options for acute renal failure over the last decade. Several different methods are now in use. They have in common a highly permeable membrane which allows removal of fluid and solutes in the presence of low driving pressures. Major advantages over IHD include: [a] continuous therapy allows more stable maintenance of volume and composition of body fluids; [b] water and electrolyte balance can be controlled; [c] unlimited hyperalimentation is possible as there are no restraints in fluid volumes which can be administered; and [d] patients are more hemodynamically stable and tolerate the procedure well. CAVHD is increasingly the first line of treatment used for acute renal failure in critically ill patients.

ACKNOWLEDGEMENTS

The author thanks Anthony Brown, M.D., and L. Taylor-Donald for their assistance in preparing this manuscript.

REFERENCES

1. Kramer P, Schrader J, Bohnsack W, Greiden G, Groan HJ, Schaler F: Continuous arteriovenous hemofiltration: A new kidney replacement therapy. Proc Eur Dial Trans Assoc, 18: 743-749, 1981.
2. Lauer A, Sacaggi A, Ronco C, Belledonne M, Glabman S, Bosch JP: Continuous arteriovenous hemofiltration in the critically ill patient. Ann Intern Med, 99: 455, 1983.
3. Kaplan AA, Longnecker RE, Folkert VW: Continuous arteriovenous hemofiltration - a report of six months experience. Ann Intern Med, 100: 358, 1984.
4. Weiss L, Danielson BG, Wikstrom B, Hedstrand U, Wahlberg J: Continuous arteriovenous hemofiltration in the treatmnet of 100 critically ill patients with acute renal failure: report on clinical outcome and nutritional aspects. Clin Nephrol, 31: 184-189, 1989.
5. Bosch JP: Continuous arteriovenous hemofiltration (CAVH): Operational characteristics and clinical use. AKF Nephrology, 3, 1986 (Letter).
6. Dickson DM, Hillman KM: Continuous renal replacement in the critically ill. Anesthes Intensiv Care, 18: 76-101, 1990.
7. Schneider NS, Geronemus RP: Continuous arteriovenous hemodialysis. Kidney Int, 5: 159-162, 1988.
8. Gibney RTN, Stollery DE, Lefebvre RE, et al: Continuous arteriovenous hemodialysis: An alternative therapy for acute renal failure associated with critical illness. Can Med Assoc J, 139: 861-866, 1988.
9. Bellomo R, Ernest D, Love J, Parkin G, Boyce N: Continuous arteriovenous hemodiafiltration: optimal therapy for acute renal failure in an intensive care setting? Aust N Zealand J Med, 20: 237-242, 1990.
10. Bartlett R, Bosch JP, Geronemus RP Paganini EP, Ronco C, Swartz R: Continuous arteriovenous hemo-filtration for acute renal failure: Workshop Summary. Trans Am Soc Art Int Org, 34: 67-77, 1988.
11. Scribner BH, Caner JEZ, Butri R, Quinton W: The technique of continuous hemodialysis. Trans Am Soc Artif Internal Organs, 6: 88-103, 1960.
12. New perspectives in hemodialysis, peritoneal dialysis, arteriovenous hemofiltration and plasmapheresis. Proc Int Symposium, Freiburg, Oct. 1988. Adv Exp Med Biol, 260: 1-213, 1989.
13. Paganini EP: Slow continuous hemofiltration and slow continuous ultrafiltration. Trans Am Soc Art Int Org, 34: 63-66, 1988.
14. Golper TA: Continuous AV hemofiltration in acute renal failure. Am J Kidney Dis, 6: 373-386, 1985.
15. Geronemus R, Schneider N: Continuous arteriovenous hemodialysis: A new modality for the treatment of acute renal failure. Trans Am Soc Art Int Org, 30: 610, 1984.
16. Mehta RL, McDonald BR, Aguilar MM, Ward DM: Regional citrate anticoagulation for continuous arteriovenous hemodialysis in critically ill patients. Kidney Int, 38: 976-981, 1990.

17. Wendon J, Smithies M, Sheppard M, Bullen K, Tinker J, Bihari D: Continuous high volume venous-venous hemofiltration in acute renal failure. Inten Care Med, 15: 358-363, 1989.

18. Sang YY, Uldall PR, Blake P, Francoeur R, Hall E, Besley M: Continuous veno-venous hemodialysis (CVVHD) in the management of complicated renal failure. J Cannt Spring 18-19, 1990.

19. Freudiger H, Levy M, Suter P, Favre H: Continuous veno-venous hemofiltration in acute renal insufficiency. Nephrologie, 11: 129-133, 1990.

20. Simpson K, Travers M, Allison M: Appropriate renal support in the management of acute renal and respiratory failure: Does early aggressive treatment improve outcome? In: "Current Concepts in Critical Care: Acute Renal Failure in the Intensive Therapy Unit" (Eds D Bihari and G Neild), Springer Verlag, New York, 1990, pp 311-318.

21. Hambroucx R, Bogaert AM, Leroy F, De Vos JY, Larno L: Go-slow dialysis instead of continuous arterio-venous hemofiltration. Intensiv Behandlung, 15: 110, 1990.

22. Olbricht CJ, Haubitz H, Habel U, et al: Continuous arteriovenous hemofiltration: *In vivo* functional characteristics and its dependence on vascular access and filter design Nephron, 55: 49-57, 1990.

23. Jenkins R, Fink J, Chen B, Thacker D: Effect of access catheter dimensions on blood flow in CAVH: Intensiv Behandlung, 15: 111, 1990.

24. Ahmad Z: Introduction of percutaneous arteriovenous femoral shunt: A new access for continuous arteriovenous hemofiltration. Am J Kidney Dis, 16: 116-117, 1990.

25. Yohay DA, Schwab SJ, Quarter LD: Parallel plates are more effective than hollow fiber dialysis in continuous arteriovenous hemodialysis (CAVHD). J Am Soc Nephrol, 1: 382, 1990.

26. Vincent HH, Vos MC, deBakkev J, Ahckhauseyn E, van Duyl WA: Continuous A-V hemodiafiltration. Filter design and blood flow rate. Intensiv Behandlung, 15: 113-114, 1990.

27. Ronco C, Brendolan A, Milan M, Feriani M, Chiaramonte S, Bragantini L, La Greca G: Importance of hollow fiber geometry in CAVH. Intensiv Behandlung, 15: 112, 1990.

28. Siegler MH, Teehan BP: Solute transport in continuous hemodialysis: A new treatment for acute renal failure. Kidney Int, 32: 562-571, 1987.

29. Jenkins RD, Kuhn RJ, Funk JE: Permeability decay in CAVH hemofilters. Trans Am Soc Art Int Org, 34: 590-593, 1988.

30. Schultehis R, Brrings W, Glockner WM, Kierdort H, Sieberth HG: Gravimetric substitution help for controlled cyclic substitution during continuous hemofiltration. Intensiv Behandlung, 15: 112, 1990.

31. Sodemann K, Niedenthal A, Weber C, Schafer GE: Automated fluid balance in continuous hemodialysis (CHD) with blood safety module (BSM) 22. Intensiv Behandlung, 15: 113, 1990.

32. Heinrichs W, Mark S, Fauth U, Halmagyi M: An automatic system for fluid balance in continuous hemofiltration with very high precision. Intensiv Behandlung, 15: 110, 1990.

33. Mason JC: The role of spontaneous and pumped hemofiltration. In: "Acute renal failure in the intensive therapy unit" (Eds D Bihari and G Neild), Springer Verlag, London, 1990, pp 319-329.

34. Siegler MH, Teehan BP: Continuous arteriovenous hemodialysis. An improved technique for treating acute renal failure in critically ill patients. In: "Clinical Dialysis" (Eds AR Nissenson, RN Fine, DR Gentile) Second Edition, Appleton and Lange, Norwalk Connecticut, 1989, pp 720-734.

35. Golper TA, Leone M: Backtransport of dialysate solutes during *in vitro* continuous arteriovenous hemodialysis. Blood Purif, 7: 223-229, 1989.

36. Kaplan AA: The predilution mode for continuous arteriovenous hemo-filtration. In: "Acute Continuous Renal Replacement Therapy" (Ed E Paganini), Boston, Martinus Nirjhoff, 1986, p 143.

37. Davies SP, Kox WJ, Brown EA: Clearance studies in patients with acute renal failure treated by continuous arteriovenous haemodialysis. Intensiv Behandlung, 15: 106, 1990.

38. McDonald BR, Mehta RL: Transmembrane flux of IL-1B and TNFα in patients undergoing continuous arteriovenous hemodialysis (CAVHD). J Am Soc Nephrol, 1: 368, 1990.

39. Golper TA, Jenkins R, Wright M, Klein JB: Tumor necrosis factor (TNF) and hemofiltration membranes. Intensiv Behandlung, 15: 119, 1990.

40. Bickley SK: Drug dosing during continuous arteriovenous hemofiltration. Clin Pharm, 7: 198-206, 1988.

41. Golper TA, Wedel SK, Kaplan AA, Saad AM, Donata ST, Paganini EP: Drug removal during continuous arteriovenous hemofiltration. Theory and clinical observations. Int J Art Org, 8: 307-312, 1985.

42. Cleary JD, Davis G, Raju S: Cyclosporine pharmacokinetics in a lung transplant patient undergoing hemofiltration. Transplantation, 48: 710-712, 1989.

43. Lau A, Kronfol N, Powell S, Adams L: Effect of dialysate flow rate on drug removal by continuous arteriovenous hemodialysis. Am Soc Clin Pharamcol Ther, 45: 161, 1990.

44. Slugg PH, Haug M, Bosworth C, Paganini EP: Comparative vancomycin kinetics in ICU patients with acute renal failure: Intermittent hemodialysis vs continuous hemofiltration/hemodialysis. Intensiv Behandlung, 15: 108, 1990.

45. Reetze R, Bohler J, Keller D, Kohler C, Schollmeyer PJ: Elimination of vancomycin in patients on continuous arteriovenous hemodialysis. Intensiv Behandlung, 15: 108, 1990.

46. Bellomo R, Ernest D, Parker G, Bryce N: Clearance of vancomycin during continuous arteriovenous hemodiafiltration. Crit Care Med, 18: 181-183, 1990.

47. Kassum D, Light RB, Brown G, Krohn J, Fine A: Tobramycin clearance during continuous arteriovenous hemofiltration. J Crit Care, 2: 109-111, 1987.

48. Cigarran-Guldris S, Brier ME, Golper TA: Tobramycin clearance during simulated continuous hemodiafiltration. Intensiv Behandlung, 15: 106, 1990.

49. Weiss LG, Cars O, Danielson BG, Gardner A, Wickstrom B: Pharmacokinetics of intravenous cefuroxime during intermittent and continuous arterio-venous hemofiltration. Clin Nephrol, 30: 282-286, 1988.

50. Przecheva M, Bengel D, Rister T: Pharmacokinetics of imipenem/cilastin during continuous arteriovenous hemofiltration (CAVH). Intensiv Behand, 15: 107-108, 1990.

51. Zusman RM, Rubin RH, Cato AE, Cocchetto BS, Crow JW, Tolkoff-Rubin N: Hemodialysis using prostacyclin instead of heparin as the sole antithrombotic agent. N Engl J Med, 304: 934-939, 1981.

52. Schrader J, Scheler F: Coagulation disorders in acute renal failure and anticoagulation during CAVH with standard heparin and with low molecular weight heparin. In: "Continuous Arteriovenous Hemofiltration", Int Conf on CAVH, Aachen Karger, Basel, 1985, pp 25-36.

53. Spinowitz BS: Anticoagulation in continuous arterioveous hemofiltration. In: "Acute Continuous Renal Replacement Therapy", Proc Third Int Symp, Ft Lauderdale, Florida, 1987, pp 106-110.

54. Ronco C, Brendolan A, Borin D, Bragantini L, Fabris A, Feriane M, Chiaramonte S, La Greca G: Continuous arteriovenous hemofiltration in newborns. In: "Continous Arteriovenous Hemofiltration" (Eds HG Sieberth, H Mann) Karger, Basel, 1985, pp 76-79.

55. King DJ, Kelton JG: Heparin-associated thrombocytopenia. Ann Intern Med, 100: 535, 1984.

56. Schrader J, Stibbe W, Armstrong VW, Kandt M, Muche R, Köstering H, Seidel D, Scheler F: Comparison of low molecular weight heparin to standard heparin in Hemodialysis/hemofiltration. Kidney Int, 33: 890-896, 1988.

57. Moriniere P, Dieval J, Bayrou B, Roussel B, Renaud H, Fournier A, Delobel J: Low molecular-weight heparin fraxiparin in chronic hemodialysis. Blood Purif, 7: 301-308, 1989.

58. Schrader J, Stibbe W, Kandt M, Warneke G, Armstrong V, Muller HJ, Scheler F: Low molecular weight heparin versus standard heparin: a long-term study in hemodialysis and hemofiltration patients. Trans Am Soc Artif Int Org, 36: 28-32, 1990.

59. Hory B, Cachoux A, Toulemonde F: Continous arteriovenous hemofiltration with low-molecular-weight heparin. Nephron, 42: 125, 1985.

60. Wynckel A, Bernieh B, Toupance O, N'Guyen Ph. Wopng T, Lavaud s, Chanard J: Guidelines in using enoxaparin in slow continuous hemodialysis. Intensiv Behandlung, 15: 117, 1990.

61. Maher JF, Lapierre L, Schreiner GE, Geiger M, Westervelt FB Jr: Regional heparinisation for hemodialysis. N Engl J Med, 268: 451-456, 1963.

62. Kaplan AA, Petrillo R: Regional heparinization for continuous arterio-venous hemofiltration. Trans Am Soc Artif Int Org, 33: 312-315, 1987.

63. Schwab SJ, Onorato JJ, Sharar LR, Dennis PA: Hemodilaysis without anticoagulation. One year prospective trial in hospitalized patients at risk for bleeding. Am J Med, 83: 405-410, 1987.

64. Sanders PW, Taylor H, Curtis JJ: Hemodialysis without anticoagulation. Am J Kidney Dis, 5: 32-35, 1985.

65. Pinnick RV, Wiegmann TB, Diedrich DA: Regional citrate anticoagulation for hemodialysis in the patient at high risk for bleeding. N Engl J Med, 308: 258-263, 1983.

66. Von Brecht JH, Flanigan MJ, Freeman RM, Lim VS: Regional anticoagulation: Hemodialysis with hypertonic trisodium citrate. Am J Kidney Dis, 8: 196-201, 1986.

67. Mehta RL, McDonald BR, Ward DM: Membrane transfer of citrate and calcium in regional citrate anticoagulation for continuous arteriovenous hemodialysis. J Am Soc Nephrol, 1: 368, 1990.

68. Mehta RL, McDonald BR, Ward DM: Regional citrate anticoagulation for continuous arteriovenous hemodialysis. Intensiv Behandlung, 15: 116, 1990.

69. Gorman RR, Hamilton RD, Hopkins NK: Prostacyclin and thromboxane A_2 biosynthesis and regulation of adenylate cyclase in human diploid cell lines. In: "Prostacyclin", (Eds JR Vane, S Bergstrom), Raven Press, New York, 1979, pp 85-102.

70. Hory B, Saint-Hillier Y, Perol JC: Prostacyclin as the sole antithrombotic agent for acute renal failure hemodialysis. Nephron, 33: 71, 1983.

71. Maurin N: Antithrombotic management with a stable prostacyclin analogue during extracorporeal circulation. Intensive Behandlung, 15: 115, 1990.

72. Zobel G, Trop M, Muntean W, Ring E, Gleispach H: Anticoagulation for continuous arteriovenous hemofiltration in children. Blood Purif, 6: 90-95, 1988.

73. Stevens PE, Riley B, Davies SP, Gower PE, Brown EA, Kox CW: Continuous arteriovenous hemodialysis in critically ill patients. Lancet, II: 150-152, 1988.

74. Journois D, Chanu D, Castelain MH: Assessment of standardized ultrafiltrate production rate using prostacyclin (PGI_2) in continuous venovenous hemofiltration (CHF). Intensiv Behandlung, 15: 115, 1990.

75. Ponikvar R, Kandus A, Buturovic J, Kveder R et al: Use of prostacyclin as the only anticoagulant during continuous veno venous hemofiltration. Intensive Behandlung, 15: 117, 1990.

76. Ota K, Kawaguchi H, Ito K: A new prostacyclin analogue: an anticoagulant applicable to hemodialysis. Trans Am Soc Art Int Org, 12: 31, 1983.

77. Taenaka N, Terada N, Takahashi H, Tachimori Y et al: Hemodialysis using gebexate mesilate in patients with a high bleeding risk. Crit Care Med, 14: 481-483, 1986.

78. Ohtake Y, Hirasawa H, Sugai T, Oda S et al: Nafamostat mesilate (NM) as anticoagulant in continuous hemofiltration (CHF) and continuous hemodiafiltration (CHDF). Intensiv Behandlung, 15: 116, 1990.

79. Costentino F, Paganini E, Lockrem J et al: Continuous arteriovenous hemofiltration (CAVH) in the adult respiratory distress syndrome (ARDS): a randomized controlled trial. Intensiv Behandlung, 15: 103, 1990.

80. Davenport A, Will EJ, Davison AM: Early changes in intracranial pressure during hemofiltration treatment in patients with grade 4 hepatic encephalopathy and acute oliguric renal failure. Nephrol Dial Transpl, 5: 192-198, 1990.

81. Marangoni R, Civardi F, Savino R, Masi F: Continuous arteriovenous hemofiltration (CAVH) improvement by adding diffusion and adsorption. Intensiv Behandlung, 15: 11, 1990.

82. Barzilay E, Kessler D, Lesmet C et al: Sequential plasma filter-dialysis with slow continuous hemofiltration: Additional treatment for sepsis induced ARF patients. J Crit Care, 3: 163-166, 1988.

83. Golper TA, Ronco C, Kaplan AA: Continuous arterivenous hemofiltration: Improvements, modifications and future directions. Semin Dial, 1: 50-54, 1988.

84. Raja R, Kramer M, Goldstein S et al: Comparison of continuous arteriovenous hemofiltration and continuous arteriovenous dialysis in critically ill patients. Trans Am Soc Art Int Org, 32: 435-436, 1986.

85. Alarabi AA, Danielson BG, Wikstrom B: Continuous dialysis in acute renal failure. Scand J Urol Nephrol, 24: 1-5, 1990.

86. Pattison ME, Lee SM, Ogden DA: Continuous arteriovenous hemodiafiltration: An aggressive approach to the management of acute renal failure. Am J Kidney Dis, 11: 43-47, 1988.

87. Paganini EP: Continuous renal prosthetic therapy in acute renal failure: an overview. Pediatr Clin North Am, 34: 165-185, 1987.

88. Di Carlo JV, Dudley TE, Sherbotie JR, Kaplan BS, Costarino AT: Continuous arteriovenous hemofiltration/dialysis improves pulmonary gas exchange in children with multiple organ system failure. Crit Care Med, 18: 822-826, 1990.

89. Bishof NA, Welch TR, Frederic Strife C, Ryckman FC: Continuous hemodiafiltration in children. Pediatrics, 85: 819-823, 1990.

90. Zobel G, Ring E, Zobel V: Continuous arteriovenous renal replacement systems for critically ill children. Pediatr Nephrol, 3: 140-143, 1989.

91. Heney D, Brocklebank JT, Wilson N: Continuous arteriovenous hemofiltration in the newlyborn with acute renal failure and congenital heart disease. Nephrol Dial Transpl, 4: 870-876, 1989.

92. Sperl W, Geiger R, Maurer H, Guggenbichler JP: Continuous arteriovenous hemofiltration in hyperammonaemia of newborn babies. Lancet, 336: 1192-1193, 1990.

93. Zobel G, Haim M, Ritschl E, Muller W: Continuous arteriovenous hemofiltration as emergency procedure in severe hyperkalemia. Child Nephrol Urol, 9: 236, 1988-89.

94. Bartlett RH, Mault JR, Dechert RE, Palmer J, Swartz RD, Port FK: Continuous arteriovenous hemofiltration: improved survival in surgical acute renal failure. Surgery, 100: 400-408, 1986.

293

95. Chima C, Heyka R, Meyer L, Bosworth C, Hummel A, Paganini E: Nitrogen balance (NB) in postsurgical patients with acute renal failure on continuous arteriovenous hemofiltration (CAVH) and total parenteral nutriton (TPN). Intensiv Behandlung, 15: 97, 1990.

96. McDonald BR, Mehta RL, Ward DM: Decreased mortality in patients with acute renal failure (ARF) undergoing continuous arteriovenous hemodialysis (CAVHD) in the intensive care unit (ICU). Intensiv Behandlung, 15: 99, 1990.

97. Kuttnig M, Zobel G, Ring E, Trop M: Parenteral nutrition CAVH in critically ill anuric children. Intensiv Behandlung, 15: 121, 1990.

98. Voerman HI, Strack von Schjindel JM, Thijs LG: Continuous arteriovenous hemodiafiltration in critically ill patients. Crit Care Med, 18: 911-914, 1990.

99. Sigler MH, Snyder S, Teehan BP, Benz RL: Amino acid removal during continuous arteriovenous hemodialysis (CAVHD) in patients with acute renal failure (ARF) receiving total parenteral nutrition. Intensiv Behandlung, 15: 100, 1990.

100. Davenport A, Roberts NB: Amino acid losses during continuous high flux hemofiltration in the critically ill patient. Crit Care Med, 17: 1010-1014, 1989.

101. Cameron JS: Acute renal failure - The continuing challenge. Q J Med, 228: 337-343, 1986.

102. Kjellstrand CM, Etten J, Davis T: Time of death, recovery of renal function, development of chronic renal failure, and need for chronic hemodialysis in patients with acute tubular necrosis. Trans Am Soc Artif Intern Organs, 27: 47-50, 1981.

103. Wilkins RG, Faragher EB: Acute renal failure in an intensive care unit: incidence, predicton and outcome. Anaesthesiology, 38: 638, 1983.

104. Knaus WA, Draper EA, Wagner DP, Zimmerman JE: APACHE II: a severity of disease classification system for acutely ill patients. Crit Care Med, 13: 818-829, 1985.

105. Dobkin JE, Cutler RE: Use of APACHE II classification to evaluate outcome of patients receiving hemodialysis in an intensive care unit. West J Med, 149: 547-550, 1988.

106. Kohen JA, Whitley KY, and Kjellstrand CM: Continuous arteriovenous hemofiltration: A comparison with hemodialysis in acute renal failure. Trans Am Soc Art Int Org, 31: 169, 1985.

107. Sieberth HG, Kierdorf H: Is continuous haemofiltration superior to intermittent dialysis and hemofiltration treatment? Adv Exp Med Biol, 260: 181-192, 1989.

108. Tam PY, Huraib S, Mahan B, Le Blanc D, Lunski CA Holtzer C, Doyle CE, Vas SI, Uldall PR: Slow continuous dialysis in the management of complicated acute renal failure in an intensive care unit. Clin Nephrol, 30: 79-85, 1988.

109. Olbricht C, Mueller C, Schurek HJ: Treatment of acute renal failure in patients with multiple organ failure by continuous spontaneous hemofiltration. Trans Am Soc Artif Intern Organs, 28: 33, 1982.

110. Klehr HU, Kascell HJ, Kuchenbecker CH, Munch HG, Spannducker N: Clinical results of continuous arteriovenous hemofiltration. In: "Continuous Arteriovenous Hemofiltration (CAVH)" (Eds HG Sieberth, H Mann) Basel, Switzerland, Karger, 1985, pp 159-165.

111. Domoto DT: Two years experience with continuous arteriovenous hemofiltration in acute renal failure. Trans Am Soc Art Int Org, 31: 581-585, 1985.

112. Frisch S, Kindler J, Schmitter H, Glockner W, Seiberth H: Performance of CAVH in ARF therapy. In: "CAVH" (Eds G La Creca et al) Milan, Wichtig Editore, 1986, pp 283-288.

113. Mault JR, Dechert RE, Lees D, Swartz RD, Port FK, Bartlett RM: Continuous arteriovenous filtration: An effective treatment for surgical acute renal failure. Surgery 101: 478-484, 1987.

114. Lieberman KV: Continuous arteriovenous hemofiltration in children. Pediatr Nephrol, 1: 330-338, 1987.

115. Alarabi A, Brendolan A, Danielson BG et al: Outcome of continuous arteriovenous hemofiltration (CAVH) in acute renal failure (ARF): double-centre comparative study. Intensiv Behandlung, 15: 96, 1990.

116. Hirasawa H, Sugai T, Ohtake Y et al: Continuous hemofiltration (CHF) and hemodiafiltration (CHDF) in the management of multiple organ failure (MOF). Intensiv Behandlung, 15: 98, 1990.

117. Schreier P, Keusch G, Binswanger U: Outcome of acute renal failure in critically ill patients treated by continuous hemofiltration. Intensiv Behandlung, 15: 100, 1990.

118. Sluiter HE, Froberg L, van Dijl J, Go G: Mortality in high-risk intensive care patients with acute renal failure treated with CAVH. Intensiv Behandlung, 15: 101, 1990.

119. Zobel G, Ring E, Kuttnig M, Grubbauer HM: CAVH vs CVVH in critically ill pediatric patients. Intensiv Behandlung, 15: 121, 1990.

120. Canaud B, Cristol JP, Berthelemy C, Beraud JJ, Mion C: Acute renal failure (ARF) associated with multiple organ failure (MOF): pump assisted continuous veno-venous hemofiltration (CVVH) the ultimate treatment modality. Intensiv Behandlung, 15: 96, 1990.

121. Korner MM, Banayosy EL, Posival H: Ventricular assist device combined with continuous high volume venous-venous hemofiltration (CVVH). Intensiv Behand, 3: 104, 1990.
122. Barzilay E, Wksler N, Kessler D et al: The use of continuous AV hemodialysis in the management of patients with oliguria associated with multiple organ failure. J Int Care Med, 14: 444-445, 1988.
123. Geronemus RP, Schneider NS, Epstein M: Survival in patients treated with continuous arteiovenous hemodialysis (CAVHD) for acute renal failure (ARF) and chronic renal failure (CRF). Intensiv Behandlung, 15: 97, 1990.
124. Keller E, Reetze P, Bohler J, Lucking FP, Schollmeyer P: Continuous arteriovenous hemodialysis (CAVHD): experience in 18 intensive care patients. Intensiv Behandlung, 15: 98, 1990.
125. Schafer GE, Sodemann K, Doring N, Schroder HM: Continuous arterio-venous (CAVHD) and veno-venous hemodialysis (CVVHD) in critically ill patients. Intensive Behandlung 15: 100, 1990.
126. Bastien O, Saroul C, Estanove S: Continuous hemodialysis in acute renal failure following cardiac surgery. Intensiv Behandlung, 15: 101, 1990.

RENAL TRANSPLANTATION

Chapter 14

IDEAL IMMUNOSUPPRESSION AFTER RENAL TRANSPLANTATION: ARE STEROIDS NEEDED?

TIMOTHY H. MATHEW

Renal Unit, The Queen Elizabeth Hospital, Woodville, South Australia

Prior to the introduction of cyclosporin in the early 1980's, it was widely held that steroids were a necessary part of immunosuppression for successful renal transplantation. The concept of using a "low dose" prednisolone approach, reported by McGeown in 1977 (1) was slow to be accepted until controlled trial evidence was forthcoming (2). Attempts to withdraw prednisolone from long term maintenance regimes even in stable, carefully selected patients (on azathioprine) were accompanied by frequent irreversible rejection episodes (3).

The introduction of cyclosporin has allowed a re-evaluation of the need for regular continuing steroids after renal transplantation. Reports of avoiding steroids from the start of transplantation or routine attempts at prednisolone withdrawal after a few months, have shown that in about half of patients continuing steroids are unnecessary. This review assesses this evidence in an attempt to define an ideal immunosuppression approach for use in the "cyclosporin era".

USE OF STEROIDS FOR REVERSAL OF ACUTE REJECTION

From the beginning of clinical renal transplantation, a boost in the dose of corticosteroids was used to reverse acute rejection episodes. This approach remains the first line treatment for acute rejection episodes at the present time. Steroids are usually administered in high dosage orally or intravenously for about 3 days. Both routes are probably equally efficacious (4). The acute use of steroids in this manner and the peri-operative administration of large boluses of methylprednisolone appears to carry little obvious morbidity. The acute use of steroids will not be mentioned further in this review.

Table 1. Results of steroid withdrawal

DOSE EFFECT	FREQUENCY %	IMPORTANCE	REVERSIBLE	DOSE RELATED	COMMENT
Weight gain	100	Moderate	Yes	Yes	Weight gain contributes to hypertension, diabetes & wo problems.
Cushingoid appearance	100	Mild	Yes	Yes	Leads to non compliance particularly when associated w hypertrichosis.
Impaired wound healing	Occasional	Mild	Yes	Yes	Usually associated with infection and poor nutritional status.
Impaired growth	100	High	?	Yes	Large problem in children.
Osteoporosis	Frequent	High	No	Yes	Increasing importance with age. Seen even with low dos
Myopathy	10	High	Yes	Yes	Disabling when severe.
Diabetes	5-10	High	Yes	Yes	Often insulin dependent while on high dose. Steroid-indu diabetes has same long term morbidity as idiopathic.
Peptic ulceration (bleeding)	5	High	Yes	Yes	Often fatal if complicated. Incidence down to zero with l dose steroids plus H$_2$ blockers.
Hypertension	75	Moderate	Yes	Yes	High incidence of hypertension even without steroids (? to cyclosporine).
Psychiatric disturbances	1.2	Mild	Yes	Yes	Psychosis difficult to manage unless steroids reduced.
Cataracts	10	Moderate	No	?	Often progressive even with low continuing steroid dose
Acne	50	Mild	Yes	Yes	Usually disappears when dose <20 mg day prednisolone
Increased infections	?	High	Yes	Yes	Bacterial and fungal infections seen much less common. current era.
Diverticulitis (perforation)	1	High	With surgery	Yes	Usually fatal complication as presentation often late and atypical.
Avascular necrosis	15	High	No	Yes	With low dose regimen this disabling complication is n seen.
Fragile skin (easy bruising)	50	Moderate	No	No	Seen in advancing years. Large skin loss with minimal trauma is frequent cause of hospital admission.

THE CASE AGAINST ROUTINE USE OF MAINTENANCE STEROIDS

High dose regimens

One of the salutary clinical experiences (before the introduction of cyclosporin) was the slow appreciation that high oral steroid dosage for the first few months after renal transplantation is not advantageous and may be deleterious to graft and patient outcome (1, 2, 5).

However an important ancillary finding in these studies was that low dose steroids (e.g. prednisolone starting at 30 mg/day) need to be accompanied by a high dose of azathioprine (2 mg/kg b.w./day) in early weeks to be highly efficacious. A low dose of steroid together with a low dose of azathioprine brings poor results (2).

There is no evidence to support a regime of high oral dosage of steroids in early months and in our unit no patient in the last 8 years has been exposed to a continuing dose of more than 30 mg/day of prednisolone (6).

Low dose regimens

The use of low dose steroids remains widespread in clinical practise in combination with cyclosporin and/or azathioprine in the belief that rejection episodes are fewer, cyclosporin nephrotoxicity may be ameliorated and that there is little morbidity incurred. If cyclosporin is not used then experience mandates the use of prednisolone with azathioprine.

Further reference to steroid regimes in this article will assume a "low dose" approach (e.g. 30 mg/day for 3 weeks followed by reduction to 10 mg/day over the next 8-12 weeks). If cyclosporin alone or with azathioprine is used, do steroids really add to clinical outcome?

The continuing long term use of prednisolone in a dose of about 10 mg/day has been frequent practise and was probably necessary pre-cyclosporin (3). However, the morbidity associated with even this low dose in the long term raises a real question of justification of the current practise.

Alternate day regimes have been promoted particularly in children (7, 8). In the adult patient, in our experience and that of others (9), alternate day regimes at the same total dosage have not been equally immunosuppressive and the cross over period is not without difficulty of rejection escape. As a consequence alternate day steroid therapy is not seen as a satisfactory solution and in the cyclosporin era appears less popular.

Side effects

It is not proposed in this review to exhaustively detail the side effects of corticosteroid therapy. It is pertinent, however, to briefly mention the problems as seen after otherwise successful transplantation. These observations on side effects are the major rationale for the pressure felt by many transplant units to devise strategies which omit or avoid corticosteroids whenever possible. Table 1 summarizes this experience.

Some points need emphasising. Most of the side effects are dose related and reversible. The most disturbing problems from steroids are those irreversible or long lasting problems such as impaired growth, avascular necrosis of the hips and cataracts. Most of the reversible morbidity is avoidable with a low dose approach. Weight gain, cushingoid appearance, myopathy and psychiatric disturbance are all uncommon when the dose does not exceed 30 mg/day.

One long term problem of importance is the thin skin syndrome (including traumatic leg ulcers) which in our unit accounts for more hospital admission bed days than any other condition in patients transplanted for more than 2 years. Other problems are osteoporosis which is difficult to prevent or stabilise in the face of even a small ongoing dose of prednisolone and cataracts which are a distressing complication particularly in young adults and children.

Mahony's review of post transplantation survivors at ten years and beyond documents hypertension in 42-65%, avascular necrosis in 11-45%, cataracts in 7-45% and diabetes in 4-9% (10). Colonic perforation, peptic ulcer and pancreatitis, traumatic leg ulcers, osteoporosis and urinary infection still occur 10 years or more after transplantation and may all be contributed to or caused by continuing steroid therapy.

The effect of steroids on lipid levels is well documented though the effect is confused post transplantation by the frequent presence of other variables such as diuretics, hypertension, glucose intolerance and obesity. It has been suggested that cyclosporin exacerbates the hyperlipidemic tendency and that low dose prednisolone with azathioprine regimens do not.(11). A recent report confirms these findings but studied only cyclosporin with prednisolone (12). A study isolating the effects of low dose prednisolone with and without cyclosporin would help clarify the issue which is of great importance as the major mortality of long standing renal transplant recipients is coronary artery disease (10).

Bacteria and fungi infection in the wound, urine, lungs and elsewhere has been blamed on steroid therapy. A recent comparison of cyclosporin/azathioprine versus cyclosporin/azathioprine/prednisolone found a significantly greater infection rate with prednisolone (13). Others have suggested a reduced severity in cytomegalovirus infection without prednisolone (14).

From the above it is not surprising that physicians have looked favourably on the possibility that transplantation could be safely performed without corticosteroid therapy.

REASONS FOR THE ROUTINE USE OF STEROIDS

Reduction of acute rejection episodes

Convincing evidence that routine use of steroids from day 1 reduced acute rejection episodes was seen in a recent Australian report: 78% of patients not on prednisolone had acute rejection compared to 25% of those patients on prednisolone (all patients also received cyclosporin/azathioprine in equivalent dosage). Interestingly the rejection process occurring without steroids was often accompanied by fever, was a more abrupt clinical event and responded promptly and well to boluses of intravenous steroids. Only 8% of the no steroid policy group needed OKT3 to treat steroid resistant rejection. Of those patients on steroids from Day 1, the rejection process although less frequent tended to be more severe and more often steroid resistant with 13% of these patients requiring anti-lymphocyte therapy (13).

Reduction in nephrotoxicity

The initial cyclosporin experience was largely with monotherapy using doses now considered high (15, 16). Maintenance steroids were added in the belief that nephrotoxicity, consistently observed in the early experience, would be modified if the addition of steroids allowed a lower dose of cyclosporin to be used. In addition it was reported that steroids reduced nephrotoxicity even without reduction in the level of cyclosporin (17).

This led to the widespread use of combination regimens and a decline in the popularity of monotherapy. Difficulty in assessing the effect of such regimens on the incidence of nephrotoxicity is a consequence of the complex ramifications of cyclosporin on the kidney.

Even in reduced initial dosage (12.5 mg/kg b.w./day) significant nephrotoxicity occurs (18). In general most observers believe that a reduced dose of cyclosporin in conjunction with either azathioprine or prednisolone or both, minimises nephrotoxicity (18-20).

STRATEGIES AVAILABLE TO ACCOMPLISH A "NO STEROID" REGIME

Cyclosporin monotherapy

Several reports of long term cyclosporin monotherapy have recently been presented (21-24). The only two randomised controlled trials show excellent results with a similar 86% and 84% twelve month primary cadaveric graft survival; 76% and 74% of patients were still on monotherapy in the long term (18, 21). In both trials the results with cyclosporin monotherapy were better (but not significantly so) than azathioprine with prednisolone. In other reports monotherapy was considered successful (23, 24) but Margreiter concludes in 20 patients given monotherapy (in an uncontrolled experience) that only 2 could stay on monotherapy and that "it is doubtful whether such an attempt (monotherapy) which may expose some patients to added risk, is worthwhile" (22).

A small but important randomised trial of cyclosporin monotherapy versus cyclosporin and steroids was conducted by the Canadian Transplant Group (25): 22 of 33 patients assigned to no steroids were in fact placed on continuous prednisolone early in their course although in almost half of these rejection criteria were not present. Reduced morbidity (acne, hypertension, diabetes, infection and ureteric problems) was experienced in the no steroid group. Outcome was similar in the 2 study groups. The conclusion was that steroids can be safely withheld except for the treatment of rejection episodes.

Cyclosporin monotherapy has been shown to be preferred in elderly patients (over 55 years). A significant improvement in results occurred with monotherapy compared to azathioprine/prednisolone treatment, in one sequential experience: 54% of these elderly patients received no steroids. The overall results with cyclosporin monotherapy were equally good in the elderly and the young (26).

Experience clearly indicates that cyclosporin alone can be used successfully and maintained in the long term in the majority of patients. There is no evidence that the doses used as monotherapy incur any greater nephrotoxicity in the long term than other regimes (18, 24).

Cyclosporin and azathioprine

The addition of azathioprine rather than prednisolone to cyclosporin has experimental support (27) and was first suggested by Salaman (23). The obvious attraction of avoiding steroids whilst allowing a low dose of cyclosporin to be used led us to use this combination in all but highly sensitized recipients of first cadaveric grafts (28). We have now used the combination in over 150 grafts with similar conclusions to those previously published (13, 28). Over one third of our patients never received maintenance steroids and by 6 months 56% of the total group was not on steroids. Overall graft success rate was 87% at 12 months. Only 16% of our patients received OKT3 as rescue therapy for acute rejection.

The number of rejection episodes in our experience was significantly higher than in a comparative series treated with triple therapy (cyclosporin/azathioprine/prednisolone) although the number of bacterial infections was significantly less (13). A similar trend towards fewer rejection episodes with added prednisolone is seen in Salaman's data (23).

Additional cyclosporin/azathioprine experience in a non-randomly allocated trial showed no benefit of added prednisolone and about 50% of patients on double therapy stayed rejection free (29). Further experience with cyclosporin/azathioprine is being gained in the second Australian multicentre trial which compares this regimen to triple therapy and to cyclosporin/prednisolone.

STEROID WITHDRAWAL

A popular regime in recent years has been to start with triple therapy (cyclosporin/azathioprine/steroids) or to induce with an antilymphocyte preparation (followed with triple therapy) and to withdraw steroids some months later (30-36). Recent experience is summarized in Table 2.

All the studies report favourably on the success of steroid withdrawal with the percentage of patients successfully withdrawing maintenance steroids averaging 55% (range 32-73). The results were similar in living related and cadaveric donor groups. Most units prefer to maintain azathioprine although in the 2 units using cyclosporin only there was no consistent difference.

The risk of rejection in response to prednisolone withdrawal remains a concern even if withdrawal is only attempted in those with stable graft function and a creatinine level of <200 µmol/l (31, 34). More intensive monitoring (e.g. weekly clinic visits) is recommended through the time of steroid withdrawal and steroid therapy is rapidly reinstituted if graft function deteriorates (34). With this policy, graft function in one series returned to baseline levels from an acute rejection episode in 75% of patients, 20% regained good stable function and about 5% of grafts were unstabilized (34). In another series no grafts were lost and no permanent loss of graft function was reported despite rejection episodes occurring leading to reinstitution of prednisolone in 25% of patients (32).

Table 2. Results of steroid withdrawal

STUDY AUTHOR (Ref. #)	NUMBER OF PATIENTS	BASIC IMMUNO-SUPPRESSION	MONTH POST TRANSPLANT WHEN PREDNISOLONE WAS WITHDRAWN	% OF ALL PATIENTS SUCCESSFULLY OFF PREDNISOLONE	COMMENTS
Tamm et al (31)	171	C (± ATG A)	4-6	32%	OK if good graft function
O'Connell et al (32)	105	C, A	6	58%	Favourable
Hariharan et al (33)	66	C, A	12	61%	Identical sibling Experience - Yes
Frei et al (34)	181	C, A	6	45%	OK if graft function stable
Kupin et al (35)	11	C, A	8	73%	Living related Experience - Yes
Cristinelli et al (36)	27	C	7	59%	Yes with caution

C = Cyclosporin; A = Azathioprine; P = Prednisolone; ATG = Anti-Thymocyte Globulin

306

The penalty of uncontrolled rejection appears real but small - in these 6 series 4/491 grafts began progressive graft failure with an attempt at steroid withdrawal.

The benefit of steroid withdrawal is more difficult to quantify. O'Connell reported catch up growth in young patients in his series (32). Hariharan et al (33) reported reduction in the number of patients needing antihypertensives (from 43% to 20%) and significant falls in plasma cholesterol and triglyceride levels. Cristinelli et al (36) documented reduction in cataracts, acne and hirsutism in his steroid withdrawal group. Kupin (35) reported significant falls in lipids, body weight and blood pressure in his small number of patients. Longer term studies presumably will document the beneficial effects on bones and skin. All these series recommend in favour of attempting steroid withdrawal, but stress the need to do so only if graft function is adequate and stable. In this circumstance over half of patients can be completely withdrawn from maintenance steroids with only a small risk of graft loss.

IS STEROID AVOIDANCE/STEROID WITHDRAWAL JUSTIFIED?

The final answer to this question must await long term controlled trials. The side effects of steroids are well documented and are summarized earlier. Removal of these side effects alone would be clearly beneficial but just what advantage will show in the morbidity and mortality at 10 and 20 years post transplantation is most important. Into the equation of cost and benefit must be put the possibility these steroid free regimes will need a higher dose of cyclosporin or the addition of an extra agent such as azathioprine or perhaps in the future mizoribine (37), RS 61443 (38), or rapamycin (39), with the inherent dangers of additional immunosuppression. To this date combination regimes of cyclosporin and azathioprine are not showing an increased risk of skin cancer above that incurred when either drug is used singly (40). If any increase in the already high risk of cancer was to be proven, enthusiasm for double or triple regimes would be severely curtailed.

The move to low dose steroid regimes, now widely accepted, was the major step in reducing side effects. Avascular necrosis, stretch marks, psychiatric episodes are a thing of the past in most units. What then is the morbidity of a few months of low dose steroids? This too remains unclear and will be difficult to clarify except in a large controlled experience. It seems likely that significant morbidity and mortality from a 6 month course of prednisolone, never exceeding 30 mg/day will be hard to demonstrate.

That excellent renal transplantation results can be achieved without maintenance steroids has been unequivocally shown in the numerous trials and papers in this review.

307

The real question is how is this best achieved - through avoidance of steroids from Day 1 or through a planned withdrawal of low dose steroids at about 6 months? A comparison of these approaches in similar units in Australia is possible (28, 32). The end result in these two reports is remarkably similar with about 55% of patients on no steroids. With a steroid avoidance protocol about·35% of patients never get steroids and 20% need a short maintenance course of steroids but then tolerate early withdrawal. With a steroid withdrawal protocol 45% of patients either have graft dysfunction, early severe rejection or became unstable with steroid reduction.

Steroid avoidance brings with it more rejection episodes which are often more clinically obvious with fever and graft swelling. These episodes seem sensitive to treatment with high dose steroid therapy. In an interesting comparison of cyclosporin/azathioprine therapy versus cyclosporin/azathioprine/prednisolone using equivalent dose regimens, routine steroids brought a significantly reduced number of rejection episodes but a higher rate of steroid resistant rejection with a consequent increase in the rate of use of OKT3 (13). Prophylactic use of antilymphocyte preparations introduces another variable which is largely untested. It is possible that as this prophylaxis reduces rejection incidence in early months (41) the need for maintenance steroids could be reduced. Steroid avoidance thus brings more frequent problems in the early course post transplant, with more uncertainty for the patient, more early clinic visits and more alterations to therapy. Steroid withdrawal in later months, however, is necessarily accompanied by uncertainty during the withdrawal period, extra clinic visits at that time and in a significant percentage of patients the need to return to steroids. In some protocols this return to steroids is followed by another attempt at withdrawal. Both courses thus have problems and incur extra costs and stresses that need to be put into the total equation.

CONCLUSION

Morris (42) and Land (43) have recently stated "there is no clear cut and prospective controlled trial showing us that addition of steroids or azathioprine (to cyclosporin) is of any proven value". This review has come to a similar conclusion. There is strong evidence that part of the long term morbidity and mortality of well functioning grafts relates to maintenance steroids (10). It is now clearly established that over half of renal recipients receiving cyclosporin can maintain long term good function without maintenance steroids. It remains uncertain whether it is preferable to get off steroids by steroid avoidance or by an early steroid withdrawal regimen. The differences in morbidity and cost between these two approaches are likely to be small and difficult to conclusively establish. Meanwhile the choice between the two best remains in the hands of the individual unit or physician.

REFERENCES

1. McGowan MG, Kennedy JA Loughridge WGG, Douglas J, Alexander JA, Clarke SD, McEvoy J Hewitt JC: One hundred transplants in Belfast City Hospital. Lancet II: 648-651 1977.
2. D'Apice AJF, Becker GJ, Kincaid-Smith P, Mathew TH, Ng J, Hardie IR, Petrie JJB, Rigby RJ Dawborn J, Heale WF, Miarch PJ: A prospective randomised trial of low dose versus high dose steroids in cadaveric renal transplantation. Transplantation 37: 373-377, 1984.
3. Lokkegaard H, Thaysen J.H: Permanent withdrawal of prednisolone in necro-kidney transplantation Proc. EDTA 13: 216-222, 1976 (Publ. Pitman Medical).
4. Gray D, Shepherd H, Daar A: Oral versus intravenous high dose steroid treatment of renal allograft rejection, Lancet I: 117-118, 1978.
5. Russ GR, May S, Jacob CK et al: Experience with cyclosporine A and azathioprine double therapy in low risk recipients of first cadaveric renal allografts. Clin Transplantation, 4: 26-32, 1990.
6. Stabile C, Vincenti F, Garavoy M, Duca R, Melzer J, Feduskant Salvaterra O, Amend WT: Is a "low" dose of prednisolone better than a "high" dose at the time of renal transplantation? Braz J Med Biol Res, 19: 355-66 1986.
7. Fine RN: Transplantation in children. In: "Kidney Transplantation" (Ed PJ Morris), Academic Press, London, 1979, p 364.
8. Dumler F, Levin NW, Szego G, Bulpett AT, Prauss WE: Long term alternate day steroid therapy in renal transplantation. Transplantation, 34: 78-82, 1982.
9. Breitenfield FV, Hebert CA, Lemann J, Pirring WR, Kaufmann WM, Sampson D, Kalfleisch J and Beres JA: Stability of renal transplant function with alternate day corticosteroid therapy. J Am Med Assoc, 244: 157-159, 1980.
10. Mahony JF: Long term results and complications of transplantation: the kidney. Transplantation Proc, 21: 1433, 1989.
11. Raine AEG, Carter R, Mann J, Chapman JR, Morris PJ: Increased plasma LDL cholesterol after renal transplantation associated with cyclosporine immunosuppression. Transplantation Proc, 19: 1820-1821, 1987.
12. Vathsala A, Weinberg RB, Schoenberg J, Grevel J, Dunn J, Goldstein RA, Van Buren CT, Lewis RM, Kahan BM: Lipid abnormalities in renal transplant recipients treated with cyclosporine. Transplantation Proc, 21: 3670-3673, 1989.
13. Bestifo AC, Petrie JJB, Rigby RJ, Hardie IR, Jacob CK, Russ GR, Mathew TH: A comparison of triple therapy with double therapy (cyclosporine/azathioprine) in low risk first cadaveric renal allograft recipients. Transplantation Proc, 21: 1604-1605, 1989.
14. Johnson RWG, Mallick NP, Bakran A, Pearson RC, Scott PD, Dyer P, Donaghue D, Morris D, Gokal R: Cadaver renal transplantation without maintenance steroids. Transplantation Proc, 21: 1581-1588, 1989.
15. Calne RY, White DJ, Thiru S, Evans DB, McMaster P, Dunn DC, Craddock GN, Pentlow BN, Rolles K: Cyclosporin A in patients receiving renal allografts from cadaver donors. Lancet, II: 1323-1327, 1978.
16. European Multicentre Trial Group: Cyclosporine in cadaveric renal transplantations. One year following of a multicenter trial. Lancet, II: 986-989, 1983.
17. Nott D, Griffin PJ, Salaman JR: Low dose steroids do not augment cyclosporine but do diminish cyclosporine nephrotoxicity. Transplantation Proc, 17: 1289-1290, 1985.
18. Hall BM, Tiller DJ, Hardie J, Mahony J, Mathew TH, Thatcher G, Miach P, Thomson N, Shiel AG: Comparison of three immunosuppressive regimes in cadaver renal transplantation, N Engl J Med, 318: 1499-1507, 1988.
19. Simmons RL, Canafax DM, Strand M, Ascher NL, Payne WD, Sutherland DR, Najarian JS: Management and prevention of cyclosporine nephrotoxicity after renal transplantation: Use of low doses of cyclosporine, azathioprine and prednisolone. Transplantation Proc, 17: 266-275, 1985.
20. Posner MP, Mendez-Picon G, King A, Nelson KP, Spicer HG, Lee HM: Is sequential low dose immunotherapy the preferred treatment in cadaveric renal transplantation. Transplantation Proc, 21: 1594-1597, 1989.

21. Johnson RW, Mallick NP, Bakran A, Pearson RC, Scott PD, Dyer P, Donaghue D, Morris D, Gokal R: Cadaver renal transplantation without maintenance steroids. Transplantation Proc, 21: 1581-1582, 1989.
22. Margreiter R, Bosmuller C, Speilberger M, Schmid TH, Konigsrainer A: Cyclosporine monotherapy after cadaveric renal transplantation. Transplantation Proc, 21: 1591-1593, 1989.
23. Griffin PJA, Salaman JR: Long term results of cyclosporine monotherapy in kidney transplantation. Transplantation Proc, 23: 992-993, 1991.
24. Klare B, Strom TM, Hahn H, Englesberger I, Muesel E, Illner XW, Adendroth D, Land W: Remarkable long term prognosis and excellent growth in kidney transplant children under cyclosporine monotherapy. Transplantation Proc, 23: 1013-1017, 1991.
25. MacDonald AS, Daloze P, Dandavino R, Jundal S, Bear L, Dossetor JB, Klassen J, Stiller CR, Lockwood B, Reeve C and the Canadian Transplant Group: A randomised study of cyclosporine with and without prednisolone in renal allograft recipients. Transplantation Proc, 19: 1865-1866, 1987.
26. Andrew J, Campistol AJ, Oppenheimer F, Ricart MJ, Vilardele J, Talbot R, Carretero P: Improved results in elderly renal transplants without prophylatic steroids. Clin Transplantation, 5: 3-6, 1991.
27. Squifflet JS, Sutherland DER, Rynasiewcz JJ, Field J, Heil J, Najarian JS: Combined immunosuppressive therapy with cyclosporin A and azathioprine. Transplantation, 41: 541-544, 1986.
28. Russ GR, May S, Jacob CK, Mathew TH, Pugsley DJ, Disney AP, Barratt LJ, Fraenkel MB, Clarkson AR, Woodroffe A: Experience with cyclosporine A and azathioprine double therapy in low risk recipients of first cadaveric renal allografts. Clin Transplantation, 4: 26-31, 1990.
29. Bry W, Warvarin V, Bohannon L, Feduska N, Straube B, Collins G, Levin B: Cadaveric renal transplant without prophylactic prednisolone therapy. Transplantation Proc, 23: 994-996, 1991.
30. Naik RB, Abdeen H, English J, Chakraborty J, Slapak M, Lee HA: Prednisolone withdrawal after 2 years in renal transplant patients receiving only this form of immunosuppression. Transplantation Proc, 11: 39-44, 1979.
31. Tamm M, Thiel G, Huser R, Brunner F, Hatsch M, Landmann J: Cyclosporine monotherapy after kidney transplantation since 1983. Transplantation Proc, 23: 997-998, 1991.
32. O'Connell PJ, D'Apice AJ, Walker RG, Francis DM, Clubie GJ, Kincaid-Smith P: Results of steroid withdrawal in renal allograft recipients in low dose cyclosporine A, azathioprine and prednisolone. Clin Transplantation, 2: 102-106, 1988.
33. Hariharan S, First MR, Munda R, Penn I, Schroeder TJ, Fidler J, Weiskittel P, Alexander JW: Prednisolone withdrawal in HLA identical living related donor transplant recipients. Transplantation Proc, 21: 1617-1619, 1989.
34. Frei D, Keusch G, Hugentobler M, Probst W, Uhlschmid G, Largiader F, Binswanger V: Withdrawal of steroids after cadaveric kidney allotransplantation on maintenance triple therapy. Transplantation Proc. 21:1620-1622, 1989.
35. Kupin et al: Steroid withdrawal in cyclosporine treated living related donor rental transplant recipients. Transplantation Proc, 21: 1623-1624, 1989.
36. Cristinelli L, Brunori G, Setti G, Manganoni A, Manganoni AM, Scolari F, Sandrini S, Scaini PS, Savoloi S, Camerini C, Maiorca R: Withdrawal of methylprednisolone on the sixth month in renal transplant recipients treated with cyclosporine. Transplantation Proc, 19: 2021-2023, 1987.
37. Osakabe T, Uchida H, Masaki Y, Yokota K, Sato K, Nakayama Y, Ohkubo M, Kumano K, Endo T, Watanabe K, Aso K: Studies on immunosuppression with low dose cyclosporine combined with mizoribine in experimental on clinical cadaveric renal allotransplantation. Transplantation Proc, 21: 1598-1600, 1989.
38. Platz KP, Eckhoff DE, Hullett DA, Gollinger HW: Prolongation of dog renal allograft survival by RS 61443 a new patient immunosuppressive agent. Transplantation Proc, 23: 497-498, 1991.
39. Kimball PM, Kerman RH, Kahan BO: Rapamycin and cyclosporine produce synergistic but nonidentical mechanisms of immunosuppression. Transplantation Proc, 23: 1027-1028, 1991.
40. Sheil AGR, Disney AP, Mathew TH, Amiss N, Excell L: Cancer development in cadaveric donor renal allograft recipients treated with azathioprine or cyclosporin or both. Transplantation Proc, 23: 111-112, 1991.
41. Kahana L, Narvate J, Ackerman J, Lefor W, Weinstein S, Wright C, de Quiesada A, Baxter J, Shires D: OKT3 prophylaxis versus conventional drug therapy. Single centre perspective of multicentre trial. Amer J Kidney Disease, 14: 5-9, 1989.
42. Morris PJ: Single or multiple therapy. Transplantation Proc, 21: 820-822, 1989.
43. Land W: Kidney transplantation - state of the art. Transplantation Proc, 21: 1425-1429, 1989.

DIAGNOSTIC METHODS IN NEPHROLOGY

Chapter 15

ANTI-NEUTROPHIL CYTOPLASMIC ANTIBODIES (ANCA): NEW TOOLS IN THE DIAGNOSIS AND FOLLOW-UP OF NECROTIZING GLOMERULONEPHRITIS AND VASCULITIS

CEES G.M. KALLENBERG AND JAN W. COHEN TERVAERT

Departments of Clinical Immunology and Nephrology, University Hospital, Oostersingel 59; 9713 EZ Groningen, The Netherlands

INTRODUCTION

Vasculitis refers to an inflammatory process affecting blood vessels. It may represent a manifestation of disorders such as systemic lupus erythematosus (SLE), rheumatoid arthritis or mixed cryoglobulinemia, or constitutes the major and primary hallmark of a number of clinical syndromes (1-7). Within the spectrum of vasculitis the latter group of the so-called idiopathic systemic vasculitides is a pathogenetically poorly understood group of diseases that can be classified according to the size of the vessels involved (6, 7) (Table 1).

The vasculitides affecting medium- or small-sized vessels, in particular, may clinically present with a variety of manifestations, frequently resulting in a delayed diagnosis. Histopathologically, these latter vasculitides are characterized by necrotizing inflammation of the vessel wall with extensive infiltration by polymorphonuclear cells. In contrast to vasculitis associated with SLE, rheumatoid arthritis or cryoglobulinemia, immune deposits are usually not detected in the vessel wall in the afore-mentioned conditions (3, 8), with the exception of Henoch-Schönlein purpura. At the level of the kidneys these disorders manifest as necrotizing crescentic glomerulonephritis (NCGN). NCGN also occurs without systemic involvement, so-called idiopathic NCGN (9), although symptoms compatible with systemic vasculitis are present in a substantial number of these cases (10, 11). Immune deposits are generally absent in these forms of glomerulonephritis (9), and the condition is designated as pauci-immune glomerulonephritis (3, 8) to discriminate it from other forms of NCGN showing immune deposits in the glomeruli. Whereas these latter forms of NCGN are apparently mediated by immune complexes as in SLE, or by anti-basement membrane antibodies as in Goodpasture's syndrome, the immunopathogenesis of idiopathic NCGN or NCGN associated with the necrotizing vasculitides is still not clarified.

Table 1. Classification of systemic idiopathic vasculitides

I.	Affecting predominantly large- and medium-sized blood vessels
	1. Takayasu's Arteritis
	2. Giant Cell Arteritis/Temporal Arteritis
II.	Affecting predominantly medium- and small-sized blood vessels
	1. Classic Polyarteritis Nodosa
	2. Churg Strauss Syndrome
	3. Wegener's Granulomatosis
	4. Polyangiitis Overlap Syndrome
III.	Affecting predominantly small blood vessels
	1. Microscopic Polyarteritis
	2. Henoch-Schönlein Purpura

Recently, autoantibodies to neutrophil cytoplasmic antigens have been described in the sera of patients with necrotizing vasculitis and/or (idiopathic) crescentic glomerulonephritis (12-20). The detection of the anti-neutrophil cytoplasm antibodies (ANCA) has greatly improved the diagnosis of these diseases. In addition, it has placed these disorders in the spectrum of autoimmune diseases and opened a new area for their study. In this review we will first describe the antigenic specificities recognized by ANCÁ and the methods for their detection. Secondly, we will discuss the clinical value of ANCA detection for the diagnosis and follow-up of patients with necrotizing vasculitis and glomerulonephritis. Finally, we will speculate about the role that ANCA may play in the pathogenesis of these diseases.

ANCA, A CLASS OF AUTOANTIBODIES DIRECTED AGAINST MYELOID LYSOSOMAL CONSTITUENTS

c-ANCA, directed against proteinase 3

In 1982 Davies et al (12) reported on the occurrence of autoantibodies to neutrophil cytoplasmic constituents in the sera of a small group of patients with segmental necrotizing glomerulonephritis following an arbovirus infection. Another report from Australia describing anti-neutrophil cytoplasm antibodies (ANCA) was published in 1984 (13).

314

These data, however, did not attract large interest until van der Woude et al (14), in 1985, in a collaborative study from the Netherlands and Denmark, demonstrated that these autoantibodies are a sensitive and specific marker for the diagnosis of Wegener's Granulomatosis (WG). In their original publication the antibodies were designated as anticytoplasmic antibodies (ACPA). Nowadays, the term anti-neutrophil cytoplasm antibodies (ANCA) has been generally accepted.

In the afore-mentioned studies ANCA were detected by indirect immunofluorescence (IIF) on ethanol fixed neutrophils, as described in detail by Wiik (21) in the proceedings of the first international workshop on ANCA. The antibodies produce a characteristic staining pattern with accentuation of the fluorescence intensity in the area within the nuclear lobes (Figure 1). As such, this pattern has been described as "classical" or "cytoplasmic" and the antibodies are designated as c-ANCA (22).

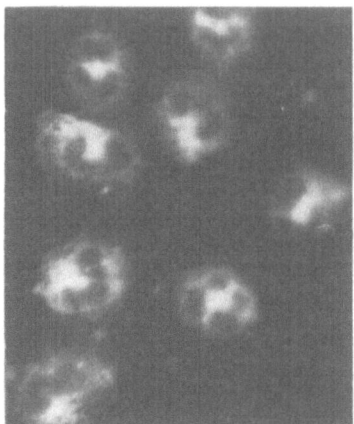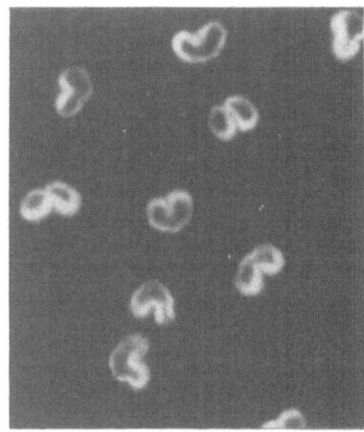

Figure 1. Staining of ethanol fixed neutrophils by indirect immunofluorescence using a serum sample from a patient with active Wegener's Granulomatosis that produces a characteristic granular pattern of fluorescence (c-ANCA, left) and a serum sample from a patient with idiopathic crescentic glomerulonephritis that produces a perinuclear pattern (p-ANCA, right). The latter serum was positive for antibodies to myeloperoxidase.

To elucidate the nature of the antigen(s) recognized by c-ANCA, four subcellular fractions were collected from neutrophils according to the method of Börregaard et al (23). These four fractions represent the azurophilic or primary granules, the specific or secondary granules, the plasmamembranes and phosphasomes, and the cytosol. Using these fractions, immunoprecipitation experiments with c-ANCA positive sera demonstrated that the antigen is a saline-soluble glycoprotein triplet of molecular weights (MW) of 29, 30.5, and 32 kD, derived from the azurophilic granules (24) (Figure 2).

315

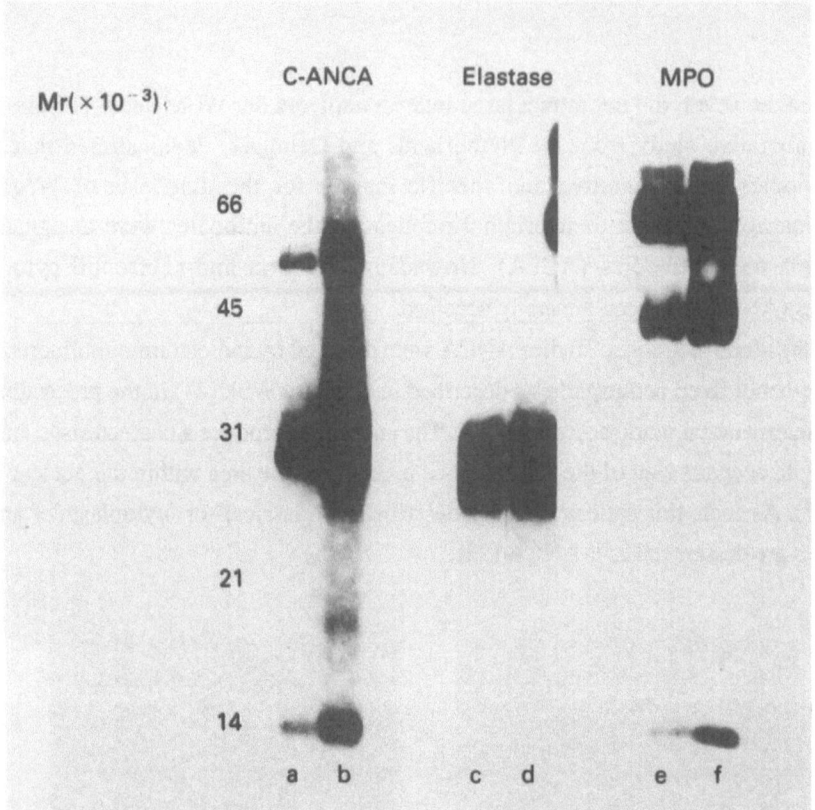

Figure 2. Immunoprecipitation of different myeloid lysosomal enzymes by mouse monoclonal antibodies (Mab) and patients' sera [Reproduced from Ref. 19: Cohen Tervaert JW, Goldschmeding R, Elema JD, van der Giessen M, Huitema MG, van der Hem GK, The TH, von dem Borne AEGKr, Kallenberg CGM: Autoantibodies against myeloid lysosomal enzymes in crescentic glomerulonephritis. Kidney Int, 37: 799-806, 1990, with permission].

a: Mab against proteinase 3
c: Mab against elastase
e: Mab against myeloperoxidase

b: c-ANCA positive serum
d: elastase antibody positive serum
f: myeloperoxidase antibody positive serum

The antigen binds di-isopropylfluorophosphate indicating that it is a serine protease, but proved different from the neutrophil serine proteases elastase and cathepsin G (24). A third leucocyte serine protease of MW 29 kD, designated as proteinase 3, had shortly before been described by Kao et al (25). Further studies (26-28) demonstrated that the antigen recognized by c-ANCA is identical to proteinase 3 as described by Kao et al (25). The triplet observed in the immunoprecipitation studies represents three isoforms of the enzyme. Its NH_2-terminal amino acid sequence was shown to be highly homologous to that of the other two serine proteases, cathepsin G and elastase (26-28) (Figure 3). Recently, a cDNA has been cloned from human bone marrow encoding the complete protein (29). Based on this cDNA proteinase 3 is predicted to consist of 228 amino acids with a MW of 25 kD for the polypeptide backbone and two potential glycosylation sites that may account for the apparent isoforms. It proved identical to two recently described proteins from azurophilic granules, namely a serine protease with broad-spectrum antimicrobial activity designated as p29b (30) and a protein described as myeloblastin based on the finding that addition of a myeloblastin antisense deoxynucleotide to the promyelocytic cell line HL-60 arrested their growth and induced their differentiation (31). Thus, c-ANCA recognizes a 29 kD glycoprotein from azurophilic granules with serine protease, antibiotic and myeloblastic activity.

```
SERINE PROTEASE            N-TERMINAL SEQUENCE

                    1      5     10     15     20
Proteinase 3        I VGGHEAQPHSRPYMASLQM R
Leucocyte elastase  - - - - R R - R - - A W - F - V - - - L -
Cathepsin G         - I - - R - S R - - - - - - - - Y - - I Q
```

Figure 3. N-terminal sequences of serine proteases from neutrophil azurophilic granules.

p-ANCA, an artifact of fixation, comprises, amongst others, antibodies to myeloperoxidase and other lysosomal constituents.

During routine IIF testing for ANCA autoantibodies different from c-ANCA were subsequently detected that produced a perinuclear to nuclear fluorescence pattern on ethanol fixed neutrophils (Figure 1). These antibodies were described as p-ANCA. A considerable number of p-ANCA positive sera from patients with vasculitis and/or glomerulonephritis were shown to contain autoantibodies to myeloperoxidase (MPO) (16, 32), whereas antibodies to human leukocyte elastase (32-34) or lactoferrin (35) were incidentally detected in p-ANCA positive sera as well (Figure 2). MPO and elastase are constituents of the alpha or azurophilic granules and lactoferrin is a constituent of the beta or secondary granules of the neutrophil. The perinuclear fluorescence produced by antibodies to these cationic granular constituents is an artifact of the ethanol fixation; the cationic proteins apparently move and attach to the negatively charged nuclear membrane during the fixation procedure. When neutrophils are fixed with cross-linking fixatives such as paraformaldehyde, the antibodies produce a granular staining of the cytoplasm (36, 37) (Figure 4).

Whereas in a selected population of patients with glomerulonephritis most p-ANCA positive sera contain antibodies to MPO (anti-MPO) (16), different results are obtained during routinely testing for ANCA in a population of patients more or less suspected for vasculitis and/or glomerulonephritis. Out of 424 sera with a p-ANCA pattern from such a population, we found antibodies to MPO in only 50 of these sera (20). This finding demonstrates that p-ANCA is not equivalent to anti-MPO and underscores the need for antigen-specific assays. This item will be dealt with in the following paragraph.

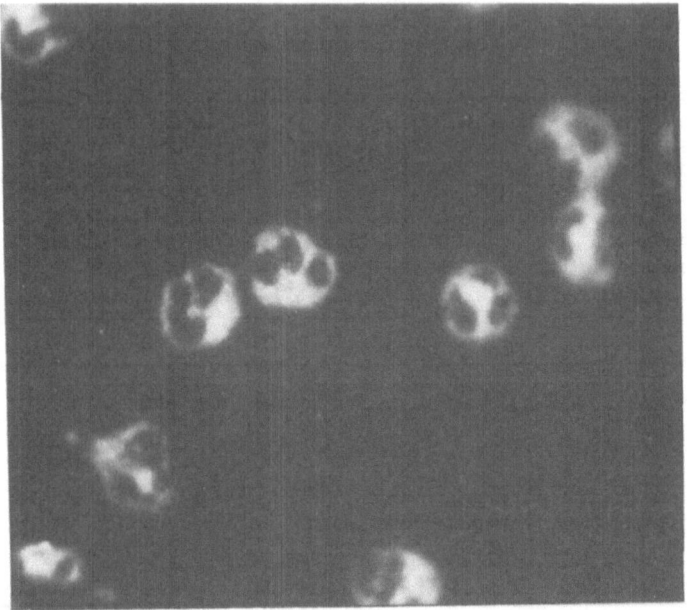

Figure 4.   Staining of neutrophils fixed with phosphate-buffered paraformaldehyde (0.5%) by indirect immunofluorescence using a serum sample containing antibodies to myeloperoxidase.

In conclusion, ANCA constitutes a class of autoantibodies directed against myeloid lysosomal constituents. Amongst these, c-ANCA are directed against proteinase 3. A (peri)nuclear pattern (p-ANCA) is, in a substantial number of sera, based on the presence of antibodies to MPO and, incidentally, to elastase or lactoferrin, and can be considered as an artifact of fixation in these cases. p-ANCA, however, is not at all equivalent with anti-MPO.

METHODS OF DETECTION FOR ANCA

Indirect immunofluorescence

Indirect immunofluorescence on ethanol-fixed granulocytes is widely accepted as the screening test for ANCA (21). The characteristic cytoplasmic fluorescence pattern

318

described as c-ANCA (Figure 1) is, in nearly all of the cases, produced by antibodies to proteinase 3 as discussed in the previous section. Very rarely, we have detected anti-proteinase 3 by ELISA (see later) in sera that produced an atypical fluorescence pattern on ethanol-fixed neutrophils.

A perinuclear to nuclear pattern (p-ANCA) might be indicative of anti-MPO. A p-ANCA pattern can, however, also be produced by antinuclear antibodies (ANA). When ANCA-testing is performed on cells from the buffy-coat as a substrate, as suggested by Wiik (21), ANA will stain the nuclei of lymphocytes whereas true ANCA will not. As a matter of fact, the presence of ANA can also be detected by using substrates such as HEp-2 cells, but a positive ANA-test does not exclude the simultaneous presence of ANCA in a certain serum. Otherwise, fixation of neutrophils with cross-linking fixatives instead of ethanol will allow the detection of true ANCA since ANCA will produce a granular fluorescence pattern on those substrates whereas ANA still produce a nuclear pattern (36-38). As stated before, p-ANCA positive sera may contain antibodies to MPO, elastase, or lactoferrin. A number of p-ANCA positive sera, that are negative for ANA, do, however, not react with either MPO, elastase or lactoferrin when tested in antigen-specific assays (see later). The nature of the antigens recognized by these sera is not yet known. Such p-ANCA of undefined specificity have particularly been described in patients with inflammatory bowel diseases such as ulcerative colitis (39) and in rheumatoid arthritis (40, 41). Thus, as it stands now, the detection of p-ANCA in a serum should be followed by the application of antigen-specific assays in order to demonstrate or to exclude the presence of antibodies to MPO and other myeloid constituents. It should be mentioned that we, incidentally, have detected anti-MPO by ELISA in sera that were negative by IIF on ethanol fixed cells (42).

ELISA systems

One of the first solid phase assays described for the detection of ANCA used an acid extract from whole neutrophils as antigenic source (15). In this radioimmunoassay positive results were obtained with c-ANCA sera but also with p-ANCA sera positive for antibodies to granular constituents other than proteinase 3, and with some ANCA-negative sera, in particular sera from patients with SLE. The non-specific binding of the latter sera could be demonstrated by including an inhibition assay with neutrophil extract as specific inhibitor. The acid extract RIA, however, still does not distinguish between the various specificities of ANCA.

A commercially available solid phase assay more specific for anti-proteinase 3 (anti-Pr3) than the former RIA has been developed by Wieslander et al (43). This ELISA uses an extract from azurophilic granules as a substrate and appears highly specific for anti-Pr3 but not highly sensitive for their detection (44).

An ELISA highly specific and sensitive for anti-Pr3 has been developed by Goldschmeding et al (45) in collaboration with our group. The ELISA uses a monoclonal antibody to Pr3 that "catches" proteinase 3 from an extract of azurophilic granules. In our first study we observed that all 21 sera positive for c-ANCA by IIF were positive as well for anti-Pr3 by this capture ELISA whereas sera negative by IIF were invariably negative by ELISA (19). Follow-up studies on c-ANCA positive patients during treatment, however, show discrepancies between IIF and ELISA in some cases: c-ANCA may turn negative by IIF when still positive by ELISA, and *vice versa*. We found a reasonable but not perfect correlation between titers of c-ANCA by IIF and the quantitative results of the ELISA (44).

Finally, anti-Pr3 can be detected by ELISA using affinity purified antigen (46). This ELISA seems to be comparable to the capture ELISA described before with respect to sensitivity and specificity for anti-Pr3. In the near future cloned proteinase 3 will become available for use in ELISA and/or RIA systems.

Antibodies to MPO, elastase or lactoferrin have been measured by ELISA using highly purified, commercially available substrates (16, 42, 47, 48), or by capture ELISA using monoclonal antibodies (19, 20, 24, 42).

In a recent study we have compared the potential of the IIF-test, both on ethanol- and paraformaldehyde-fixed neutrophils, with that of the capture ELISA and the ELISA using directly coated MPO for the detection of anti-MPO antibodies in the sera of patients with vasculitis (42). As already discussed, the perinuclear pattern on ethanol-fixed cells changed into a granular cytoplasmic pattern when paraformaldehyde fixation was used. In addition, some sera positive for anti-MPO by ELISA were negative by IIF on ethanol-fixed cells. The capture ELISA and the directly coated ELISA performed equally well in detecting anti-MPO.

What may be concluded from these data for clinical practice? Screening for ANCA should be done by IIF on ethanol-fixed neutrophils. A c-ANCA pattern is indicative of anti-Pr3. When a p-ANCA pattern is found, antigen-specific tests for anti-MPO (and possibly also for anti-elastase and anti-lactoferrin) should be performed; in addition, a test for ANA, and, preferably, an ANCA-test on paraformaldehyde-fixed neutrophils should be done to confirm or exclude the presence of true ANCA. In case of a strong clinical suspection, IIF on paraformaldehyde-fixed cells and antigen-specific ELISAs may be indicated also when ANCA-testing by IIF on ethanol-fixed neutrophils is negative.

DIAGNOSTIC VALUE OF C-ANCA IN GLOMERULONEPHRITIS/VASCULITIS

As already discussed c-ANCA were first described in 1982 in 8 patients with pauci-immune necrotizing and/or crescentic glomerulonephritis (12). All patients additionally had symptoms compatible with a multisystem disease, including respiratory symptoms in four of them. Another four patients with c-ANCA were described by Hall et al (13). Three of these four patients had necrotizing glomerulonephritis, and all four had a multisystem disease with pulmonary involvement. In 1985, van der Woude et al (14) described the occurrence of c-ANCA in 25 of 27 serum samples from patients with active generalized and biopsy-proven Wegener's granulomatosis (WG), i.e. patients with (necrotizing and/or crescentic) glomerulonephritis, vasculitis, and granulomatous inflammation of the respiratory tract (49). In these initial studies more than 15,500 serum samples from controls were reported to be negative for c-ANCA (12-14). These controls consisted of healthy persons and disease controls, including patients with various forms of glomerulonephritis and/or vasculitis (14). The high specificity of c-ANCA for active generalized WG as observed in these studies was confirmed by Lüdemann and Gross (50), who detected c-ANCA in all of their patients with active generalized WG but not in 300 healthy and 600 disease controls. Following these (retrospective) studies, a prospective study was reported from the UK (15). In this study, 22 of 23 patients with active generalized WG or microscopic polyarteritis (MPA) appeared to be positive for c-ANCA, whereas only 2 of 60 patients without WG/MPA were definitely positive for c-ANCA. Thus, it can be concluded from the afore-mentioned studies that almost all patients with c-ANCA have necrotizing and/or crescentic glomerulonephritis (NCGN) as part of either WG or MPA.

Whereas the Dutch-Danish (14) and the German (50) studies showed c-ANCA to be specific for WG, the studies from Australia (12, 13) and UK (15) suggested that granulomatous inflammation of the respiratory tract is not always found in patients with c-ANCA. Before the "ANCA era" it was already recognized that MPA shares many features with WG (51). The most important difference between the two disorders is the presence of prominent upper airway lesions or pulmonary granulomatous inflammation in WG and its absence in MPA (51). It has been known for a long time that a number of patients who initially present with MPA develop full blown WG during a relapse of the disease (52, own observation). As extensive ear, nose and throat evaluation, including nasal biopsies, frequently is required in order to demonstrate or exclude WG, it has been suggested that MPA might be diagnosed and WG overlooked in cases where the clinical condition necessitates the prompt institution of immunosuppressive treatment. Such an extensive ear, nose and throat evaluation may even be deleterious in a patient who presents with rapidly progressive glomerulonephritis in combination with alveolar lung hemorrhage as it delays the start of treatment. Otherwise, the presence of granulomatous inflammation in nasal biopsies may easily be missed due to sampling errors. Multiple repeated biopsies frequently disclose granulomatous inflammation in these cases. This is, however, hardly feasible in cases of NCGN or systemic vasculitis when immunosuppressive treatment has to be instituted immediately. Taken together, MPA might be considered a variant of WG.

Table 2. Sensitivity and specificity of c-ANCA for active Wegener's granulomatosis and/or microscopic polyarteritis.

Ref. #	No.[a]	Sensitivity[b] % with pos. results	No.[c]	Specificity[b] % with neg. results
14	27 [d]	93%	190	100%
50	18	56%	600	98.5%
15	23	96%	63	96%
53	11	91%	n.t.[e]	
54	19	84%	140	98.5%
55 [f]	14	86%	n.t.	
56	58 [d]	78%	116	98%
57	35	77%	205	95%
17	112	91%	539	98%
18	45	93%	58	97%
58	31	71%	159	95.5%
59	20	75%	n.t.	
20	77	84%	171	97.5%
60	30	47%	90	97.5%
61	51	78%	649	99%

[a] number of patients with active Wegener' granulomatosis or microscopic polyarteritis tested for the presence of c-ANCA.
[b] nosological sensitivity and nosological specificity (Wulff HR: Rational diagnosis and treatment. 2nd Ed. Oxford, Blackwell, 1981, pp 80-102).
[c] number of patients with related disorders
[d] number of serum samples tested (number of patients not reported)
[e] n.t. = not tested.
[f] in this study only patients with Wegener's granulomatosis without renal involvement (i.e., limited Wegener's granulomatosis) were studied.

At present, the sensitivity of c-ANCA for *active* WG/MPA has been demonstrated in many studies (median, 81%; range 47% to 96%) (14, 15, 17, 18, 20, 50, 53-61), (Table

2). An extremely low percentage (47%) of positive serum samples was found in one study (60). This might have been due to the method used for ANCA detection. A drop of whole blood spread over a pre-cleared glass slide and directly fixed in 100% ethanol was used as a substrate in that study. When ANCA-testing is performed on cells from a buffy-coat as a substrate, as recommended by the first international workshop on ANCA (21), more positive results probably will be observed. Also, the first study from Kiel reported a low incidence of c-ANCA in active WG (50). In this study patients were divided into two groups, one with limited and the other with extensive disease. Whereas c-ANCA was found in all (n = 7) patients with active generalized WG, only 3 of 11 patients with limited WG were positive for c-ANCA. These results are in contrast with our findings in limited WG as we found c-ANCA in 86% of our patients (55). A later study from the Kiel group (17) reported a much higher prevalence of c-ANCA in active limited WG (75%). Thus, some 80% of patients with WG and/or MPA are positive for c-ANCA by IIF and positive for anti-Pr3 by ELISA and simultaneously negative for anti-MPO. Interestingly, we found that nearly all patients with active WG who lack proteinase-3 antibodies are positive for MPO antibodies (20).

Table 3. Occurrence of c-ANCA in vasculitis-associated or idiopathic necrotizing and/or crescentic glomerulonephritis and in other renal lesions.

Ref. #	Prevalence of c-ANCA in necrotizing and/or crescentic glomerulonephritis with or without systemic vasculitis		Prevalence of c-ANCA in other renal lesions	
	No.[a]	% with pos. results	No.[a]	% with pos. results
16	35	54%	n.t.[b]	
62	37	57%	n.t.	
8	76	38%	79	0
19	32	66%	44	0
63	56	50%	61	0
67	46	35%	n.t.	

[a] number of patients tested; [b] n.t. = not tested

c-ANCA is not only observed in patients with systemic vasculitis, whether WG or MPA, but also, occasionally, in patients with idiopathic NCGN (8, 19). From the total group of patients with pauci-immune NCGN, either idiopathic or vasculitis-associated, about 40 to 60% are positive for c-ANCA (8, 16, 19, 62-64) (Table 3). Recently, we found that patients with NCGN and c-ANCA/anti-Pr3 but without biopsy proven WG have more prominent otorhinolaryngeal involvement than those patients with NCGN who lack anti-Pr3 and are positive for anti-MPO (65). This suggests that c-ANCA/anti-Pr3 is associated with a distinct clinical syndrome even when a diagnosis of definite WG can not be made.

Finally, a minority of patients with anti-glomerular basement membrane disease are positive for c-ANCA (66, 67): This subgroup has clinical and histological features of both anti-glomerular basement membrane disease and vasculitis (67).

ANCA have also been reported in children with Kawasaki disease (68). Since the cytoplasmic fluorescence pattern of ANCA in this disease seems to differ from the pattern described as c-ANCA, the former antibodies may not necessarily be directed against proteinase-3. So, further studies with respect to the antigenic specificity of ANCA in Kawasaki disease are needed.

In summary, about 80% of the patients with active WG or MPA, and about 30% of patients with idiopathic (?) pauci-immune NCGN, are positive for c-ANCA. Since nearly all patients with c-ANCA have chronic nasal inflammation, a clinical diagnosis of WG is strongly suspected in these latter patients. They may, in fact, be diagnosed as WG when less strict criteria are used (69).

DIAGNOSTIC VALUE OF p-ANCA IN GLOMERULONEPHRITIS/VASCULITIS

p-ANCA were first described in 1959 in patients with rheumatoid arthritis (70). These so-called granulocyte-specific antinuclear antibodies (GS-ANA) produce a perinuclear staining pattern on ethanol fixed donor granulocytes. Recently, it has been shown that their perinuclear pattern turns into a cytoplasmic one when neutrophils are fixed with cross-linking fixatives (38). GS-ANA are common in rheumatoid arthritis and are only rarely absent in Felty's syndrome (41). In addition to their occurrence in rheumatoid arthritis, p-ANCA have been described in drug-induced lupus erythematosus, juvenile chronic polyarthritis, chronic ulcerative colitis, myasthenia gravis and chronic active hepatitis (39, 41). Following the detection of c-ANCA in WG and related conditions, p-ANCA were also detected in systemic vasculitis and idiopathic crescentic glomerulonephritis (16, 19, 20). Finally, p-ANCA are detected in 1% of the serum samples of 20 to 60 years old normal blood donors, and in 8% of the serum samples of normal controls above the age of 60 years (41). Thus, a positive p-ANCA test is, at present, of restricted diagnostic value. As already discussed the antigenic specificity of most of these p-ANCA positive sera is unknown (20, 41). Possible candidates are myeloperoxidase (16, 32), elastase (32-34), and lactoferrin (35). Whereas the clinical significance of elastase antibodies and lactoferrin antibodies is probably restricted, the clinical significance of MPO antibodies is widely accepted and will be reviewed here.

Anti-MPO antibodies were first described in patients with idiopathic and/or vasculitis-associated crescentic glomerulonephritis (8, 16, 19). At present, one third of the patients with anti-MPO have NCGN without extrarenal disease and a substantial number presents with a pulmonary-renal syndrome with progressive dyspnea, pulmonary infiltrates and/or alveolar lung hemorrhage (8, 19, 20, 71, 72). The remaining patients present with a systemic illness with constitutional symptoms, arthralgias, purpura and/or otorhinolaryngologic symptoms, most frequently nasal polyposis and chronic rhinosinusitis (20). Although a clinical diagnosis of WG is suspected in many of these patients granulomatous inflammation of the respiratory tract is observed only infrequently (8, 20). A substantial number of these patients have Churg Strauss Syndrome (20, 73).

Table 4.   Occurrence of anti-myeloperoxidase (MPO) antibodies in vasculitis-associated or idiopathic necrotizing and/or crescentic glomerulonephritis and in other renal lesions.

Ref. #	prevalence of anti-MPO antibodies in necrotizing and/or crescentic glomerulonephritis		prevalence of anti-MPO antibodies in other renal lesions	
	No.([a])	%([b])	No.([a])	number of positives
16	35	63%	32	3
19	32	34%	44	-
63	56	32%	61	-
64	46	28%	n.t. ([c])	

([a]) number of patients tested
([b]) percentage positive for anti-MPO antibodies
([c]) not tested

In Table 4 the prevalences of anti-MPO in vasculitis-associated and idiopathic NCGN is summarized. About 30-40% of these patients have anti-MPO. As already discussed, 40-60% of patients with NCGN have c-ANCA (see Table 3). Since c-ANCA and anti-MPO do not occur simultaneously it can be concluded that the majority of patients with pauci-immune NCGN have one of both ANCAs (19).

To assess the combined sensitivity of anti-MPO and anti-Pr3 for necrotizing arteritis and/or NCGN we tested the serum samples of 130 consecutive patients with biopsy proven idiopathic necrotizing arteritis or pauci-immune NCGN for the presence of these autoantibodies (65) (Table 5). Anti-MPO were particularly found in patients with Churg Strauss Syndrome (characterized by asthma, eosinophilia and necrotizing arteritis), idiopathic NCGN, and in patients with necrotizing arteritis or NCGN with either asthma or eosinophilia (who may be considered as incomplete Churg Strauss Syndrome).

Table 5. Disease pattern in relation to the presence of antineutrophil cytoplasmic autoantibodies (ANCA).

Disease entity	anti-proteinase-3 antibodies	anti-myeloperoxidase antibodies	None
Polyarteritis nodosa (n = 10)	1	2	7
Polyangiitis overlap syndrome (n = 10)	4	2	4
Churg Strauss Syndrome (n = 13)	1	10	2
Wegener's granulomatosis (n = 48)	43	3	2
Necrotizing and/or crescentic glomerulonephritis with respiratory symptoms (n = 41)	30	11	-
Idiopathic necrotizing and/or crescentic glomerulonephritis (n = 8)	2	6	-

Recently, anti-MPO have also been detected in the sera of 6 patients with hydralazine induced lupus (48). Anti-MPO were accompanied in these cases by anti-elastase antibodies, which are not found in patients with idiopathic and/or vasculitis-associated NCGN (19).

The specificity of anti-MPO for NCGN has been studied with respect to various renal disorders (Table 4). Anti-MPO, however, are found also in patients with polyarteritis or Churg Strauss Syndrome without renal involvement (20, 73). Therefore, the specificity of anti-MPO for systemic vasculitis and idiopathic NCGN has further been tested in selected groups of patients with closely related diseases with and without renal involvement. Two out of 144 patients had anti-MPO resulting in a specificity of 99% (20). In one study, 21% of sera from patients with systemic lupus erythematosus were found positive for anti-MPO, although usually in low titer (48). There has been some debate about the possible interaction of anti-histone antibodies in the ELISA for measuring anti-MPO. Histones derived from disrupted cells in sera can bind to negatively charged MPO. As a result anti-histone antibodies may give false positive results in the ELISA. This item has to be studied in more detail. As it stands now, the occurrence of anti-MPO in patients with SLE cannot be excluded.

In summary, anti-MPO are present in the majority of the patients with idiopathic crescentic glomerulonephritis or the Churg Strauss Syndrome. In addition, these antibodies can be found in patients with WG or MPA who lack anti-Pr3 antibodies, and in a minority of patients with classic polyarteritis nodosa or polyangiitis overlap syndrome (Table 6).

Table 6. ANCA and disease associations (Summary).

| Disease entity | Sensitivity of | |
	anti-proteinase 3 (anti-Pr3) antibodies	anti-myeloperoxidase (anti-MPO) antibodies
Idiopatic crescentic glomerulonephritis	30%	70%
Microscopic polyarteritis (MPA)	50%	50%
Wegener's granulomatosis (WG)	80%	20%
Churg Strauss Syndrome	10%	70%
Classic polyarteritis nodosa	10%	20%
Polyangiitis overlap syndrome	40%	20%

THE VALUE OF MEASURING LEVELS OF ANCA FOR THE FOLLOW-UP OF PATIENTS WITH WEGENER'S GRANULOMATOSIS (WG) AND RELATED DISORDERS

As discussed in the preceding section, c-ANCA are both sensitive and specific for active WG or MPA. In the first paper on ANCA by Davies et al (12) it was already mentioned that ANCA disappeared during immunosuppressive treatment but reappeared during recurrent disease in two of their patients. In 1985, van der Woude et al (14) described the first prospective study from Groningen (the Netherlands) on 19 patients with WG. ANCA titers were, generally, strongly related to the activity of the disease, although high ANCA titers were also observed in some patients with inactive disease (14). These findings were confirmed by Lüdemann and Gross (50). They recognized, however, that clinical improvement was not always exactly paralleled by decrease of ANCA titer or by its disappearance. Specks et al (56) described decreasing titers in 10 patients in whom remission was induced and increasing titers in 4 patients during a relapse of WG. Minor titer increases, not directly associated with an increase of the disease activity of WG, were reported in 3 cases. Nölle et al (17) reported that median ANCA titers increased in patients with WG during relapses but not during intercurrent infections without signs of reactivation of WG.

In 1989, we reported the results of the second prospective study from Groningen (18). In 13 patients with newly diagnosed generalized WG, ANCA titers declined in all of them during immunosuppressive treatment, and ANCA were not detectable any more after 11 weeks of treatment (range: 4 to 20 weeks). Another 35 patients already known with WG were followed for a mean period of 16 months. Eight major and 9 minor relapses were observed in 12 out of these 35 patients. Each relapse was preceded by a significant rise of the ANCA titer, i.e. an increase of at least two titer steps (fourfold) compared with a previous sample that had been obtained within a period of 4 weeks (Figure 5). The mean period between the time the ANCA titer had risen and the moment a relapse was clinically diagnosed was 49.5 days (range: 9 to 106 days). During the study period 23 patients had persistently inactive disease. In only one of these patients significant increases of the ANCA titer without reactivation of the disease were observed.

Egner and Chapel (74) reported a prospective study of 2 years duration in which 10 ANCA-positive patients with WG, MPA or unclassified vasculitis were followed. Six relapses were observed in 4 patients and every relapse was preceded by a significant increase of c-ANCA during the preceding 2-15 weeks. Increase in c-ANCA titer was accompanied by minor symptoms of the disease in one patient, and occurred in one patient without signs of reactivation. Thus, relapses of WG (or MPA) are preceded by recurrence or increase in titer of c-ANCA, but a rise in ANCA titer is not entirely specific for an ensuing relapse.

The close correlation between a rising ANCA titer and the ensuing disease reactivation may allow early treatment or even prevention of relapses. In 1990 we reported our third prospective study in WG (75) in which patients were randomised to treatment or no treatment once a significant rise of ANCA had occurred. In this study 58 patients with WG were prospectively screened for clinical evidence of disease activity at least every 3 months, whereas ANCA measurements were performed every month. Over an observation period of 24 months titers of ANCA rose in 20 patients. Nine of them were randomly assigned to start immunosuppressive treatment at the time ANCA had risen, and 11 patients were left untreated at that time but were treated when a clinical relapse occurred. Nine out of the 11 untreated patients relapsed, whereas no relapses occurred in patients randomized to treatment. Patients receiving no treatment at the time of ANCA rise took significantly more cyclophosphamide and prednisolone than patients who were randomly assigned to treatment.

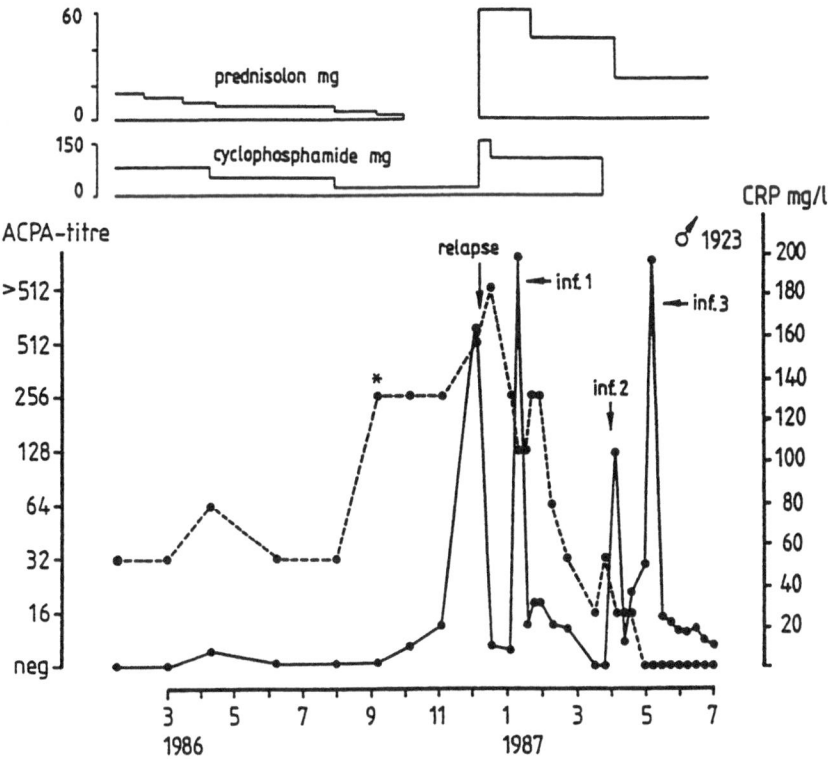

Figure 5.   Antineutrophil cytoplasm antibody (ANCA) titers (ACPA, dotted line), levels of C-reactive protein (CRP, solid line), and relapsing disease activity in a patient with Wegener's Granulomatosis. A significant rise in ACPA titer (September 1986) was followed by a clinical relapse in December 1986, coinciding with a rise in level of CRP. During immunosuppressive treatment, ANCA titers decreased while levels of CRP increased another three times concomitantly with three episodes of infection. In March 1987, cyclophosphamide treatment was discontinued because of Pneumocystis carinii pneumonia and cytomegalovirus infection. Asterisk indicates significant rise of ANCA titer [Reproduced from Ref. 18: Cohen Tervaert JW, van der Woude FJ, Fauci AS, Ambrus JL, Velosa J, Keane WF, Meijer S, van der Giessen M, The TH, van der Hem GK, Kallenberg CGM: Association between active Wegener's Granulomatosis and anticytoplasmic antibodies. Arch Intern Med, 149: 2461-2465, 1989, with permission. Copyright 1989, American Medical Association].

So, quantitation of c-ANCA seems useful for predicting disease activity in patients with WG or MPA, since relapses are usually preceded by a significant rise in ANCA. Moreover, relapses can be prevented by early treatment based on changes in ANCA titers.

With respect to levels of anti-MPO and disease activity, we found higher levels in sera obtained during active disease compared with those obtained during remission (20). In addition, we observed increases in levels of anti-MPO prior to disease relapses (20). However, at present no prospective studies have been described in patients with anti-MPO. Since anti-MPO associated diseases seem to relapse at a much lower frequency than anti-

Pr3 associated WG/MPA, collaborative studies will probably be needed to evaluate the significance of anti-MPO for following or predicting disease activity.

ANCA: PATHOPHYSIOLOGICAL SIGNIFICANCE?

The strong association between anti-proteinase 3 antibodies and Wegener's Granulomatosis suggests that the autoantibodies are pathophysiologically involved in the disease process. Although the pathogenetic role of the autoantibodies with respect to the disease manifestations of WG has not been clearly demonstrated, there are some recent data that may support a pathogenetic role for anti-Pr3.

Anti-Pr3 can activate primed neutrophils *in vitro* to the release of oxygen radicals and lysosomal enzymes (76), probably because these primed neutrophils express the antigens temporarily on their cell surface. Expression of Pr3 on the cell surface of neutrophils has, indeed, been demonstrated by electron microscopy (77). It has been recognized for a long time that disease exacerbations of WG are frequently associated with or preceded by infections, especially infections of the upper respiratory tract (78, 79). Neutrophils, primed as a result of infection, may be further activated by the autoantibodies. In normal physiology, tissue destruction by neutrophils is restricted by the inactivation of proteinases by anti-proteinases. Very recently, it has been shown that the autoantibodies do not bind to the active site of Pr3 but to the site of interaction with alpha1-anti-protease (van der Wiel, personal communication). As a result, Pr3 might escape its physiological inactivation and contribute to the extensive tissue destruction as seen in WG. Additionally, a local T-cell proliferative response to Pr3 might be involved in granuloma formation, a characteristic feature of the inflammatory process in WG. The occurrence of T-cells recognizing Pr3 in the peripheral blood of patients with WG has, indeed, been suggested by *in vitro* studies (80).

How to explain the development of crescentic glomerulonephritis (CGN) in WG in relation to the presence of anti-Pr3? Pr3, as already discussed, is a cationic serine protease and may localize to the polyanionic GBM. The development of CGN without immune deposits may be explained by a cellular immune response to Pr3 in analogy with studies of Oite et al (81) and Rennke et al (82). Oite et al (81) planted trinitrophenyl (TNP)-BSA in the kidney of rats that had been sensitized with the TNP hapten 7 days before. These rats developed transient glomerulonephritis without antibody deposition. Rennke et al (82) induced CGN with granuloma formation in rats sensitized to azobenzene-arsonate (ABA), a substance that elicited a T-cell restricted immune response, by *ex vivo* perfusion of the kidney with ABA. A comparable mechanism might be operative in CGN in the case of WG associated with an immune response to Pr3 (83). Experimental data to support this hypothesis are, however, lacking until now.

With respect to the pathogenetic role of anti-MPO, it has been demonstrated that anti-MPO, comparable to anti-Pr3, also can activate (primed) neutrophils *in vitro* (76). In addition, a T-cell mediated immune response to MPO might result in CGN according to mechanisms described above for the immune response to Pr3. Again, experimental data are lacking in this respect. In addition, it is not clear from the foregoing discussion why WG is specifically associated with anti-Pr3 whereas the presence of anti-MPO is not only associated with idiopathic CGN but also with different forms of necrotizing vasculitis some of which without kidney involvement. Experimental models are probably needed to clarify this issue.

CONCLUSION

The identification of ANCA and their several antigenic specificities has opened a new area for the study of the necrotizing vasculitides and glomerulonephritides. The presence of anti-Pr3 is highly sensitive and specific for the diagnosis of active Wegener's Granulomatosis. In addition, titration of anti-Pr3 is helpful for the monitoring of disease activity in WG. Changes in titre of anti-Pr3 may be used as a guideline for treatment. The detection of anti-MPO in the serum of a patient with clinical signs of glomerulonephritis suggests the presence of (idiopathic) necrotizing and/or crescentic glomerulonephritis or one of the necrotizing systemic vasculitides, in particular Churg Strauss Syndrome. Anti-MPO may be present in these latter conditions also when kidney involvement is lacking. Anti-elastase and anti-lactoferrin have been reported incidentally, but the clinical significance of these autoantibodies probably is restricted. It might be expected that more specificities of ANCA will be described in the near future. The pathogenetic significance of ANCA for the several diseases with which they are associated, awaits further study.

REFERENCES

1. Fauci AS, Haynes BF, Katz P: The spectrum of vasculitis: clinical, pathologic, immunologic and therapeutic considerations. Ann Intern Med, 89: 660-676, 1978.
2. Conn DL: Update on systemic necrotizing vasculitis. Mayo Clin Proc, 64: 535-543, 1989.
3. McCluskey RT, Fienberg R: Vasculitis in primary vasculitides, granulomatoses and connective tissue diseases. Hum Pathol, 14: 305-315, 1983.
4. Bacon PA: Vasculitis-clinical aspects and therapy. Acta Med Scand, Suppl 715: 157-163, 1987.
5. Alarcón-Segovia D: Classification of the necrotizing vasculitides in man. Clin Rheum Dis, 6: 223-231, 1980.

6. Lie JT: The classification and diagnosis of vasculitis in large and medium-sized blood vessels. Pathol Annu, 22: 125-162, 1987.

7. Lie JT: Classification and immunodiagnosis of vasculitis: a new solution or promises unfulfilled (Editorial). J Rheumatol, 15: 728-732, 1988.

8. Jennette JC, Wilkman AS, Falk RJ: Antineutrophil cytoplasmic autoantibodies-associated glomerulonephritis and vasculitis. Am J Pathol, 135: 921-930, 1989.

9. Stilmant MM, Bolton WK, Sturgill BC, Schmitt GW, Couser WG: Crescentic glomerulonephritis without immune deposits: clinicopathologic features. Kidney Int, 15: 184-195, 1979.

10. Crocker BP, Lee T, Gunnells JC: Clinical and pathological features of polyarteritis nodosa and its renal limited variant: primary crescentic and necrotizing glomerulonephritis. Hum Pathol, 18: 38-44, 1987.

11. Velosa JA: Idiopathic crescentic glomerulonephritis or systemic vasculitis? Mayo Clinic Proc, 62: 145-147, 1987.

12. Davies DJ, Moran JE, Niall JF, Ryan GB: Segmental necrotizing glomerulonephritis with antineutrophil antibody: possible arbovirus aetiology? Br Med J, 285: 606, 1982.

13. Hall JB, Wadham BMcN, Wood CJ, Ashton V, Adam WR: Vasculitis and glomerulonephritis: a subgroup with an antineutrophil cytoplasmic antibody. Aust N Z J Med, 14: 277-278, 1984.

14. Van der Woude FJ, Rasmussen N, Lobatto S, Wiik A, Permin H, van Es LA, van der Giessen M, van der Hem GK, The TH: Autoantibodies to neutrophils and monocytes: a new tool for diagnosis and a marker of disease activity in Wegener's Granulomatosis. Lancet, II: 425-429, 1985.

15. Savage COS, Winearls CG, Jones SJ, Marshall PD, Lockwood CM: Prospective study of radioimmunoassay for antibodies against neutrophil cytoplasm in diagnosis of systemic vasculitis. Lancet, 8: 1389-1393, 1986.

16. Falk RJ, Jennette JC: Anti-neutrophil cytoplasmic autoantibodies with specificity for myeloperoxidase in patients with systemic vasculitis and idiopathic necrotizing and crescentic glomerulonephritis. N Engl J Med, 318: 1651-1657, 1988.

17. Nölle B, Specks V, Lüdemann J, Rohrbach MS, De Remee DA, Gross WL: Anticytoplasmic autoantibodies: their immunodiagnostic value in Wegener's Granulomatosis. Ann Int Med, 111: 28-40, 1989.

18. Cohen Tervaert JW, van der Woude FJ, Fauci AS, Ambrus JL, Velosa J, Keane WF, Meijer S, van der Giessen M, The TH, van der Hem GK, Kallenberg CGM: Association between active Wegener's Granulomatosis and anticytoplasmic antibodies. Arch Intern Med, 149: 2461-2465, 1989.

19. Cohen Tervaert JW, Goldschmeding R, Elema JD, van der Giessen M, Huitema MG, van der Hem GK, The TH, von dem Borne AEGKr, Kallenberg CGM: Autoantibodies against myeloid lysosomal enzymes in crescentic glomerulonephritis. Kidney Int, 37: 799-806, 1990.

20. Cohen Tervaert JW, Goldschmeding R, Elema JD, Limburg PC, van der Giessen M, Huitema MG, Koolen MI, Hené RJ, The TH, van der Hem GK, von dem Borne AEGKr, Kallenberg CGM: Association of autoantibodies to myeloperoxidase with different forms of vasculitis. Arthritis Rheum, 33: 1264-1272, 1990.

21. Wiik A: Delineation of a standard procedure for indirect immunofluorescence detection of ANCA. APMIS, 97 (S6): 12-13, 1989.

22. Van der Woude FJ, Daha MR, van Es LA: The current status of neutrophil cytoplasmic antibodies. Clin Exp Immunol, 78: 143-148, 1989.

23. Borregaard N, Heiple JM, Simons FR, Clark RA: Subcellular localisation of the b-cytochrome component of the human neutrophil microbicidal oxidase translocation during activation. J Cell Biol, 97: 52-61, 1983.

24. Goldschmeding R, van der Schoot CE, ten Bokkel Huinink D, Hack CE, van den Ende ME, Kallenberg CGM, von dem Borne AEGKr: Wegener's Granulomatosis autoantibodies identify a novel diisopropylfluorophosphate-binding protein in the lysosomes of normal human neutrophils. J Clin Invest, 84: 1577-1587, 1989.

25. Kao RC, Wehner MG, Skubitz KM, Gray BH, Hoidal JR: Proteinase 3. A distinct human polymorphonuclear leucocyte proteinase that produces emphysema in hamsters. J Clin Invest, 82: 1963-1973, 1988.

26. Niles JL, McCluskey RT, Ahmad MF, Arnaout MA: Wegener's Granulomatosis autoantigen is a novel serine proteinase. Blood, 74: 1888-1893, 1989.

27. Lüdemann J, Utecht B, Gross WL: Anti-neutrophil cytoplasm antibodies in Wegener's Granulomatosis recognize an elastinolytic enzyme. J Exp Med, 171: 357-362, 1990.

28. Dolman KM, Goldschmeding R, van den Ende ME, Sonnenberg A, von dem Borne AEGKr: The antigen recognized by Wegener's Granulomatosis autoantibodies is a fourth protease of azurophilic granules (proteinase 4). Kidney Int (in press) (Abstract).

29. Campanelli D, Melchior M, Fu Y, Nakata N, Shuman H, Nathan C, Gabay JE: Cloning of cDNA for proteinase 3: a serine protease, antibiotic, and autoantigen from human neutrophils. J Exp Med, 172: 1709-1715, 1990.

30. Campanelli D, Detmers PA, Nathan CF, Gabay JE: Azurocidin and a homologous serine protease from neutrophils. Differential antimicrobial and proteolytic properties. J Clin Invest, 85: 904-915, 1990.

31. Bories D, Raynal MC, Solomon DH, Darzynkiewicz Z, Cayre Y: Down-regulation of a serine protease, myeloblastin, causes growth arrest and differentiation of promyelocytic leukemia cells. Cell, 59: 959-968, 1990.

32. Goldschmeding R, van der Schoot CE, Cohen Tervaert JW, Mason DY, von dem Borne AEGKr, Kallenberg CGM: Autoantibodies against myeloid lysosomal enzymes: a novel class of autoantibodies associated with vasculitic syndromes. Kidney Int, 34: 558-559, 1988 (Abstract).

33. Goldschmeding R, Cohen Tervaert JW, van der Schoot CE, van der Veen C, Kallenberg CGM, von dem Borne AEGKr: ANCA, anti-myeloperoxydase and anti-elastase: three members of a novel class of autoantibodies against myeloid lysosomal enzymes. APMIS, 97 (S6): 48-49, 1989.

34. Cohen Tervaert JW, Huitema MG, Dolman KM, Goldschmeding R, The TH, Kallenberg CGM: The clinical significance of autoantibodies to human leucocyte elastase. Academic thesis, Groningen, the Netherlands, pp 59-66, 1990.

35. Thomson RA, Lee SS: Antineutrophil cytoplasmic antibodies. Lancet, I: 670-671, 1989 (Letter).

36. Pryzwansky MB, Martin LE, Spitznagel JK: Immunocytochemical localization of myeloperoxidase, lactoferrin, lysozyme, and neutral proteases in human monocytes and neutrophilic granulocytes. J Reticuloendothel Soc, 24: 295-310, 1978.

37. Charles LA, Falk RJ, Jennette JC: Reactivity of anti-neutrophil cytoplasmic autoantibodies with HL-60 cells. Clin Immunol Immunopathol, 53: 243-253, 1989.

38. Mulder AHL, Horst G, van Leeuwen MA, Limburg PC, Kallenberg CGM: Granulocyte-specific antinuclear antibodies are directed against a granular compound of the granulocyte. Clin Rheumatol, 9: 578, 1990 (Abstract).

39. Saxon A, Sharahan F, Landers C, Ganz T, Targan S: A distinct subset of antineutrophil cytoplasmic antibodies is associated with inflammatory bowel disease. J Allergy Clin Immunol, 86: 202-210, 1990.

40. Farber V, Elling P: Leucocyte-specific anti-nuclear factors in patients with Felty's syndrome, rheumatoid arthritis, systemic lupus erythematosus, and other diseases. Acta Med Scand, 179: 257-267, 1966.

41. Wiik A: Granulocyte-specific antinuclear antibodies. Allergy, 35: 263-289, 1980.

42. Cohen Tervaert JW, Brouwer E, Mulder AHL, Limburg PC, Kallenberg CGM: The detection of myeloperoxidase antibodies: a comparison of four different techniques. Am J Kidney Dis (in press) (Abstract).

43. Wieslander J, Rasmussen N, Bygren P: An ELISA for ANCA and preliminary studies of the antigens involved. APMIS, 97 (Suppl 6): 42, 1989.

44. Kallenberg CGM, Rasmussen N: Solid phase assays for ANCA. Neth J Med, 36: 132-136, 1990.

45. Goldschmeding R, van der Schoot CE, van der Snoek MA, von dem Borne AEGKr: A monoclonal antibody against the 29 kD ANCA-antigen: application as catching antibody in a sandwich-ELISA for ANCA detection. APMIS, 97 (suppl 6): 47, 1989.

46. Lüdemann J, Utecht B, Gross WL: Detection and quantitation of anti-neutrophil cytoplasm antibodies in Wegener's granulomatosis by ELISA using affinity-purified antigen. J Immunol Meth, 114: 167-174, 1988.

47. Lee SS, Adu D, Thompson A: Anti-myeloperoxidase antibodies in systemic vasculitis. Clin Exp Immunol, 79: 41-46, 1990.

48. Nässberger L, Sjöholm AG, Jonsson H, Sturfelt G, Äkessen A: Autoantibodies against neutrophil cytoplasm components in systemic lupus erythematosus and in hydralazine-induced lupus. Clin Exp Immunol, 81: 380-383, 1990.

49. Godman GC, Churg J: Wegener's Granulomatosis. Pathology and review of the literature. Arch Pathol, 58: 533-553, 1954.

50. Lüdemann G, Gross WL: Autoantibodies against cytoplasmic structures of neutrophil granulocytes in Wegener's granulomatosis. Clin Exp Immunol, 69: 350-357, 1987.

51. Savage COS, Winearls CG, Evans DJ, Rees AJ, Lockwood CM: Microscopic polyarteritis: presentation, pathology and prognosis. Q J Med, 56: 467-483, 1985.
52. Woodworth TS, Abuelo JG, Austin HA, Esparza A: Severe glomerulonephritis with late emergence of classic Wegener's granulomatosis. Report of 4 cases and review of the literature. Medicine, 66: 181-191, 1987.
53. Parlevliet KJ, Henzen-Logmans SC, Oe PL, Bronsveld W, Balm AJM, Donker AJM: Antibodies to components of neutrophil cytoplasm: a new diagnostic tool in patients with Wegener's granulomatosis and systemic vasculitis. Q J Med, 66: 55-63, 1988.
54. Harrison DJ, Simpson R, Neary C, Wathen CG: Renal biopsy and antineutrophil antibodies in the diagnosis and assessment of Wegener's granulomatosis. Br J Dis Chest, 82: 398-404, 1988.
55. Cohen Tervaert JW, Goldschmeding R, Hené RJ, Kallenberg CGM: Neutrophil cytoplasmic antibodies and Wegener's granulomatosis. Lancet, I: 270, 1989 (Letter).
56. Specks V, Wheatley CL, McDonald TJ, Rohrbach MS, DeRemee RA: Anticytoplasmic autoantibodies in the diagnosis and follow-up of Wegener's granulomatosis. Mayo Clin Proc, 64: 28-36, 1989.
57. Harrison DJ, Simpson R, Kharbanda R, Abernethy VE, Nimmo G: Antibodies to neutrophil cytoplasmic antigens in Wegener's granulomatosis and other conditions. Thorax, 44: 373-377, 1989.
58. Andrassy K, Koderisch J, Rufer M, Erb A, Waldherr R, Ritz E: Detection and clinical implication of antineutrophil cytoplasm antibodies in Wegener's granulomatosis and rapidly progressive glomerulonephritis. Clin Nephrol, 32: 159-167, 1989.
59. Ferraro G, Meroni PL, Tincani A et al: Anti-endothelial cell antibodies in patients with Wegener's granulomatosis and micropolyarteritis. Clin Exp Immunol, 79: 47-53, 1990.
60. MacIsaac AI, Moran JE, Davies DJ, Murphy BF, Georgiou T, Niall JF: Antineutrophil cytoplasm antibody (ANCA) associated vasculitis. Clin Nephrol, 34: 5-8, 1990.
61. Venning MC, Quinn A, Broomhead V, Bird AG: Antibodies directed against neutrophils (c-ANCA and p-ANCA) are of distinct diagnostic value in systemic vasculitis. Q J Med, 77: 1287-1296, 1990.
62. Nässberger L, Sjöholm AG, Bygren P, Thysell H, Højer-Madsen M, Rasmussen N: Circulating anti-neutrophil cytoplasm antibodies in patients with rapidly progressive glomerulonephritis and extra-capillary proliferation. J Intern Med, 225: 191-196, 1989.
63. Nässberger L, Sjöholm AG, Thysell H: Antimyeloperoxidase antibodies in patients with extracapillary glomerulonephritis. Nephron, 56: 152-156, 1990.
64. Savige JA, Gallicchio M, Georgiou T, Davies DJ: Diverse target antigens recognized by circulating antibodies in anti-neutrophil cytoplasm antibody-associated renal vasculitides. Clin Exp Immunol, 82: 238-243, 1990.
65. Cohen Tervaert JW, Elema JD, Huitema MG, Kallenberg CGM: Autoantibodies against myeloid lysosomal enzymes in systemic vasculitis: a useful adjunct to classification. Am J Kidney Dis, 1991 (in press) (Abstract).
66. O'Donogue DJ, Short CD, Brenchley PEC, Lawler W, Ballardie FW: Sequential development of systemic vasculitis with anti-neutrophil cytoplasmic antibodies complicating anti-glomerular basement membrane disease. Clin Nephrol, 32: 251-255, 1989.
67. Jayne DRW, Marshall PD, Jones SJ, Lockwood CM: Autoantibodies to GBM and neutrophil cytoplasm in rapidly progressive glomerulonephritis. Kidney Int, 37: 965-970, 1990.
68. Savage COS, Tizard J, Jayne D, Lockwood CM, Dillon MJ: Antineutrophil cytoplasm antibodies in Kawasaki disease. Arch Dis Child, 64: 360-363, 1989.
69. Leavitt RY, Fauci AS, Bloch DA et al: The American College of Rheumatology 1990 criteria for the classification of Wegener's granulomatosis. Arthritis Rheum, 33: 1101-1107, 1990.
70. Calabresi P, Edwards EA, Schilling RF: Fluorescent antiglobulin studies in leukopenic and related disorders. J Clin Invest, 38: 2091-2100, 1959.
71. Andrassy K, Koderisch J, Schäfer A, Waldherr R: Idiopathic rapidly progressive (crescentic) glomerulonephritis with myeloperoxidase antibodies: a new entity linked to female sex? Nephron, 56: 99-100, 1990 (Letter).
72. Nada AK, Torres VE, Rye JH, Lie JT, Holley KE: Pulmonary fibrosis as an unusual clinical manifestion of a pulmonary-renal vasculitis in elderly patients. Mayo Clin Proc, 65: 847-856, 1990.
73. Cohen Tervaert JW, Goldschmeding R, Elema JD, von dem Borne AEGKr, Kallenberg CGM: Antimyeloperoxidase antibodies in the Churg-Strauss Syndrome. Thorax, 46: 70-71, 1991.
74. Egner W, Chapel HM: Titration of antibodies against neutrophil cytoplasmic antigens is useful in monitoring disease activity in systemic vasculitides. Clin exp Immunol, 82: 244-249, 1990.

75. Cohen Tervaert JW, Huitema MG, Hené RJ, Sluiter WJ, The TH, van der Hem GK, Kallenberg CGM: Prevention of relapses in Wegener's granulomatosis by treatment based on antineutrophil cytoplasmic antibody titre. Lancet, 336: 709-711, 1990.

76. Falk RJ, Terell RS, Charles LA, Jennette JC: Anti-neutrophil cytoplasmic autoantibodies induce neutrophils to degranulate and produce oxygen radicals *in vitro*. Proc Natl Acad Sci, 87: 4115-4119, 1990.

77. Csérnok E, Lüdemann J, Gross WL, Bainton DF: Immunocytochemical localization of proteinase 3, the target antigen of anti-cytoplasmic antibodies circulating in Wegener's Granulomatosis, in normal human neutrophils and monocytes. Clin Rheumatol, 9: 107, 1990 (Abstract).

78. Pinching AJ, Rees AJ, Pussell BA, Lockwood CM, Mitchison RS, Peters DK: Relapses in Wegener's Granulomatosis: the role of infection. Br Med J, 281: 836-838, 1980.

79. DeRemee RA: The treatment of Wegener's Granulomatosis with trimethoprim/sulfamethoxazole: illusion or vision? Arthritis Rheum, 31: 1068-1072, 1988.

80. Van der Woude FJ, van Es LA, Daha MR: The role of the c-ANCA antigen in the pathogenesis of Wegener's Granulomatosis. A hypothesis based on both humoral and cellular mechanisms. Neth J Med, 36: 169-171, 1990.

81. Oite T, Shimizu F, Kagami S, Morioku T: Hapten-specific cellular immune response producing glomerular injury. Clin exp Immunol, 76: 463-468, 1989.

82. Rennke HG, Klein PhS, Mendrick DL: Cell-mediated immunity in hapten-induced interstitial nephritis and glomerular crescent formation in the rat. Kidney Int, 37: 428, 1990 (Abstract).

83. Kallenberg CGM, Cohen Tervaert JW, van der Woude FJ, Goldschmeding R, von dem Borne AEGKr, Weening JJ. Autoimmunity to lysosomal enzymes: new clues to vasculitis and glomerulonephritis? Immunol Today, 12: 61-64, 1991.

Chapter 16

MICROSCOPIC EXAMINATION OF THE URINARY SEDIMENT TO DIFFERENTIATE HIGH FROM LOW RENAL BLEEDING

G. BERRY SCHUMANN AND JANET L. SCHUMANN

Cytopathology and Cytotechnology Department of Pathology, University of Alberta, Edmonton, Canada

INTRODUCTION

Normal adults excrete small numbers of erythrocytes in their urine; individual reports vary but, in general, up to 3% of adults will routinely shed small numbers of erythrocytes (from occasional to three red cells per high power field or up to 1,000 red cells/ ml) if examined using standardized urinalysis systems (1). Hematuria is defined as the excretion of abnormal numbers of red cells in urine on more than one occasion (i.e., greater than 3 red cells per high power field) (1). There are over 100 different medical and surgical causes for hematuria (2) affecting an estimated 13% of the U.S. population (3), and accounts for an estimated 20% of all primary physicians office visits (4). Gross hematuria, the appearance of blood in urine, is a startling discovery usually identified by the patient whereas microscopic hematuria is usually asymptomatic, found subsequent to a routine physical examination, hospital admission, or visit to the physician for some other symptom or complaint. Persistent microscopic hematuria in adults or children is an abnormal finding whose source must be identified. A method that would indicate the anatomic source or location of urinary bleeding would facilitate the work-up and subsequent diagnostic evaluation of patients with hematuria (3).

This chapter will describe the anatomic locations of hematuria and its clinical implications, review the theories of erythrocyte migration into urine, describe the routine and specialized microscopic methods used in detecting, characterizing and evaluating upper (glomerular), lower renal (tubular) and lower urinary tract hematuria. The diagnostic value of dysmorphic erythrocytes as a urine sediment aid in detecting glomerular bleeding and its comparison with other urinary sediment parameters indicative of renal bleeding will be reviewed. An algorithm for the laboratory evaluation of individuals with hematuria will be presented.

ANATOMIC LOCATION OF HEMATURIA

Hematuria may occur at any site along the entire expanse of the urinary system from the glomerulus to the distal urethra. The direction and magnitude of the clinical evaluation is dependent, to a large extent, on the age and sex of the patient. Urinary tract infection must always be excluded as the cause of urinary tract symptoms and hematuria (5). Lower urinary tract cancer must also be considered in all patients, particularly in those with gross hematuria in the third to sixth decades (6).

CLINICAL CONSIDERATIONS OF HEMATURIA

Lower urinary tract bleeding may be caused by infection, trauma, stones, inflammatory, hematologic or systemic disease processes, therapeutic regimens or neoplasms. The clinical evaluation of gross or microscopic hematuria begins with a thorough history, physical examination and laboratory data supplied by routine urinalysis, urine culture and urine cytology. These initial findings are important to guide subsequent investigations. Intravenous pyelograms, cystourethroscopy, renal function tests and renal biopsy may follow these initial studies. The microscopic examination of urinary sediment is a laboratory method which would aid in the localization of the site of hematuria and thereby greatly facilitate the extensive and very costly work-up of hematuria and avoidance of needless urologic procedures (3, 7).

The presence of significant proteinuria (greater than 2+), dysmorphic red cells and blood casts is strong evidence for renal parenchymal bleeding (most probably glomerular), although clinical and laboratory experiences have shown that dysmorphic red cells and blood casts may, in fact, occur in patients with non-glomerular, lower renal (tubular) bleeding (7, 8).

MECHANISMS OF ERYTHROCYTE MIGRATION INTO URINE

Numerous disease processes involving lower urinary tract may cause small to large vessel damage and subsequent bleeding or hemorrhage into the urinary stream. Bleeding originating in the lower urinary tract has been described as "isomorphic" showing a uniform, homogeneous population of normochromic oval and bi-concave cells (Figure 1).

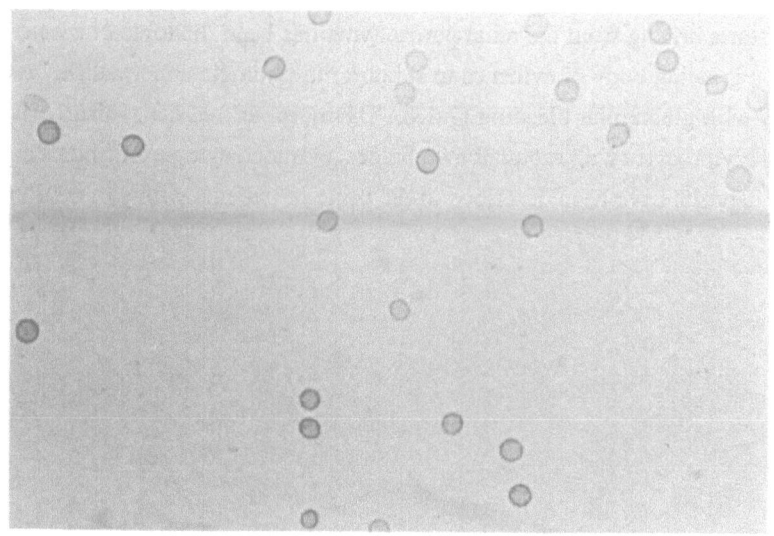

Figure 1. Normal (isomorphic) erythrocytes in urine. Brightfield microscopy.

Red cells occurring as the result of extrarenal bleeding may loose their hemoglobin content and appear as "ghost cells". These cells should be considered as normal variants and of no diagnostic consequence. Crenated red cells, products of the tonicity of hypertonic urine may also be found in associated with various lesions of the lower urinary tract (Figure 2).

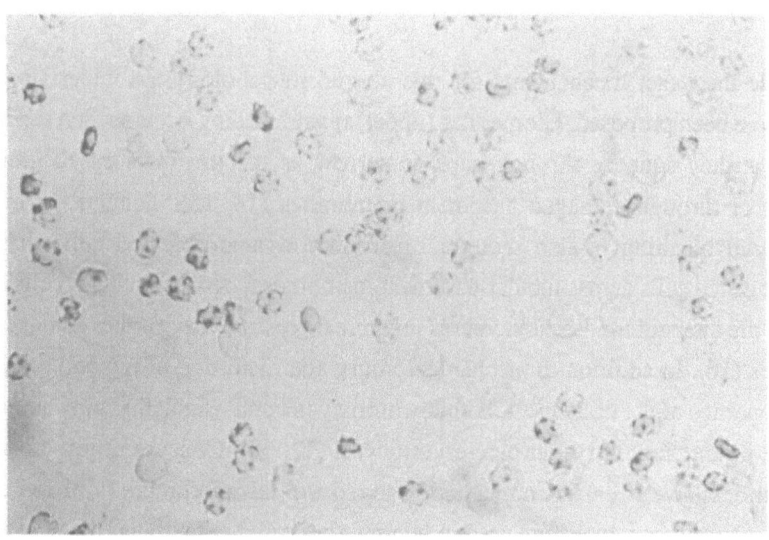

Figure 2. Crenated erythrocytes in urine. Brightfield microscopy.

Hematuria arising from the renal parenchyma has been the topic of recent interest because of a growing body of evidence to support morphologic abnormalities associated specifically with glomerular bleeding (7-13). "Dysmorphic" red cells, bizarre, irregular, fragmented erythrocytes with ruptured membranes, extruded cytoplasmic blebs and dense membrane deposits have been described in the urine of patients with glomerulonephritis (Figure 3).

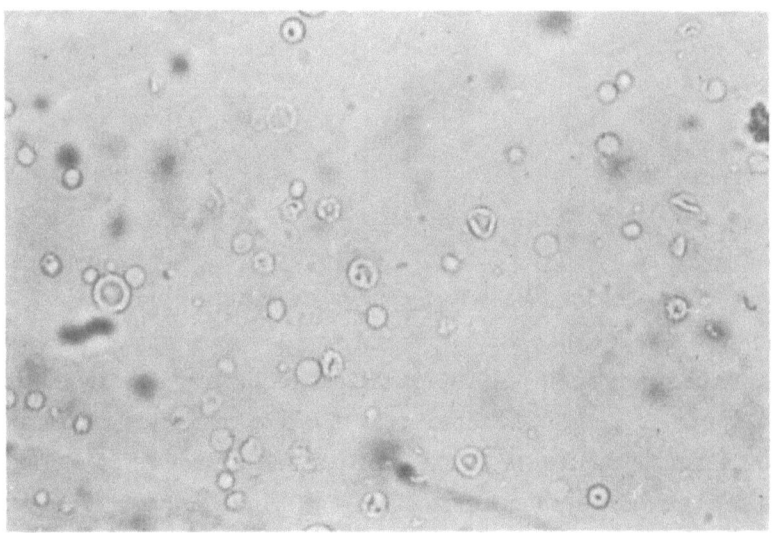

Figure 3. Dysmorphic erythrocytes in urine. Brightfield microscopy.

While the exact mechanisms for this altered morphology are uncertain, several theories have been proposed. Glomerular (upper) renal bleeding occurs when red cells are damaged as they squeeze through gaps as narrow as 0.3 μm in diseased glomerular capillaries or through damaged basement membranes (14, 15). Tubular or interstitial (lower) renal bleeding is also thought to produce dysmorphic red cells due to the movement of red cells across tubular basement membranes, between tubular cells and into and out of the interstitium. Local increases in luminal pressure may further damage red cell membranes (16). In addition to mechanical injury and distortion of red cell membranes, certain properties of the urine itself, both low urinary pH and osmolality, play an important role in the production of dysmorphic erythrocytes (17, 18). Concurrent urine osmolality determinations have been recommended to avoid the misinterpretation of red cell size especially when autoanalysers are used to interpret red cell distribution (18). Goldwasser et al (19) provided evidence that objective data regarding red cell sizing could be obtained by

340

the use of a hematology analyzer. This method appears to be a simple, highly accurate method by which to differentiate glomerular from non-glomerular hematuria. However, this study did not include cases of lower renal (non-glomerular) etiologies of renal bleeding such as tubular or interstitial disease processes. Some patients display a "mixed" pattern of erythrocyte morphology, which may likely represent concurrent disease processes. Patients with infections, renal calculi, and high fluid intake may present with "mixed" hematuria. Chang (7) described such a mixed pattern of hematuria occurring in a patient with lupus nephritis and concurrent lower urinary tract infection. The incidence and quantitation of erythrocyte morphology found in the various categories of renal parenchymal diseases, i.e. glomerular, tubular, interstitial and vascular lesions, require further studies.

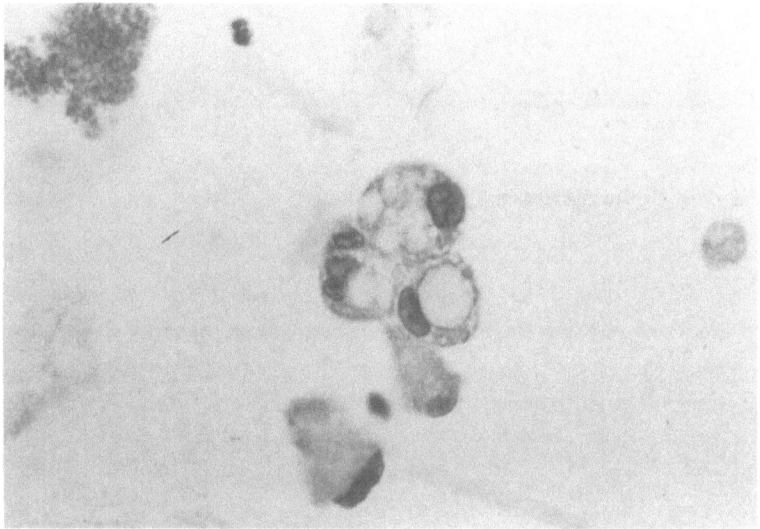

Figure 4.   Lipid-laden foamy renal cell. Papanicolaou stain.

THE ROLE OF MICROSCOPIC EXAMINATION OF URINARY SEDIMENT IN DETECTION AND LOCALIZATION OF RENAL HEMATURIA

Microscopic examination of urine sediment in conjunction with a reagent-strip chemical test for intact red cells, free hemoglobin or myoglobin, is important in the initial assessment of hematuria. The presence of moderate proteinuria (greater than 2+ by macroscopic urinalysis) and three specific types of renal casts, i.e. blood (hemoglobin), erythrocytic, and fibrin, represents important morphologic evidence of glomerulopathy or renal parenchymal bleeding (20, 21).

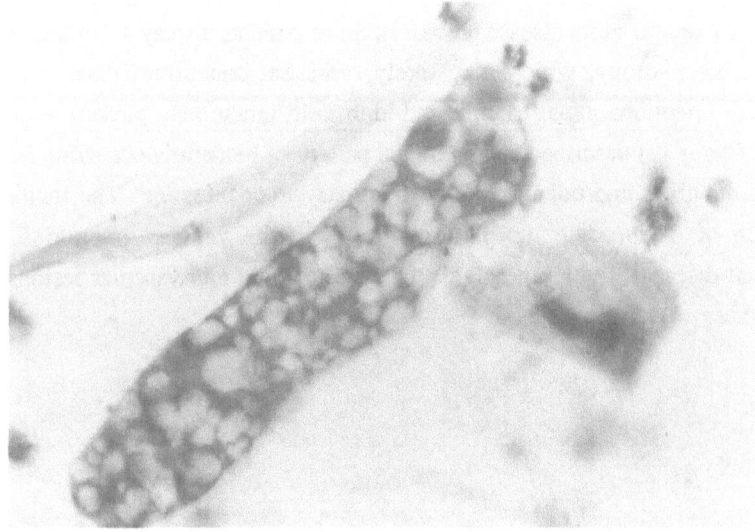

Figure 5.   Fatty cast. Papanicolaou stain.

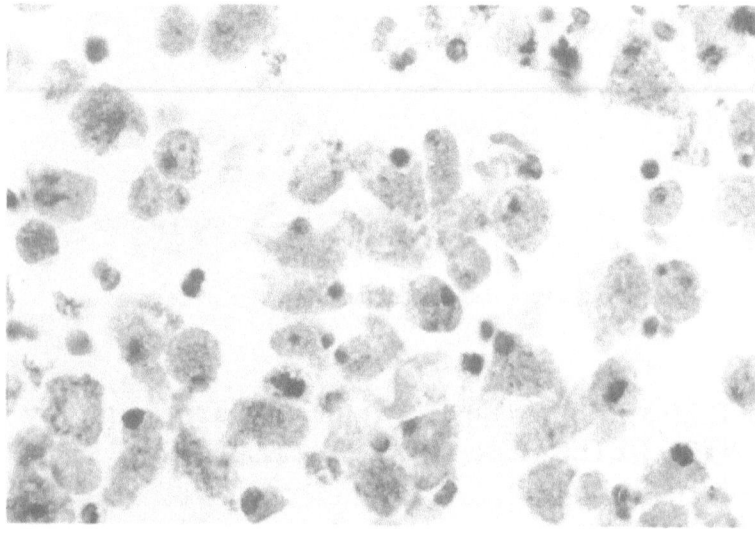

Figure 6.   Convoluted renal tubular cells. Papanicolaou stain.

The characteristic urine sediment findings in patients with nephrotic syndrome includes lipiduria and the identification of fat droplets, renal epithelial foam cells (Figure 4) (oval fat bodies See Figure 4) and fatty casts (Figure 5) (21). Dysmorphic red cells can also be associated with these sediment findings. Increased numbers of renal tubular cells are indicative of renal tubular injury or damage and when found with hematuria imply renal parenchymal bleeding (20, 21). Convoluted renal tubular cells (Figure 6) and collecting duct cells (Figure 7) are often found in a variety of renal tubular and interstitial disease processes. Exfoliated renal fragments represent severe tubular basement membrane disruption and parenchymal ischemia (21).

All of these urinalysis findings indicate active renal disease, and their absence infers an extrarenal or lower urinary tract disease or condition as a source for the hematuria. Two microscopic urinalysis methods which can be used to detect and characterize renal bleeding are described below.

MICROSCOPIC URINALYSIS METHODS FOR DETECTING RENAL BLEEDING

Routine urinalysis

Wet, unstained brightfield microscopy can be used to detect and confirm erythrocytes as the etiology of a positive hemoglobin reaction on the reagent-strip test. Red urine in the absence of red blood cells implies the presence of food color, drugs or myoglobin.

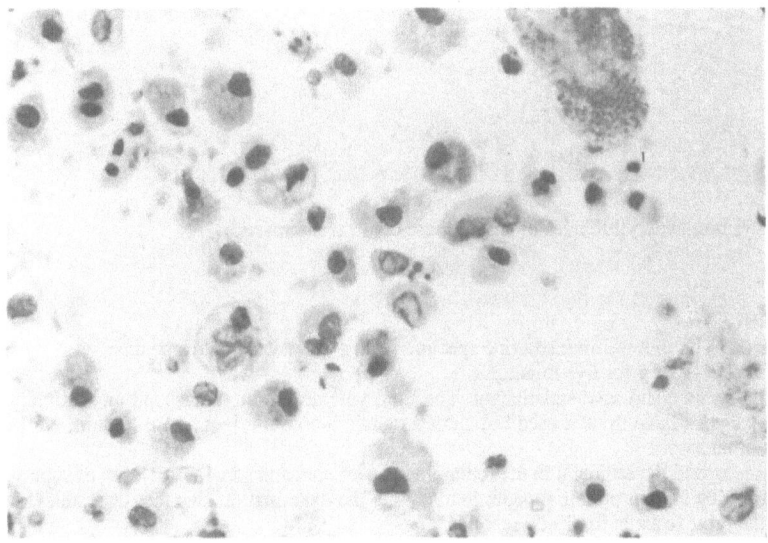

Figure 7.   Collecting duct renal tubular cells. Papanicolaou stain.

343

A reduced light source is recommended and supravital stains may be used to enhance morphologic detail. Standardized microscopic urinalysis systems are available and superior to the conventional glass slide and coverlip method. Interference and phase contrast microscopy provide improved discrimination of urinary sediment elements including dysmorphic red cells (Figure 8) and casts (Figure 9) but require specialized attachments to the microscope and personnel trained in the interpretation of this microscopic method (22). Wright's stain has also been used on air dried material for improved erythrocyte morphology (7).

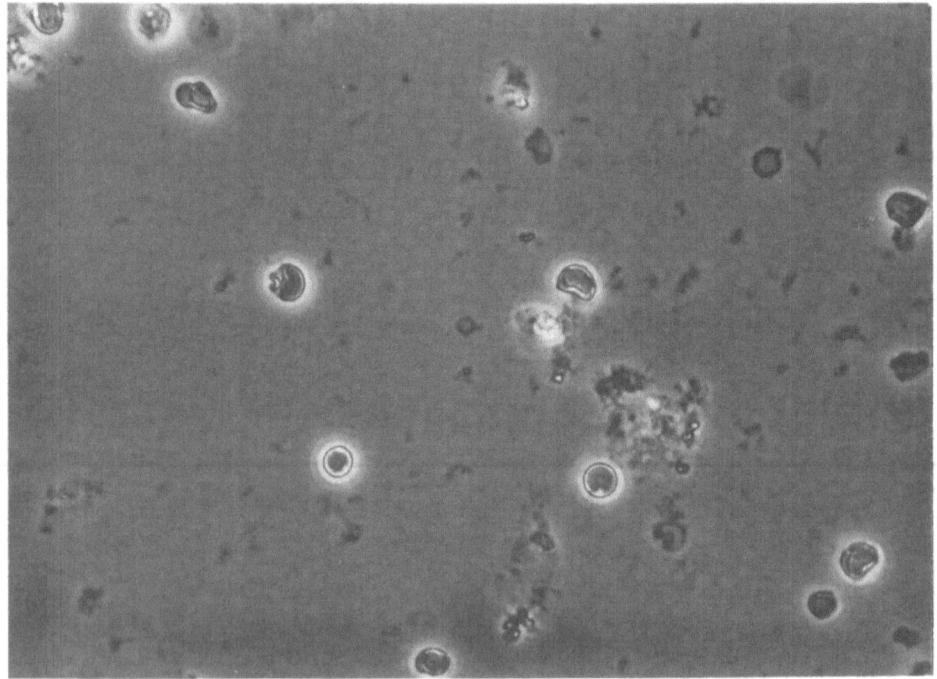

Figure 8. Dysmorphic erythrocytes in urine. Phase contrast microscopy.

PROCEDURE (22)
1. Pour 10 or 15 ml of a well-mixed urine specimen into a graduated centrifuge tube.
2. Centrifuge at 450 x g for five minutes.
3. Carefully remove and save supernatant. The final volume used to resuspend the sediment may vary with the standardized system used but should remain a constant [e.g., 1 ml, 0.5 ml, etc.] within any given laboratory.
4. Gently resuspend the sediment in the remaining supernatant and add 1/2 to 1 drop of supravital stain if desired. Using an appropriate pipette, load/charge the examination chamber of a standardized slide. Allow the urine to settle for 30-60 seconds.
5. Examine with low- and high-power objectives. Subdued light or phase-contrast illumination will be required to detect sediment entities with a low refractive index, i.e. hyaline casts. The fine focus should

be varied continuously while scanning. Systemically progress around the entire examination chamber, being careful to examine along edges for casts.

6. Count the number of casts in at least 10 low-power fields, average, and report the number of casts per low-power field (lpf). A reasonable range may be used in reporting [i.e., 0-2, 2 to 5, 5 to 10, etc.] Use high power to identify casts by type. Casts will not be missed if phase-contrast or supravital stains are used.

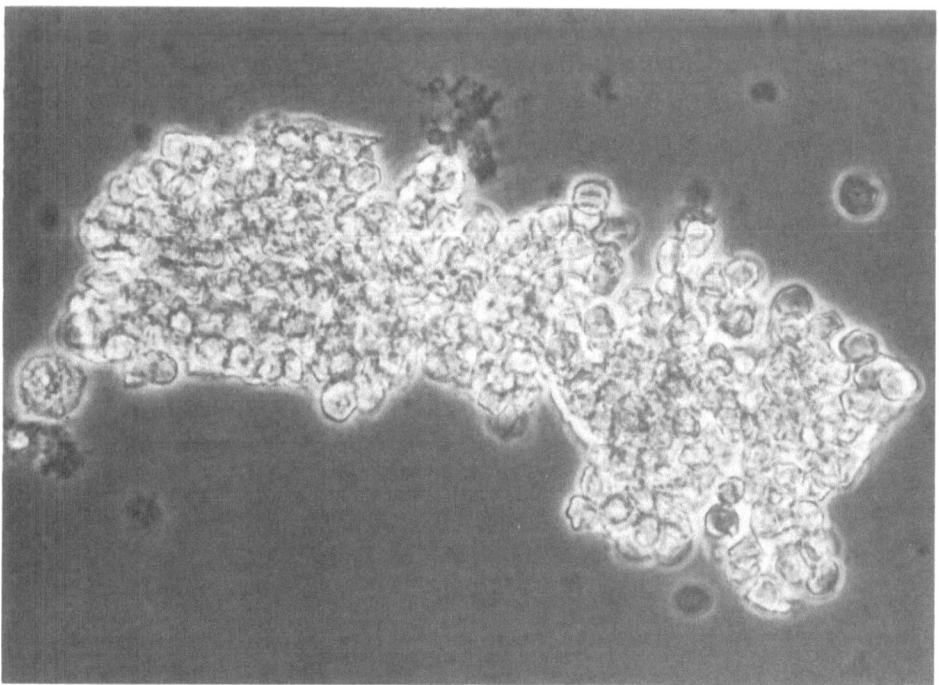

Figure 9. Erythrocytic cast in urine. Phase contrast microscopy.

7. Identify and count erythrocytes, leukocytes and renal epithelial cells using a high power objective. Count at least 10 high-power fields (hpf), average, and report as cells/hpf. A reasonable range may be used for reporting.

8. Comment on the presence of dysmorphic or isomorphic erythrocytes. An assessment of the amount or percentage of dysmorphic erythrocytes is desired.

9. The authors recommend confirming the following abnormal sediment results with cytodiagnostic urinalysis.
    a. More than 2 renal epithelial cells/hpf
    b. Pathologic casts
    c. Tissue fragments
    d. Atypical mononuclear cells
    e. Pathologic crystals

10. Review entire report, including physical, chemical and microscopic data, and correlate with available clinical information. Discrepancies should be resolved before releasing report.

     Normal values for the procedure:
       0 to 10 isomorphic erythrocytes (RBCs)/hpf
       0 to 10 leukocytes (WBCs)/hpf
       0 to 2 hyaline casts/hpf
    Note: Values will vary, depending on standardized microscopic system used.

CYTODIAGNOSTIC URINALYSIS

Cytodiagnostic urinalysis includes a semiquantitative, cytocentrifuged/Papanicolaou stained sediment examination. Cytologic analysis of urine which has been found to be the most sensitive method for detecting erythrocytes, more so than the reagent-strip (23, 24). Cytologic techniques are time-consuming and require trained personnel. Cytodiagnostic urinalysis, while not the procedure of choice for the initial detection of hematuria and dysmorphic erithrocytes, is far superior in the accurate identification and characterization of erythrocyte morphology (Figure 10), pathologic casts and typing of exfoliated renal epithelial cells (25, 26). Using this method of urine examination, renal cells are readily distinguished from leukocytes and smaller deep urothelial cells, a common problem in traditional brightfield microscopy (21). Cytodiagnostic urinalysis allows documentation of progressive and regressive renal parenchymal injury (26).

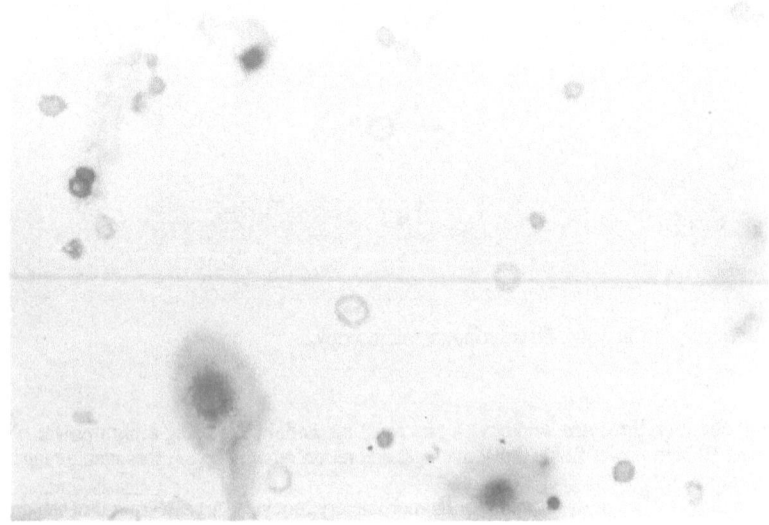

Figure 10. Dysmorphic erythrocytes in urine. Papanicolaou stain.

PROCEDURE (22)
1. Pour 10 ml of urine into an optically clear centrifuge tube.
2. Perform a macroscopic urinalysis using a multiparameter reagent-strip test.
3. Centrifuge capped tubes at 1500 rpm (490 x g) for 10 minutes.
4. Remove supernatant. Perform SSA test for protein. Specific gravity may also be performed at this time.
5. Add saline to bring urine sediment and remaining supernatant to exactly 1 ml.
6. Using a cytocentrifuge, prepare four slides using 250 µl of suspended sediment per chamber. Cytocentrifuge at 750 rpm (65 x g) for 6 minutes. If the sediment is hypercellular, use a smaller amount of sediment (125 µl, 60 µl, 30 µl) and decrease cytocentrifugation time (4, 3, 2 minutes).

7. After cytocentrifuging, discard filter card and immediately add one to two drops of Parlodion to the cell button.
8. Fix slides for 15 minutes in Saccomanno's fixative or in 95% ethanol.
9. Stain slides using conventional Papanicolaou method which can be found in standard cytology textbooks. A modified, rapid (7 minute) staining procedure is also available. Manual or automated staining methods take approximately 20 minutes.
10. Screen all four slides completely, noting background pattern, cellularity, viral inclusions, tissue fragments, and abnormal cells.
11. Count erythrocytes, neutrophils, lymphocytes, eosinophils, casts, and renal tubular epithelial cells in 10 hpfs. Casts and renal cells are differentiated by type.
12. Review the report, including physical, chemical, and microscopic data, and correlate with the clinical history. Discrepancies must be resolved before reporting.
13. Sign-out report with pathologist/M.D. specialist.

DYSMORPHIC ERYTHROCYTES AS A RELIABLE INDICATOR OF GLOMERULAR BLEEDING

The observation of dysmorphic red cells have been confirmed in numerous studies using phase-contrast microscopy (27, 28), light microscopy with (7, 29) or without staining (8, 30), and electron microscopy (30, 31). Recently, utilization of red cell volume and the use of red cell analyzers have been advocated to provide a rapid, objective screen for glomerular bleeding (32-36).

The application of strict morphologic criteria to differentiate isomorphic from dysmorphic erythrocytes as an indicator for glomerular versus lower urinary tract disease, has a reported sensitivity approaching 100% and specificity ranging from 90 to 100% (19). Urine specimen quality, skill levels of observers, inaccessibility to high quality microscopes or phase contrast enhancers are factors which have influenced reports of less success with this method.

COMPARISON OF DYSMORPHIC ERYTHROCYTES WITH OTHER URINARY SEDIMENT PARAMETERS OF RENAL BLEEDING

In 1986 Thal et al studied the prevalence of dysmorphic erythrocytes in 5,128 urines specimens from urology, nephrology, general medicine and renal transplant services. Blood, erythrocytic, or fibrin casts, proteinuria, and significant number of exfoliated renal tubular epithelial cells (RTCs) were also noted in the concentrated urine sediments. Of the 510 samples found to contain pathologic casts, 15% had dysmorphic erythrocytes, 60% had proteinuria, 71% had RTCs, and 12% had no other abnormality. Of the 186 samples containing dysmorphic erythrocytes, 55% had pathologic casts, 42% had proteinuria, 71% had RTCs, and 13% had no other abnormality. While this study did not correlate renal function studies, renal biopsy results, clinical history or follow-up of patients with evidence of renal bleeding to document glomerulopathies from other etiologies of lower renal (tubular, interstitial, vascular) disease processes, it was nevertheless suggested that renal hematuria can best be evaluated by examination of all four of these urinary sediment parameters of renal bleeding rather than using a single parameters for diagnosis, specifically dysmorphic red cells. Clearly, other sediment elements (dysmorphic red cells, fibrin, blood casts and renal tubular cells from various portions of the nephron) can be expected in cases of advanced renal disease.

Initially, our laboratory supported the use of the criteria suggested by Fassett (12) that when more than 80% of erythrocytes are dysmorphic, this should be considered upper (glomerular) or lower (tubular) hematuria, and when more the 80% of the erythrocytes are isomorphic or undistorted, this should be considered evidence of lower urinary tract bleeding. However, we now feel that proteinuria combined with the microscopic detection of as low as 10% dysmorphic red cells can be used to suggest upper (glomerular) bleeding. Careful scrutiny of the urine sediment for the presence of additional indicators of renal disease such as erythrocytic, blood or fibrin casts and increased renal tubular cells indicate concurrent lower renal (tubular/interstitial) bleeding. If dysmorphic erythrocytes are the only abnormality found, the patient should still be considered to be at risk for the development of renal disease, but may be followed and monitored at regular intervals using microscopic examination of urine sediment.

In the mid 1980's while at the University of Utah Cytopathology Laboratory, we began to incorporate a statement on the presence of dysmorphic red cells as a part of the cytologic report. This finding appeared to increase in referrals from the urologic service in patients with hematuria who were found to be cystoscopically negative for a source of lower urinary tract bleeding. At that time we recommended to urologists that a renal source of the bleeding be investigated if the hematuria persisted or progressed. We performed a retrospective analysis of 535 specimens accompanied by a urologic history, most often being hematuria. Renal parenchymal bleeding, defined by the presence of dysmorphic red cells and/or hemoglobin, erythrocytic or fibrin casts were reported in 54 (10%) of these cases. We then reviewed 28 available medical records from 43 patients for subsequent clinical and/or histological evidence of renal disease. Eleven of these patients were referred to nephrologists for follow-up studies and/or renal biopsies. Glomerulopathies were identified in five of the eleven patients, one had amyloidosis, one had renal cystic disease, one had renal lithiasis and one was found to have a renal mass of undetermined origin. Chronic renal disease was identified in the remaining two patients.

In 1991 a correlative study performed at the University of Alberta compared the findings using cytodiagnostic urinalysis with renal biopsy in 33 consecutive patients.

Results of this prospective study revealed that dysmorphic red cells were present in 17/18 (94%) biopsy confirmed glomerular lesions, 2/14 (14%) tubulointerstitial lesions and in 0/1 vascular lesions. Pathologic renal casts (erythrocytic, hemoglobin or fibrin) were found in 9/18 (50%) of glomerular lesions, 12/14 (86%) of tubulointerstitial lesions and in 1/1 (100%) vascular lesions. Renal tubular injury, as evidenced by the presence of renal tubular cells per 10 hpf using cytodiagnostic urinalysis techniques showed a mean count of 130 renal cells in glomerular lesions, 344 in tubulointerstitial lesions and 1,140 in the vascular lesions.

Macroscopic profiles of theses 33 cases showed that the glomerular lesions were characterized by 2+ protein (confirmed by SSA technique) and trace blood on reagent-strip testing (BMC Chemstrip 9). Tubulointerstitial lesions were characterized by trace protein and trace blood, and the vascular lesion was characterized by trace protein and trace blood.

The authors experience with both of these studies suggest that renal bleeding, upper (glomerular) and lower (tubulointerstitial), can be separated from lower urinary tract bleeding and that dysmorphic red cells are a reliable morphologic marker of glomerular bleeding.

Dysmorphic red cells may, also yet less frequently, be found in tubular or interstitial disease processes. Proteinuria found increased in glomerular disease is a helpful functional marker of glomerular damage. Pathologic casts (especially blood, erythrocytic and fibrin) are present in both glomerular and tubular disease, however, when found with increased numbers of renal epithelial cell points to a lower renal parenchymal lesion.

AN ALGORITHM FOR THE LABARATORY WORK-UP OF RENAL HEMATURIA

The evaluation of hematuria has been extensively examined and numerous algorithms had been proposed (2, 3, 5, 37, 38). In evaluating any abnormality, especially microscopic hematuria, the physician must weigh the benefits of a diagnosis against the cost (physical, mental, and monetary) to achieve it (38).

The physician must carefully decide which patients should undergo potentially harmful and invasive procedures, such as cystoscopy, arteriography or renal biopsy.

Table 1 outlines a 3 level, multi-step approach for the laboratory work-up of renal hematuria. Following a thorough history (including medications, familial history and other risk factors), the first laboratory step would be to detect, confirm on more than one occasion, categorize and subclassify the type of hematuria by conventional routine brightfield or phase contrast microscopy.

349

Table 1. Laboratory work-up of renal hematuria.

INITIAL LABORATORY STUDIES

STEPS

Level "A"

1. *Detect hematuria*
   (Determine if intermittent or persistent)
2. *Categorize type of hematuria*
   Gross (Inspection)
   Macroscopic (Reagent-strip Test)
   Microscopic (Morphologic Test)
3. *Categorize red cell morphology*
   Determine the following:
   Isomorphic (Non-glomerular/lower urinary tract)
   Dysmorphic (Glomerular/Renal Parenchymal)

CONFIRMATORY LABORATORY STUDIES

STEPS

Level "B"

1. *Cytodiagnostic urinalysis test*
   Aim: Exclude urine sediment findings of lower urinary tract disease and
   determine urine sediment findings of:
   A. Renal bleeding
   B. Renal parenchymal injury / damage
   C. Document progression/regression of injury
2. *Renal function tests*
   Aim: Establish:
   A. Renal dysfunction
   B. Document progression / regression of function

ADDITIONAL CONFIRMATORY LABORATORY STUDIES

Level "C"

Aim: Classify & determine severity of the renal condition
   A. Cytodiagnostic Urinalysis
   B. Immunology
   C. Renal biopsy

Urine color is very important: pseudohematuria caused by food color, drug additives or therapy, urate concentration, or myoglobin should be distinguished from gross hematuria and microscopic hematuria. Clots imply the source of the blood is of lower urinary origin (6). If dysmorphic erythrocytes are identified in the microscopic urinalysis, a more sensitive urinalysis, i.e. cytodiagnostic urinalysis, and renal function tests should be used (Table 1 - Level "B"). Level "C" involves adjunctive, costly and invasive techniques for classifying and assessing the severity of the renal lesion(s). The suggested algorithm provides a straightforward and logical approach to the laboratory assessment of renal hematuria.

CONCLUSION

The examination of urinary sediment remains an irreplaceable, front-line procedure for the initial detection of renal hematuria. The identification of dysmorphic erythrocytes in a non-anemic patient is an important morphologic marker for the localization of renal disease, and probable glomerulopathy. To discriminate upper renal (glomerular) from lower renal (tubular/interstitial) hematuria, additional urine sediment parameters of renal parenchymal bleeding, injury or damage should be documented (Table 2). Cytodiagnostic urinalysis is a specialized confirmatory method and is complementary to conventional renal functional studies and should precede invasive techniques, such as renal biopsy. While addition of prospective studies to separate upper renal (glomerular) from lower renal (tubular) bleeding are needed, it appears that the microscopic examination of the urinary sediment will allow the differentiation of high from low renal bleeding.

Table 2. Important urinalysis findings in distinguishing upper from lower renal parenchymal hematuria.

URINALYSIS FINDINGS	RENAL PARENCHYMAL LESIONS	
	Glomerular	Tubular/Interstitial
Protein (>2+)	***	-/*
Blood	***	***
Lipid	***	-/*
URINE SEDIMENT ENTITIES		
Dysmorphic red blood cells	***	-/*
Erythrocytic casts	**	**
Fibrin casts	**	**
Hemoglobin casts	**	**
Fatty casts	***	-/*
Foamy lipid-laden cells	***	-/*
Renal tubular cells	*	***
Renal tubular fragments	-	***

REFERENCES

1. Schaeffer AJ, Del Greco F: Other renal diseases of urologic significance. In: "Campbell's Urology", 5th Edition, Vol. 3, WB Saunders, Philadelphia, 1986, p 2342.
2. Spirnack JP: Hematuria. In: "Decision making in urology" (Eds MJ Resnick, AA Caldamore and JP Spirnack), BC Decker Inc, Philadephia, 1985, p 4.
3. Corwin LH, Silverstein MD: Microscopic hematuria. Clinics Lab Med, 8: 601-609, 1988.
4. Mariani AJ, Mariani MC, Macchinoni C, et al: The significance of adult hematuria: 1,000 hematuria evaluations including a risk-benefit and cost-effectiveness analysis. J Urol, 141 (2): 350-355, 1989.
5. Brewer ED, Benson GS: Hematuria: Algorithms for diagnosis. I. Hematuria in the child. JAMA, 246 (8): 877-880, 1981.
6. Gillenwater JY, Grayback JT, Howards SS, et al: Adult and Pediatric Urology. Mosby, St. Louis, 2nd Edition, 1991, p 68-71.
7. Chang BS: Red cell morphology as a diagnostic aid in hematuria. JAMA, 252 (13): 1747-1749, 1984.

8. Fairley KF, Birch DF: Hematuria. A simple method for identifying glomerular bleeding. Kidney Int, 21: 105-108, 1982.
9. Schifferli JA: Hematuria: Glomerular or non-glomerular. Lancet, II: 1014, 1979.
10. Pellet H, Minaire E: Red cells in the urine. Lancet, I: 24, 1980.
11. Jacobellis V, Fabiano A, Tallarigo C: A new technique to localize the origin of idiopathic microscopic hematuria. J Urol, 127: 475-476, 1981.
12 Fassett M, Horgan BA, Matheus TH: Detection of glomerular bleeding by phase contrast microscopy. Lancet, I: 1432-1434, 1982.
13. Kincaid Smith P: Haematuria and exercise-related haematuria. Br Med J, 285: 1677-1678, 1982.
14. Mouradian JA, Sherman K: Passage of an erythrocyte through a glomerular basement membrane gap. N Eng J Med, 293: 940-941, 1975.
15. Burkholder PM: Ultrastructure demonstration and perforation of glomerular capillary basement membrane in acute proliferative glomerulonephritis. Am J Pathol, 56: 251-266, 1969.
16. Nadasy T, Nagy KK, Csajbok E, et al: Hematuria of tubular origin. Ultrastructural Pathol, 13: 63-68, 1989.
17. Briner VA, Reinhart WH: *In vitro* production of "glomerular red cells": Role of pH and osmolality. Nephron, 56: 13-18, 1990.
18. Turitzin SN, Rotellar C, Winchester JF, et al: Effect of urine osmalality on urinary red cell morphology. Nephron, 55: 344-355, 1990.
19. Goldwasser P, Antignani A, Mittman N: Urinary red cell size: Diagnostic value and determinants. Am J Nephrol, 10: 148-156, 1990.
20. Thal M, De Bellis C, Iversun A, et al: Comparison of dysmorphic erythrocytes with other urinary sediment parameters of renal bleeding. Am J Clin Pathol, 86: 784-787, 1986.
21. Schumann GB: Urine sediment examination. Williams & Wilkins, Baltimore, 1980.
22. Schumann GB, Schweitzer SC: Examination of urine. In: "Clinical diagnosis and management by laboratory methods" (Ed JB Henry), 18th Edition, WB Saunders, Philadelphia, 1991.
23. Freni SS, Heeederik GJ, Hol C: Centrifugation techniques and reagent-strips in the assessment of microhematuria. J Clin Pathol, 30: 336-340, 1977.
24. Shenoy UA, Schumann GB, De Bellis CC: Incidence of MH in urothelial neoplasia. J Clin Pathol, 85: 80-82, 1986.
25. Schumann GB, Schumann JL, DeBellis C: Cytodiagnostic urinalysis: The method and its applications. Lab Management, 11: 36-40, 1985.
26. Schumann GB: Cytodiagnostic urinalysis for the nephrology practice. Sem Nephrol, 6: 308-345, 1986.
27. Rizzoni G, Braggion F, Zacchello G: Evaluation of glomerular and non-glomerular hematuria by phase-contrast morphology. J Pediat, 130: 370-374, 1983.
28. De Santo NG, Nuzzi F, Capodicasa G, et al: Phase contrast microscopy of the urine sediment for the diagnosis of glomerular and non-glomerular bleeding - data in children and adults with normal creatine clearance. Nephrol, 45: 35-39, 1987.
29. Hauglustaine D, Bollins W, Michielsen P: Detection of glomerular bleeding using a simple staining method for light microscopy. Lancet II: 761, 1982 (Letter).
30. Birch DF, Fairley KF, Whitworth JA: Urinary erythrocyte morphology in the diagnosis of glomerular hematuria. Clin Nephrol, 20: 78-84, 1983.
31. Fassett RG, Horgan B, Gove D, et al: Scanning electron microscopy of glomerular and non-glomerular red blood cells. Clin Nephrol, 20: 11-16, 1983.
32. Docci D, Baldrati L, Turci F, et al: Microcytic hematuria is an indicator of glomerular bleeding. Am J Nephrol, 8: 344-345, 1988.
34. Chung WY, Lee SY: The mean cellular volume (MCV) and red cell distribution (URBC) for determination of glomerular bleeding in children with hematuria. IX International Congress of Nephrology, 1990, Tokyo, (Abstract).
35. de Caestecher MP, Gower PE, Ballardie FW: Improved urinary erythrocyte morphology using red cell analysers. IX International Congress of Nephrology, 1990, Tokyo, (Abstract).
36. Goldwasser P, Antignani A, Norbergs A, et al: Urinary red cell volume differentiates glomerular and non-glomerular hematuria. Kidney Int, 33: 191, 1988.
37. Ng RCK, Seto DSJ: Hematuria. A suggested work-up strategy. Postgrad Med, 75, 1: 139-144, 1984.
38. Bloom KJ: An algorithm for hematuria. Clin Lab Med, 8: 577-583, 1988.

INDEX

[Page numbers following (T) refer to Tables; page number following (F) refer to Figures]

abortion 180; 201
abruptio placentae (T) 20
ACE = Angiotensin-Converting-Enzyme 97
ACE-I = Angiotensin-Converting-Enzyme
    Inhibitor (T) 98; (T) 154
ACE-inhibitors 95-113; 132; 133; (T) 143; 156;
    187
acebutalol 184
acetylcholine 129
acne (T) 300; 304; 307
ACPA = AntiCytoPlasmic Antibodies 315; (F)
    329
acromegaly 78
ACT = Activated Clotting Times 277; 280; 281;
    (T) 283
acute renal failure 4; (T) 4; 18-21; 26; (T) 39; 40;
    271; (T) 286; (T) 287
acute tubular necrosis 18; 19-21; (T) 20
adenosine-diphosphatase 12; (T) 17
adenosine-diphosphate 9
ADP 9; 10; 12
ADPase 12
ADPKD = Autosomal Dominant Polycystic
    Kidney Disease 199-207; (T) 200; (F) 203
AER = Albumin Excretion Rate 145
AIDS 265
AII = Angiotensin II 79-80; 124; 165
albumin excretion 141; 145; 148; 156
albuminuria 101; 103; 141
aldosterone 126
Aleutian disease (T) 4
alkaline phosphatase 248
alpha-adrenergic blockers 187
alpha-adrenergic receptors 171
ALT 260; 261; 263; 265
aminoacid infusion 77; 78; 79; 81; 83; (T) 84;
    85; (T) 86
aminoacid metabolism 234
aminoacid supplementation 231
aminoacids 75; 76; 81; 83; 85; 232; 235; 236;
    (T) 237
AN-69 274
ANA = AntiNuclear Antibodies 320
ANCA = Anti-Neutrophil Cytoplasmic
    Antibodies 313-335; (F) 315; (F) 316; (T) 322;
    (T) 323; (T) 326; (T) 327; (F) 329
ancrod 26
anemia 27
ANF = Atrial Natriuretic Factor 80
angiotensin 9; (T) 78; 79-80; 97; 102; 104; 105;
    106; 107; 109; 123; 124; 165; 173; 189

angiotensin-converting-enzyme inhibitors 95-113;
    132; (T) 179; 187
anthropometric measurements 239
anthropometry (T) 238; (T) 239
anti-CD3 monoclonal antibody 35-36
anti-GBM antibodies 24
anti-GBM glomerulonephritis 21-23
anti-GBM GN 22; 23; (T) 39
anti-lymphocyte therapy 303
anti-neutrophil cytoplasmic antibodies 313-335
anticoagulant agents 26
anticonvulsant drugs 175
antilymphocyte preparations 308
antineoplastic drugs (T) 28
antiplatelet agents 26
antiproteinuric effect of ACE inhibitors 95-113
antithrombin III 6
arachidonic acid 13
ARF = Acute Renal Failure 18; (T) 39; 271-295
arginine 78
arginine-vasopressin 9
ARPKD = Autosomal Recessive Polycystic
    Kidney Disease 201; 202
arteritis (T) 314
aspirin 31; 32; 33; (T) 191; (T) 192; 188-192
AT III 6
atenolol 104; 182; 183; (T) 185; (T) 186
ATG = Anti-Thymocyte Globulin (T) 306
atherosclerosis 130-131; 132
ATN = Acute Tubular Necrosis 18; 19-21; (T) 20
ATPase 62
atrial natriuretic factor (T) 78
autoantibodies 314
azathioprine 299; 301; 302; 303; 304; 305; (T)
    306; 307; 308

Babinski signs 60
BCN = Bilateral Cortical Necrosis 19-21
benazepril (T) 98
benzodiazepines 177-178
Berger's disease 25
beta-adrenergic blockers 182-186
beta-adrenergic inhibitors (T) 179
betablocker (T) 84; 103; 104; 132; 156; (T) 179
betablocking agents (T) 185; (T) 186
bilateral cortical necrosis (T) 4; 19-21
biliary cirrhosis 256
bleeding, peptic ulceration (T) 300
blood casts 338; 348
blood urea nitrogen 284
bradykinin 82; 107; 129; 132

brain dehydration 56; 63; 67
brain demyelination 55
brain edema 59-60
BUN = Blood Urea Nitrogen 284

C3 24; 26
calcitriol 245-252; (F) 249
calcium 245; 246; 247; 248; (F) 249; 250
calcium antagonist (T) 154
calcium carbonate 234
calcium channel blockers 132
calcium channel blocking agents 172-174
calcium-oxalate monohydrate (T) 213
cancer (T) 20; 307; 338
CAPD 271
captopril (T) 98; 105; 132
carbohydrate intolerance 234
carcinoma 260
cardiac decompensation 145; 166
cardioselective beta-blocking agents 182
casts 338; (F) 342; 343; 344; 345; 347; 348;
    349; (T) 351
cataracts (T) 300; 302; 307
catecholamines 165; 171
catheters 273; 274; 285
CAVH = Continuous ArterioVenous
    Hemofiltration 271-295; (T) 272; (T) 286
CAVHD = Continuous ArterioVenous
    HemoDialysis 271-295; (T) 272; (T) 277; (F)
    278; (T) 287
CAVHDF = Continuous ArterioVenous Hemo
    DiaFiltration 272; (T) 272; 275; 276; 286; 287
CCPD 271
ceftazidime (T) 277
cefuroxime (T) 277
CEI = Converting Enzyme Inhibitors 79; (T) 84;
    (T) 86
cellulose 271
central pontine myelinolysis 63-65
cerebral edema 55; 56; 57; 59; (F) 59; 60; 61; 62;
    67; 71
cerebrovascular accidents 166
Cheyne-Stokes respiration 60
cholesterol 130; 131; 132; 133; 156; 232; 307
chronic renal failure 36-37; 84; 85; 148; 229-242
Churg Strauss syndrome (T) 314; 325; 326; (T)
    326; 327; (T) 327; 331
ciprofloxacin (T) 277
cirrhosis 256; 260
citrate (T) 283
citrate anticoagulation 280
clonidine 124; (T) 179
coagulation 6-9; 109
coagulation in renal diseases 3-54
coagulation system 5; 20
cocaine "crack" inhalation 28
colitis 319; 324
coma 60; 61; 62; 65
compliance 237; 238; 240

consumption coagulopathy 4; 27
continuous arteriovenous hemofiltration/dialysis
    271-295
contraceptives (T) 28
converting enzyme inhibitors 83; (T) 84; 85; (T)
    86; 87
convulsions 177
cortical necrosis 19; 20; 26; 27
corticosteroids 299; 302
cortisol 234
Coxsackie virus echovirus (T) 28
CPM 63; 65; 68; 70
crescentic glomerulonephritis 18; 23; 314; (F)
    315; 321; (T) 323; (T) 325; (T) 326; 327; (T)
    327; 330
crescentic GN 25; (T) 39; 40
CRF = Chronic Renal Failure 229-242; (T) 233
cryoglobulinemia 313
CSF = CerebroSpinal Fluid (F) 58
CT = Computed Tomography 60; 63; 67
CUPID = Continuous Ultrafiltration Plus
    Intermittent hemo-Dialysis 273; 288
cuprophane 271
cushingoid appearance 302
CVVH = Continuous Veno-Venous
    Hemofiltration 272; (T) 272; 276; 282; (T)
    286
CVVHD = Continuous Veno-Venous Hemo
    Dialysis 272; (T) 272; 273; 281; (T) 287
CVVHDF = Continuous Veno-Venous Hemo
    DiaFiltration 273
cyclooxygenase 13; 30
cyclophosphamide 329; (F) 329
cyclosporin (T) 28; 34-35; 40; 299; (T) 300; 301;
    302; 303; 304; 305; (T) 306; 307; 308
cystic disease 201; 348
cystic fibrosis 205
cystic kidneys (T) 200
cystine (T) 237
cystine stones (T) 213; (T) 215; 218
cystoscopes 218
cytodiagnostic urinalysis 346-347; 348; 349; 350;
    (T) 350; 351
cytokines 18; 260
cytomegalovirus 253; 303; (F) 329

D3 250
DDAVP (F) 66
defibrotide 26
delirium 58
diabetes 87; 117; 122; 125; 141; 144; (T) 300;
    302; 304
diabetes mellitus 9; 75; 84; (T) 84; (T) 86; 132;
    (T) 154
diabetic nephropathy 97; (T) 98; 141; 143; (T)
    143; 145; 148; 149; 153; 156; 232
dialysis   32; 149; 245; 246; 247; 248; 250;
    253-270; (T) 262; 271-295
diazepam 177; 178

354

diazoxide (T) 169; 174
DIC = Disseminated Intravascular Coagulation 18; 19; 20; 21; 24; 31; 32; (T) 39
dietary calcium supplementation 187
dietary protein intake 234
dietary protein restriction 234; 239; (T) 239; (T) 240
dietary treatment of CRF 235-237
digoxin 276
diltiazem 132
dipyridamole 32; 33
disseminated intravascular coagulation 4; (T) 4; (T) 20; (T) 39
diuretics 68; (T) 84; 100; 108; 132; 156; 174; (T) 179; 187; 302
diverticulitis (T) 300
DNA 24; 254
dopamine 76; 77; (T) 84
doxycycline (T) 277

EACA = Epsilon-AminoCaproic Acid 19; 24
eclampsia 164; 166; 176; 177; 178
edema 165
EDRF = Endothelial-Derived Relaxing Factors 81; 129
EEG 175
elastase 318; 319; 320; 325; 326; 331
elderly 304; 219
ELISA 255; (T) 255; 256; 257; 262; (T) 262; 263; 264; 319; 320; 321; 323; 327
enalapril (T) 98; (F) 103; 104
encephalopathy, post-anoxic 67-68
end-stage-renal disease 141; 205
end-stage-renal failure (T) 142; 144; (F) 147; 149; 245-246
endorphin 234
endoscopic stone surgery 211
endoscopy 217
endothelial-derived relaxing factor 78; (T) 78
endotoxins 28; 29
Epstein Barr virus (T) 28; 253
erythrocytes in urine 337-352; (F) 339; (F) 344; (F) 346
erythrocytic cast in urine (F) 345
erythrocytic casts (T) 351
erythropoietin 234; 265
Escherichia coli 28; (T) 28
ESRF = End-Stage-Renal-Failure 141; (T) 142; (T) 143; (F) 147
essential hypertension 117-138; 165
ESWL = Extracorporeal Shock Wave Lithotripsy 211-226; (T) 212; (T) 213; (T) 215
extracapillary glomerulonephritis (T) 4; 15
extracapillary GN 26; 37
extracorporeal shock wave lithotripsy 211-226

fatty casts (T) 351
Felty's syndrome 324
fetal growth retardation 165

fibrin 3; (T) 4; (T) 7; (T) 39; 349
fibrin casts 347; 348; (T) 351
fibrin degradation products 27
fibrin-related antigen 3
fibrinolysis 4; 5; 6-9; 16; (T) 17; 21-26; 30; 32
fibrinolytic activity 18
fibrinolytic system 7; (T) 7; (F) 8; 12-16; 19; 23
fibronectin 9; (T) 17; 27
fluoroscopy 216; 218; 220; 221; 222
frusemide 178
FUN = Fluid Urea Nitrogen 284

gentamicin (T) 277
GH = Growth Hormone 78-79; 80
ghost cells 339
giant cell arteritis (T) 314
glomerular bleeding 347-352
glomerular endotheliosis 165
glomerular hemostasis system 3-54; (T) 39
glomerular hypertension 75; 85; 86; 87
glomerular sclerosis 26; 96
glomerular thrombosis 26
glomerulonephritides 3; 21-26
glomerulonephritis (T) 4; (T) 39; 230; 313; 317; 321; (T) 323; 327; 330; 340
glomerulonephritis, rapidly progressive 322
glomerulopressin 79
glomerulosclerosis 16; 97; 125
glomerulotubular balance 83
glucagon (T) 78; 79; 234
glucose intolerance 302
glycerol (T) 4; 19; (T) 39; 40
glycine 62; 75; 77; 78; 83
glycine infusion 83; 85; 86
GN = GlomeruloNephritis 3; 4; 16; 22; 23; 24; 25; (T) 39; (T) 98
Goldblatt hypertension 86; (T) 86
Goodpasture's syndrome 314
grand mal 67
growth (T) 300; 302
growth factor 78
growth hormone 78-79; (T) 78; 232; 234
growth retardation 185; 191
GS-ANA = Granulocyte-Specific AntiNuclear Antibodies 324
GSP = Generalized Shwartzman Phenomenon 18; 19; 39

HBV = Hepatitis B Virus 259; 263; 265
HCV = Hepatitis C Virus 253-270; (T) 262
HCV infection 255-258; (T) 255 prevention of, 265-266
HDL-cholesterol 131; 132; 133
heart disease 286
hematuria 190; 337-352
hemodialysis 250; 253; 271; 281; 282; 284; 285; 286; 287; 288
hemofiltration 271-295
hemoglobin 339; 341; 343; 349

hemoglobin casts (T) 351
hemoglobinuric acute renal failure (T) 4
hemolysis 19; 165
hemolytic anemia (T) 20; 26
hemolytic uremic syndrome (T) 4; 9; 18; 26-33; (T) 28
hemoperfusion 284
hemophiliacs 257
hemorrhage 166; 169; 190
hemostasis system 3-54
Henoch-Schönlein purpura 313; (T) 314
heparan sulfate (T) 17
heparin 21; 26; 31; 33; 39; 277-279; (F) 278; 281; 282; (T) 283
heparin-free anticoagulation 280
heparinization, regional 280
hepatic failure 284
hepatitis 253-270; 324
hepatitis B 253; 261
hepatitis C 253; 258-261
    in hemodialysis patients 261-263
    in renal transplant recipients 263-265
hepatitis E 253
Heymann's nephritis 24; 37
hirsutism 307
histamine 129
histidine (T) 237
HIV = Human Immunodeficiency Virus 259
HLA 34; 36
human immunodeficiency virus 28
Huntington's disease 205
HUS = Hemolytic Uremic Syndrome 26-34; (T) 28
hydatidosis 256
hydralazine (T) 169; 170-172; 174; 178; (T) 179; 182; 326
hydroxylase 250
hyperammonemia 286
hypercalcemia 246; 247; 249; 250
hyperfiltration 76; 85; 87; 96; 141; (T) 142; (T) 143; 144-145; 156
hyperinsulinemia 117; 122; 123; (T) 123; 124; 125; 127; 130-131
hyperkalemia 108; 109; 286
hyperlipidemia 96; 108
hyperlipidemic tendency 302
hypernatremia 55; 56
hyperparathyroidism 231; 234; 245-252
hyperperfusion 75
hyperphosphatemia 248; 250
hypertension (T) 28; 33; 34; (T) 84; 85; 86; 87; 98; 104; 117-138; (F) 121; (T) 125; (T) 142; 153; 154-156; 163-196; (T) 169; (T) 179; (T) 185; (T) 186; (T) 191; (T) 200; 212; (T) 212; 214; 219; 231; (T) 300; 302; 304
hypertension during pregnancy 163-196
hypertrichosis (T) 300
hypocalcemia 246; 248; 250
hypocalciuria 187

hyponatremia 55-74; (F) 57; (F) 58; (F) 59; (F) 65; (F) 66
hyponatremia correction 69-72
hypotension 109; 284

IDDM = Insulin Dependent Diabetes Mellitus (T) 84; 145; 150; (F) 150; (F) 151; (F) 153; 154-156; (T) 154
IgA nephropathy (T) 4; 25
IGF-1 = Insulin-like Growth Factor 1 80; 130
IgG 24
IgM 26
IHD = Intermittent HemoDialysis 271; 289
IL1 = Interleukin 1 11; 12; 16; 22; 27; 34; 276
immune complex GN 23-24
immunosuppression 299-310; (T) 306
immunosuppression for renal transplantation 299-310
immunosuppressive therapy 34-36
indomethacin 97; (F) 99; 108
infection (T) 300; 304
insulin 117; (F) 118; (F) 121; (T) 123; (F) 128; (T) 143; 232; 233
insulin-dependent diabetes mellitus (T) 84; 145; (F) 150; (F) 151; (T) 154; (F) 153
insulin-dependent diabetic patients 141-160
insulin-like growth factor 1 (T) 78; 130
insulin resistance (F) 121; (T) 125
insulin resistance in essential hypertension 117-138
interferon-α 260; 261; 263
interleukin 1 11; 276; 289
interleukin 6 289
isoleucine (T) 237
IVBF = InterVillous Blood Flow 171

jaundice 260

kallikrein (F) 5; 34
kallikrein-kinin system 81
Kawasaki disease 324
keratin 15
ketoanalogues 232
kinin (T) 78; 81; 82; 107; 129; 132
kininogen (F) 5

labetalol (T) 169; 174; (T) 179; 183; 184; 185; (T) 186
LACI 6; 11
lactoferrin 318; 319; 320; 325; 331
LDL 130
LDL cholesterol 132
leucine (T) 237
leukemia (T) 20; 259
linoleic acid 232; (T) 233
lipid and carbohydrate restriction in CRF 232-234
lipid composition of erythrocyte membrane (T) 233

lipid metabolism 229-230
lipid-laden cells (T) 351
lipiduria 342
lipoprotein lipase 232
lipoprotein-associated coagulation inhibitor 6
lipoproteins 230; 236
lipoproteinuria 230
lipoxygenase 13
lisinopril 97; (T) 98; (F) 99; 100; (F) 101; 102; 108
lithium clearance 82; 83
lithotripsy 211-226; (T) 213; (T) 220
lithotripter 212; 213; 216; 218; (T) 220; 221; 222
liver 85; 165; 172; 250
liver dysfunction 253
low-protein diet 231-232; (T) 230; 233; (T) 233; 234; 235; 236; (T) 237; 238; (T) 239; (T) 240
LpA = ultrafiltration coefficient 77; 78
LPD (T) 230
LPS 18; 27
lupus erythematosus (T) 28; 97; 324; 326
lupus GN 25; 37
lupus nephritis (T) 4; 26; 40; 341
lupus-like nephritis 23-24
lysine (T) 237

magnesium sulphate 171; 175-177; 178
magnesium-ammonium phosphate 219
malaria 256
malnutrition 238-240
mannitol 62
MAP = Mean Arterial blood Pressure (F) 153; 154; (T) 154; (F) 155; 156
Masugi's nephritis 21
membranous GN 25
mercuric chloride (T) 4; 24-25
methionine (T) 237
methyldopa 103; 168; 179-182; (T) 179; 184; 185; (T) 185; (T) 186
methylprednisolone 299
metoprolol (F) 103; 182; 183
microalbuminuria 96; 141; (T) 142; (T) 143; 144; 145-147; 148; 149; 150; 152; (T) 152; 153; (F) 153; 154; (T) 154; 156
microangiopathic hemolytic anemia 165
microscopic polyarteritis (T) 314; (T) 322; (T) 327
minimal change disease 95; 100
minoxidil (T) 84
mitomycin C 26; 28
mizoribine 307
monoclonal antibodies (F) 316
MPA = Microscopic PolyArteritis 321; 322; 323; 324; 327; (T) 327; 328
MPO = MyeloPerOxidase 317; 318; 319; 320; 323; (T) 325; 326; (T) 327; 329; 330; 331
MRI = Magnetic Resonance Imaging 64; 68

myasthenia gravis 324
myelinolysis 66; 67; 68; 69
myeloperoxidase (F) 315; (F) 316; (F) 318; 325; (T) 325; (T) 327
myoglobin 341; 343
myopathy (T) 300; 302

nafomostat mesilate 282; (T) 283
NANBH = Non-A, Non-B Hepatitis 253-270
NCGN = Necrotizing Crescentic GlomeruloNephritis 313-335
necrosis, avascular (T) 300; 302; 307
necrotic GN 25
necrotizing arteritis 325
necrotizing glomerulonephritis 313-335; (T) 323; (T) 325; (T) 326
necrotizing vasculitis 313-335
nephrectomy 219; 231
nephrocalcinosis (T) 215; 217
nephrolithiasis 214
nephrostomy (T) 212; 214; 220
nephrotic syndrome 4; 37-39; 96; 107; 230; 231; 342
nephrotoxicity 301; 303; 304
neuropathy (T) 142
nicardipine 172; 173
NIDDM = Non-Insulin Dependent Diabetes Mellitus (T) 84; 117; 119; 120; 121; (F) 121; 122; 124; 131; 132; (T) 154
nifedipine (T) 84; 132; (T) 169; 172; 173; 174; (T) 179; 186
nitric oxide (T) 78; 80; 81
nitroprusside (T) 169
non-A, non-B hepatitis 253-270
norepinephrine 124; 129
NS = Nephrotic Syndrome 4; 37
NSAID = Non Steroidal Anti-Inflammatory Drugs 80; 97; 107; 108; 109
nutritional status (in CRF) (T) 238; (T) 239; (T) 240

obesity 117; 119; 120; (F) 121; 122; 123; 124; (T) 125; 126; 131; 212; 302
OKT3 35-36; 303; 305; 308
OKY 046 37
OKY 1581 37
opisthotonos 60
OPL = Oral Protein Load 76; 77; (T) 84; 85
osmotic demyelination syndrome 55; 63-68; 70
osteitis fibrosa 245-252
osteomalacia 177
osteoporosis (T) 300; 302
oxalic acid 234
oxprenolol 180; 181; 182; 185; (T) 186
oxytocin 61

PA 7; (T) 7; 8; 9; 12-16; (T) 17; 18; 23; 32; 33; 34

357

PA-R (T) 7
pacemakers (T) 212
PAF = Platelet Activating Factor 9; 10; (T) 17; 35
PAI (T) 7; 9; 15; (T) 17; 18; 25; 32; 35
PAN membrane 274
pancreatitis 20; (T) 20; 302
paraproteinemia 256
parathyroid hormone 232; 235; 245
parathyroidectomy 250
PCA = ProCoagulant Activity 33; 35
PCR = Polymerase Chain Reaction 257
PCWP = Pulmonary Capillary Wedge Pressure 170; 171
penicillamine (T) 4; 24-25
pentoxifylline 40
peptic ulcer 302
percutaneous renal surgery (T) 215; 217; 218-219
percutaneous stone surgery 211; 214
PG = ProstaGlandin 80
PGE$_2$ 9; 35; (T) 78; 80; 132
PGI$_2$ (T) 17; 29; 30; 31; 33; 35; (T) 78; 80; 281; 282
phenylalanine (T) 237
phenytoin 178; 276
pheochromocytoma 187
phosphate 245
phosphate restriction 231
phosphaturia 231
phospholipase A$_2$ 13
phospholipase C 11
pindolol 182
plasma exchange 32
plasma infusion 32; 33
plasmapheresis 284
plasmin (T) 7; 8
plasminogen 7; (T) 7; 8; 21; 30; 34
plasminogen activation 7
plasminogen activator (T) 7; 8; 12-16
plasminogen activator inhibitor (T) 7; 9
plasminogen activator receptor (T) 7
platelet activating factor 9; (T) 17
platelet adhesion (T) 17
platelet agglutinating factor 31
platelet aggregation 9; 12; 17; (T) 17; 22; 172
platelet-derived growth factor 3
PMA = Phorbol Myristate Acetate 13; 15
polyacrylonitrile 271
polyamide 271; 274
polyangiitis overlap (T) 326
polyangiitis overlap syndrome (T) 314; 327; (T) 327
polyarteritis (T) 314; (T) 322; 326
polyarteritis nodosa (T) 314; (T) 326; 327; (T) 327
polyarthritis 324
polycystic kidney disease 199-207
polysulphone 271; 273; 274
prazosin 133; (T) 179

pre-eclampsia 163; 164; 165; 170; 171; 174; 176; 177; 178; 180; 182; 187; 188; 189; 190; 191
pre-eclamptic toxemia (T) 20
prednisolone 299; (T) 300; 301; 302; 303; 304; 305; (T) 306; 308; 329
pregnancy 75; 163-196; (T) 167; (T) 169; (T) 179; (T) 185; (T) 186; (T) 191; (T) 200; 201; 204; 205; (T) 212; 218
pregnancy-associated HUS (T) 28
progression of CRF 229-242
progression of renal diseases 36-37; 75; 87
propranolol 182
prostacyclin 9; 16; 17; (T) 17; 26; 27; 30; 34; 165; 176; 188; 189; 281; (T) 283
prostacyclin analogues 281-282
prostaglandin 80; 107; 129; 132
prostaglandin E$_2$ 80
prostanoids 78; (T) 78; 80-81
prostatectomy 70
protamine 279
protein administration 78; (T) 78; 80; 81
protein and phosphate restriction 231
protein intake 75; 76; 77
protein kinase A 15
protein kinase C 13; 15
protein load 75; 77; 83; 85
protein metabolism 234
protein restricted diet 233
protein restriction 231; 232; 234
proteinase 3 316; 318; 319; 320; (T) 327
proteinuria 95-113; (T) 98; (F) 103; 141; (T) 142; (T) 143; 146; 148; 149; 150; 153; 154; 155; 164; 165; 184; 191; (T) 191; 230; 231; 234; 235; 338; 341; 347; 349
prothrombin (F) 5; 6
prothrombinase (F) 5; 6
psychiatric disturbance (T) 300; 302
psychiatric episodes 307
psychosis (T) 300
PTH 245-252; (F) 249
PUFA = PolyUnsaturated Fatty Acids 232; (T) 233
pyelonephritis 213; 215; 219

RAAS = Renin-Angiotensin-Aldosterone-System 99; 100; 102; 104; 106; 110
rapamycin 307
rejection (T) 4; (T) 28; 33-34; (T) 39; 40; 299; 303; 304; 305; 307; 308
renal biopsies 150
renal bleeding 337-352; (T) 350
renal cell (F) 341
renal functional reserve 75-91; (T) 84; (T) 86
renal hemodynamics 76-84
renal hematuria 348; 350; (T) 350
renal transplantation 33-36; 299-310
renal tubular cells (F) 342; (F) 343; (T) 351
renin 19; 79; 102; 106; 234
renin-angiotensin system 19; 127; 234

358

renin-angiotensin-aldosterone system 172
renovascular hypertension 83; 106
respiratory distress syndrome 40; 284
retinopathy (T) 142; 152
retrograde intrarenal surgery 216-218
RFR = Renal Functional Reserve 75; 76; 81; (T) 84; 86; (T) 86
rheumatoid arthritis 256; 313; 319; 324
RIBA = Recombinant ImmunoBlot Assay (T) 255; 256; 257; 262; 264
ribavirin 261
RIRS = Retrograde Intrarenal Surgery 216-218
RPF 80

Salmonella (T) 28
saralasin 19; 106
schistosomiasis 256
scleroderma (T) 28
Scribner shunt 273
SCUF = Slow Continuous Ultra-Filtration 272; (T) 272; 288
seizures 55; 59; 60; 61; 62; 63; 64; 65; 67; 175; 176; 177; 178
sepsis (T) 20
septic abortion (T) 20
septicemia (T) 20
serine protease inhibitors 9
serine proteases (F) 317
serotonin 79; 129
serpin 9
serum nephritis (T) 4
serum sickness (T) 4; 35
serum sickness nephritis 23-24
Shiga toxin 29
Shiga-like toxins 28
Shigella 27; 28; (T) 28
SHR = Spontaneously Hypertensive Rat 127; 128
shunt 273
Shwartzman phenomenon (T) 4; 27; (T) 39
sickle cell disease 75
SLE = Systemic Lupus Erythematosus (T) 98; 313; 314; 319
SLT 28
SNGFR = Single Nephron GFR 78; 85; (T) 86
SNPF = Single Nephron Plasma Flow 78
SOD = SuperOxide Dismutase 254; 257
sodium nitroprusside 175
somatostatin 79; 124; 128; (T) 143
sorbitol 62
staghorn stones 213; 214; (T) 215; 224
status epilepticus 177
steroid 299-310; (T) 300; (T) 306
    withdrawal (after transplantation) 305-309
stone disease (T) 215
stone-burden 212; 213; (T) 213; 216
stone-cracker's no-mansland 221
stones 211-226; (T) 213; (T) 215
Streptococcus Pneumoniae 28; (T) 28
streptokinase 7; 23; 33

streptozotocin 83
streptozotocin-induced diabetes mellitus 75
struvite (T) 215
struvite stone 219
sympathetic nervous system 127

Takayasu's arteritis (T) 314
temporal arteritis (T) 314
testosterone 233
TGF = TubuloGlomerular Feedback system 78; 82-84
TGF ß = Transforming Growth Factor ß 15
thalassemia major 259
theophylline 276
thiazide 132; 174; (T) 179
thiazide-induced hyponatremia 68
threonine (T) 237
thrombin 3; (T) 4; 6; 9; 11; 15; 16; 18; 19; 27; 38; (T) 39
thrombocytopenia 26; 27; 31; 182; 278; 279; 281
thrombomodulin 6; 12; (T) 17; 35
thrombophlebitis 5
thromboplastin (T) 4; (F) 5; 10; 11; 16; (T) 17; 18; 22; 34; 40
thrombospondin 9; (T) 17
thrombotic thrombocytopenic purpura 27
thromboxane 6; 16; 17; (T) 17; 22; 34; 37; 40; 165; 188; 189
thromboxane A$_2$ 9; 10; (T) 17
thromboxane B$_2$ 9
thromboxane synthetase 23
thromplastin 6
thyroid hormone 233; 234
TNF = Tumor Necrosis Factor 11; 12; 16; 27; 276; 289
TNF α 18; 34; 35
tobramycin 276; (T) 277
toxemia of pregnancy (T) 4
transfusion 253; 254; 255; 259; 262; 264
transplant recipients 263
transplantation 149; 218; 264; 265; 299-310
triglyceride 131; 132; 133; 232; 307
tryptophan (T) 237
TTP 27; 28; 29; 30; 31; 32
tubular necrosis 19
tubuloglomerular feedback system (T) 78; 82-84
tumor 260
tumor necrosis factor 11; 276
Tx = Thromboxane 6
TxA$_2$ 6; 19; 29; 31; 34; 35; 36
TxB$_2$ 34; 35; 36
tyrosine (T) 237

UAE = Urinary Albumin Excretion (T) 143; 145; (F) 147; (F) 153
UAER = Urinary Albumin Excretion Rate (T) 142; 145; 156
ultrasonography (T) 200; 201
uremia (T) 142; 153

uremic toxins 234
ureteral stones 219-224; (T) 220
ureteric problems 304
ureteroscopes 218
ureteroscopic lithotripsy 221
ureteroscopy 211; 217; 220; 223; 224
urinalysis 337-352; (T) 351
    methods for detecting renal bleeding 343-345
urinary albumin excretion 141; (F) 146; (F) 153
urinary diversion (T) 215; 217-218; 224
urinary infection 302
urinary protein excretion 148; 149
urinary sediment 337-352; (T) 351
urinary stones 211
urinary tract infection 145; 338; 341
urokinase (T) 7; 8; (F) 14; 33
urokinase-type plasminogen activator (T) 7

vaccine 258

valine (T) 237
vancomycin 276; (T) 277
vascular access 273
vasculitides 313; (T) 314
vasculitis 18; 313-335; (T) 323; (T) 325
verapamil (T) 86; 132; 172
verotoxin 28
vitamin D 245-252
VLDL triglyceride 131; 132
von Willebrand factor 9; (T) 17; 31
VT = VeroToxins 29
vWF = von Willebrand Factor 30; 31; 32; 35

water intoxication 57; 60; 61; 62; 63; 71
Wegener's granulomatosis (T) 314; (F) 315; 321;
    (T) 322; (T) 326; 327-330; (T) 327; (F) 329
WG = Wegener's Granulomatosis 315; 321; 322;
    323; 324; 327; (T) 327; 328; 330; 331